Manual of
Home
Health Care
Nursing

Joleen Walsh, R.N., M.S.N., Ed.D.

Associate Professor
West Texas State University
Canyon, Texas

Carol Batten Persons, R.N., M.S.N., Ed.D.

Special Assistant to the Chief of Staff
Veterans Administration Hospital
Amarillo, Texas

Lynn Wieck, R.N., M.S.N.

Director of Special Projects and Planning and
Director of Quality Assurance
Northwest Texas Hospital
Amarillo, Texas

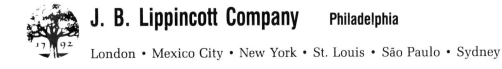 **J. B. Lippincott Company**   Philadelphia

London • Mexico City • New York • St. Louis • São Paulo • Sydney

Manual of

Home Health Care Nursing

Acquisitions Editor: Patricia L. Cleary
Manuscript Editor: Lee Henderson
Indexer: Alberta Morrison
Design Director: Tracy Baldwin
Design Coordinator: Anne O'Donnell

Production Supervisor: Carol A. Florence
Production Assistant: Kathleen R. Diamond
Compositor: Circle Graphics
Printer/Binder: The Murray Printing Company
Cover Printer: Philips Offset

6   5   4   3   2

Library of Congress Cataloging-in-Publication Data
Walsh, Joleen.
  Manual of home health care nursing.

  Includes bibliographies and index.
  1. Home nursing.   2. Critically ill—Home care.
3. Nursing.   I. Persons, Carol Batten.   II. Wieck,
Lynn.   III. Title. [DNLM: 1. Home Care Services.
2. Nursing Process—methods.   WY 115 W225m]
RT120.H65W35   1987   610.73   86-20173
ISBN 0-397-54616-5

The authors and publisher have exerted every effort to ensure that drug selection and dosage set forth in this text are in accord with current recommendations and practice at the time of publication. However, in view of ongoing research, changes in government regulations, and the constant flow of information relating to drug therapy and drug reactions, the reader is urged to check the package insert for each drug for any change in indications and dosage and for added warnings and precautions. This is particularly important when the recommended agent is a new or infrequently employed drug.

To Rita and Hubert, who, facing life and death, gave strength to us all
Joleen

To my daughters, Meredith and Ashleigh
Carol

To my husband, Steve, and our boys, Joey, Scott, and Doug, for their support and infinite patience
Lynn

Preface

The move by Medicare to a prospective reimbursement system from a retrospective system has changed health-care delivery patterns in the United States. The advent of Diagnosis-Related Groups (DRGs) as a basis for reimbursement for hospitalized Medicare patients has motivated hospitals to discharge patients sooner. The demand for home health-care services has risen dramatically, and a large proportion of home health services is provided to Medicare patients.

The change in practice patterns has precipitated the need for practitioners to adapt acute-care techniques to the home care setting. The emphasis is on teaching the client and family members to assume as many self-care activities as possible. Caring for Hickman catheters or giving intravenous antibiotics is now commonplace in the rapidly advancing field of home health nursing, whereas previously this care would have been provided in the hospital setting. The home health movement has not only given professional nurses the opportunity to adapt complex nursing skills to the home environment, but has increased the need for astute assessment and counseling skills. Home health is the newest expanded role for the professional nurse.

Manual of Home Health Care Nursing was written to fill a gap in the literature on adapting acute-care nursing techniques to the home setting. Presenting these techniques is not meant to limit the creativity of the practitioner. The professional nurse will be in the position to adapt techniques to the particular situation and will be able to call on a variety of clinical experiences.

One of the most obvious changes from the hospital to the home is adapting sterile technique to aseptic or clean technique in many instances. There are two reasons for this apparent departure from accepted practice. The biggest problem in infection control in hospitals is nosocomial infection because of the prevalence of antibiotic-resistant organisms. Resistant organisms do not usually occur in the home, although the practitioner can very easily become a carrier from client to client if appropriate precautions are not taken. As in the hospital setting, effective handwashing is the most effective infection control technique in the home. The second reason for adapting sterile techniques is that in the home, the family is involved as much as possible in giving care. Sterile technique requires extensive training for people who have not been exposed to the concept before. Teaching a "no touch" technique is just as effective for preventing infection.

The book has been written within the framework of the nursing process and uses accepted nursing diagnoses to focus each technique. Some techniques, like Holter monitoring and bedmaking, have been presented with the idea of teaching the family, rather than providing instructions to the professional nurse. Each technique is presented in the following outline format:

Background
Assessment of Self-Care Potential
Client/Family Assessment
Physical Assessment
Environmental Assessment
Planning Strategies
Potential Nursing Diagnoses
Expected Outcomes
Health Promotion Goals
• The client/family will . . .
Equipment
Interventions/Health Promotion
ACTION   RATIONALE/AMPLIFICATION
Related Care
Education/Communication
• Teach the client and family to . . .
Referrals and Consultations
Evaluation of Health Promotion Activities
Quality Assurance/Reassessment
DOCUMENTATION
Charting for the Home Health Nurse
Records Kept by the Client/Family
Health Teaching Checklist
Product Availability
Selected References

Only those headings that apply to the particular technique are included, so not all sections appear in all techniques. The background section provides information that the clinician requires prior to implementing the technique. The assessment phase includes not only assessment of the family's capability of assuming self-care activities, but also physical assessment of the client and environmental assessment.

Potential nursing diagnoses are listed and will guide the clinician in writing individualized care plans and client-centered outcomes and goals. Interventions are presented in a two-column format, with rationale provided as necessary. Age-specific modifications have been included in techniques when appropriate. The documentation section should be particularly useful to the home health nurse, and suggestions are given for record keeping for both the family and the nurse. The health teaching checklist can be used to record teaching activities, and in some cases could be adapted to serve as a checklist for the motivated family. The product availability section will assist the home health nurse to locate home health vendors, as well as products or equipment necessary to provide care in the home. Selected references have been provided to guide the clinician seeking additional background information on the technique.

The appendix was carefully designed to provide additional information and referral sources available to the clinician. Techniques for promoting an environment for the sight-impaired client, teaching strategies, and an extensive list of publications, special interest groups, and referral agencies are among the highlights.

Infection control standards as published by the Centers for Disease Control have been included in an appendix. The home health nurse should adapt these guidelines to the individual situation. Good handwashing and proper waste disposal will be the best protection for other family members. Keep in mind, however, that in most cases the client has already been in close contact with family members.

Although Medicare regulations guide home health practices to a large extent, it is with design that these regulations have not been included. Frequent changes in the regulations make it difficult to provide up-to-date information in a textbook.

In the mushrooming field of home health nursing, necessity will precede invention. We would be grateful if clinicians wish to share creative solutions to the problems of caring for clients in the home.

Joleen Walsh, R.N., M.S.N., Ed.D.
Carol Batten Persons, R.N., M.S.N., Ed.D
Lynn Wieck, R.N., M.S.N.

Acknowledgments

A number of people have contributed to make this book a reality. We wish to acknowledge the contributions made by the publishing team at Lippincott. They have put in many hours helping us to refine and improve the manuscript.

Many of the photographs for this book were taken by Robert Bradshaw, R.N., and Ernie Farino, Chief of Medical Media, Veterans Administration Hospital, Amarillo, Texas. Steve Akeroyd graciously consented to process photographic film and produce prints for yet another project.

Valuable consultations were provided by Tom Brown, R.N., M.S.N.; Wayne Woodward, C.R.T., R.N., M.S.N.; and Jerry Johnson, R.N., B.S.N., of Amarillo Area Hospital Home Health Care, and Jimmy Bryant, R.R.T., of Glasrock Home Health Agency.

Contents

Activity/Rest

Circulation

Elimination

Food/Fluid

Hygiene

Monitoring/Surveillance

Safety

Teaching/Learning

Ventilation

Appendices

Index

Activity/Rest

1 Active and Passive Range-of-Motion Exercises

Background

Range-of-motion exercises are those that take the body joints through their extent of movement. Their purpose is to maintain joint function and muscle tone. Range-of-motion exercises are categorized according to the independence of performance, that is, the amount of assistance required in their performance.

Active range-of-motion exercises: Those performed independently by the client

Assisted range-of-motion exercises: Those that the client can partially perform but that require some assistance for the total performance

Passive range-of-motion exercises: Those exercises the client is totally unable to perform and that require total assistance from another person

Assessment of Self-Care Potential

Client/Family Assessment

- Determine if a family member is willing and capable (has the strength and available time) to assist the client with those exercises the client is unable to perform independently.

Physical Assessment

- Assess the flexibility of each joint to determine which exercises can be performed independently and which will require assistance.

Environmental Assessment

- Determine if there is adequate space in the home in an easily accessible place for the exercises to be performed properly.
- If passive exercises are to be done, space must be available for the assisting person to stand on either side of the client.

Planning Strategies

Potential Nursing Diagnoses

Mobility, impaired physical

Expected Outcomes

Maintenance or restoration of maximum range of motion of all joints within the constraints of existing physical limitations

Maintenance or restoration of muscle tone in extremities

Health Promotion Goals

- The client and family will
  Demonstrate proper technique for range-of-motion exercises
  Achieve an increased level of active range-of-motion exercises within the physical limitations of the client
  Perform recommended number of range-of-motion exercises on a regular, consistent basis
  Discontinue exercises and notify the nurse if pain is felt or resistance is encountered in the process of performing the exercises

Interventions/Health Promotion

ACTION

1. Encourage independent range-of-motion exercises to the extent the client is capable.

2. Flex, extend, rotate *neck* (Fig. 1-1). If passive, support head and move it.

RATIONALE/AMPLIFICATION

Perform all exercises in a rhythmic, slow fashion. If pain or resistance occurs, discontinue the exercise and consult the physician or physical therapist.

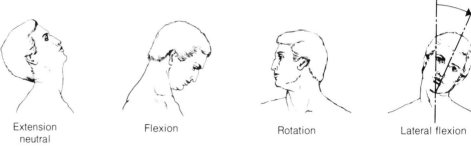

Figure 1.1

3. *Shoulder:* Lying in prone position, stabilize shoulder girdle and move arm. Perform flexion, extension, abduction, adduction, internal and external rotation, and hyperextension (Fig. 1-2).

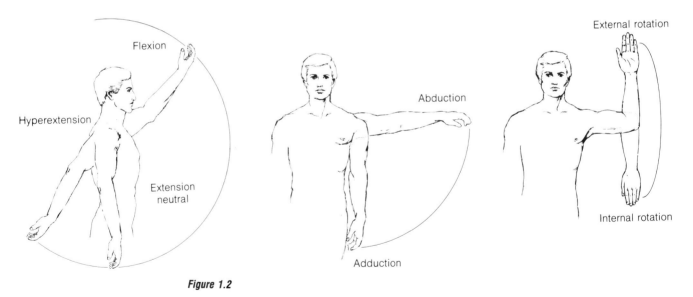

Figure 1.2

ACTION   **RATIONALE/AMPLIFICATION**

4. *Elbow:* Stabilize upper arm and move the forearm. Perform flexion, extension, supination, and pronation (Fig. 1-3).

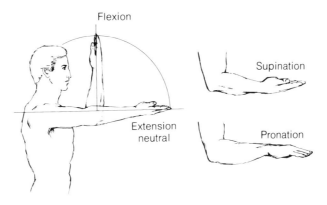

Flexion

Supination

Extension
neutral

Pronation

Figure 1.3

5. *Wrist:* Stabilize forearm and move the hand. Perform flexion, extension, ulnar deviation, and radial deviation (Fig. 1-4).

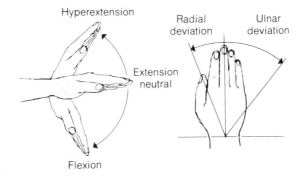

Hyperextension

Radial deviation   Ulnar deviation

Extension neutral

Flexion

Figure 1.4

6. *Joints of fingers:* Stabilize the hand and move the fingers (Fig. 1-5).

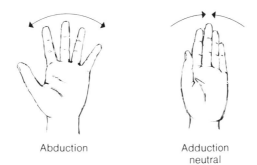

Abduction

Adduction neutral

Figure 1.5

ACTION   **RATIONALE/AMPLIFICATION**

7. *Thumb:* Stabilize fingers and
   wrist. Flex, extend, adduct,
   abduct, and bring thumb to finger
   (Fig. 1-6).

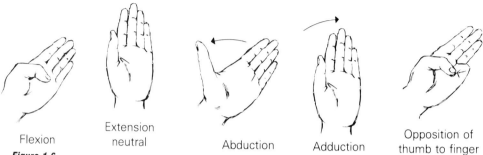

Flexion   Extension   Abduction   Adduction   Opposition of
                 neutral   thumb to finger
Figure 1.6

8. *Hip:* Stabilize the pelvis and
   move the thigh (Fig. 1-7). Do this
   in prone position.

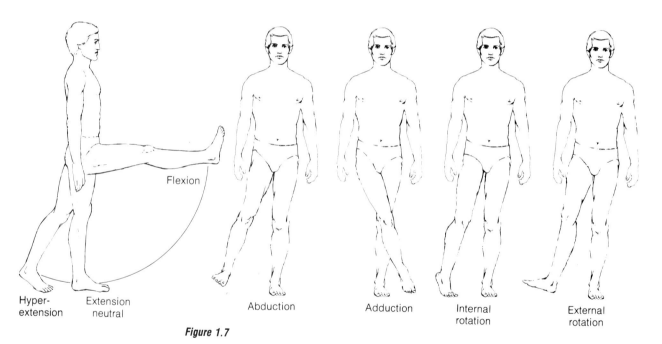

Hyper-   Extension   Abduction   Adduction   Internal   External
extension   neutral   rotation   rotation

Figure 1.7

ACTION   **RATIONALE/AMPLIFICATION**

9. *Knee:* Stabilize the thigh and
   move the leg (Fig. 1-8). Do this in
   prone position.

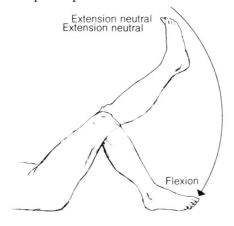

Extension neutral
Extension neutral

Flexion

Figure 1.8

10. *Ankle:* Stabilize leg and move
    the foot (Fig. 1-9).

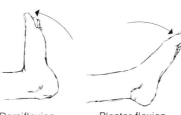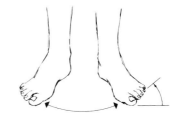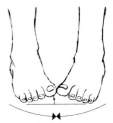

Dorsiflexion   Plantar flexion   Eversion   Inversion

Figure 1.9

11. *Toes:* Stabilize foot and move
    toes. Spread toes and return to
    relaxed position (Fig. 1-10).

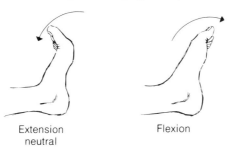

Extension   Flexion   Adduction   Abduction
neutral   neutral

Figure 1.10

Education/ Communication	• Teach the client and family to
	  Perform each exercise accurately
	  Perform each exercise with as much independence as possible, progressing toward total independence as soon as is possible, and advancing to strength-building or aerobic exercises if desired and if possible
	  Perform the exercises consistently; arrange the daily life schedule to allow a specified time for the exercises; perform the exercises slowly and in the same sequence each time
	  Perform the same number of exercises on each side of the body
	  Discontinue the exercises if resistance is encountered or if pain is experienced
	  Integrate the exercises into other daily activities, such as bathing, watching television, or playing games.

Referrals and Consultations	• Consult a physical therapist for further exercises or for questions concerning the exercise program and for guidance in progression toward independence. • Consult a physician if problems arise.

Evaluation of Health Promotion Activities

Quality Assurance/ Reassessment	• Visit the home regularly during the time the exercises are being performed to ensure that they are being performed correctly. • Periodically reassess the client to determine if greater independence in exercise performance is possible.
DOCUMENTATION	***Charting for the Home Health Nurse*** • Document the teaching of the exercise protocol. • Document any limitations to the full performance of the exercises. • Record the client's adherence to the prescribed exercise program. • Document any adverse responses as indicated by the client and/or family. ***Records Kept by the Client/Family*** • Record any problems encountered in the performance of the prescribed exercises. • Develop a schedule for recording the performance of the exercises.

Health Teaching Checklist

Name of Care Provider _____

Relationship to Client _____ Telephone #_____

Taught by _____ Date _____

	EXPLAINED	DEMONSTRATED
Exercise routine	_____	_____
Indications for discontinuing exercises	_____	
Indications to consult the nurse	_____	

Product Availability

No special products are needed.

2 Body Mechanics

Background

The term *body mechanics* refers to movements used to lift and move objects or persons in a manner that is efficient and preventive of muscle and/or back strain. Family members caring for a client in the home are often required to perform lifting maneuvers or other movements requiring good body mechanics to ensure safe and efficient use of muscle groups. Since the family members will be performing these maneuvers in the absence of the health-care provider, principles of good body mechanics must be taught to all family members who will be assisting the client.

Assessment of Self-Care Potential

Client/Family Assessment

- Identify all persons who will be assisting with lifting, turning, or other major muscle-use procedures.
- Assess each identified person for willingness and ability to learn proper body mechanics.

Physical Assessment

- Assess each person being taught body mechanics for
  Joint mobility: Joint flexion is required to perform many lifting procedures.
  Physical growth and development
  Pain or any disease processes that would prohibit strenuous lifting or moving
  Posture and body alignment

Environmental Assessment

- Assess the environment for availability of aids to lifting and moving:
  Wheelchair
  Cart
  Dolly
  Casters on heavy items
  Adjustability of height of chairs and beds
- Assess the height of objects that must be lifted in relation to the person lifting.
- Assess the height of the bed in relation to height of wheelchair if the client is to be moved from the bed to the wheelchair (or between any two surfaces).
- Assess the adequacy of space in which moving and lifting will take place.

Planning Strategies

Potential Nursing Diagnoses

Potential for physical injury

Expected Outcomes

Performance of required lifting and moving maneuvers without muscle strain or back injury

Health Promotion Goals

- The client and family will
  Demonstrate good body mechanics in the process of lifting heavy objects
  Use the force of pushing rather than pulling
  Use available assistive devices for moving the client or heavy objects
  Hold items being carried close to the body
  Work at waist height

Equipment
Dolly
Cart
Casters or rollers under heavy objects
Transfer board or mechanical lift to assist in moving client if needed

Interventions/Health Promotion

ACTION

RATIONALE/AMPLIFICATION

1. Begin any movement with good body alignment (Fig. 2-1).

The body is aligned vertically, with the center of gravity of the head, arms, and body in a plane slightly posterior to the hip joints and slightly anterior to the knee joints. Minimal muscular effort is necessary in this position since the weight of the head, arms, and trunk locks the hip and knee joints.

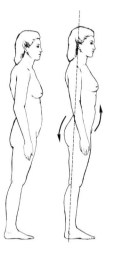

Figure 2.1
The figure on the left shows a "slouched," relaxed position. The figure on the right shows good body alignment. The abdominal muscles give a feeling of upward pull, and the gluteal muscles give a feeling of downward pull. Note the vertical plane line.

2. Adjust the working area to waist height, and arrange items in the work area as close to the body as possible.

Stretching, straining, and unnecessary reaching use energy unnecessarily and alter the center of gravity, producing instability.

3. When lifting, flex the knees and hips in a squatting position, keeping the upper body straight and holding the object being lifted close to the body (Fig. 2-2).

This lowers the body's center of gravity, thus using energy more efficiently.

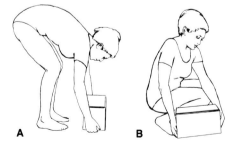

A   B

Figure 2.2
(A) Wrong position for lifting. Pull is exerted on the back muscles and leaning causes the center of gravity to fall beyond the base of support. (B) Correct position for lifting. The long and strong muscles of the legs and arms are used, and holding the object close to the body permits the line of gravity to be within the base of support.

ACTION	**RATIONALE/AMPLIFICATION**
4. When possible, push rather than pull (Fig. 2-3).	When pushing, the body weight is used as a force against the object being moved.

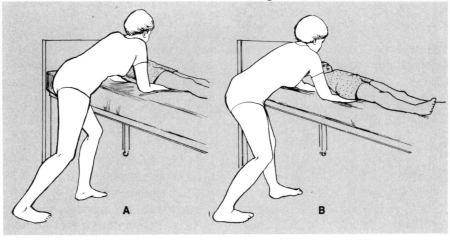

Figure 2.3
Technique for moving a client to the edge of the bed. (A) Provide a broad support; slide your arms as far as possible under the client, and lean close to the client. (B) Rock backward, using your bodyweight to assist in moving the client to the edge of the bed.

5. Push or pull rather than lift.	Lifting involves directly counteracting gravity, thus requiring more force.
6. Face the direction of the move when moving a heavy object.	This keeps the spine straight and prevents the need for spinal twisting or torsion.
7. Use a smooth surface when moving an object.	Reducing friction reduces the energy required to move an object.
8. Intersperse rest periods between work periods.	Continuous muscle exertion causes muscle fatigue and predisposes to muscle strain.
9. Obtain assistance or use an assistive device for moving heavy objects.	Various available devices (casters, carts, mechanical patient lifts, etc.) can assist in preventing muscle strain.

Related Care

1. Engage in a consistent exercise program.	Moderate, consistent exercise improves body mechanics. Exercises can be performed in a structured program or in the home through videotapes, cycling, walking, jogging, or using mechanical devices. Direct focus toward increasing flexibility, increasing strength, and learning safe muscle-group movements.
2. Keep body weight within acceptable limits.	Body mechanics and alignment are improved with appropriate body weight.

ACTION	RATIONALE/AMPLIFICATION
3. If indicated, learn one of a variety of stress-reduction methods.	If the care of the client is proving stressful to the family member, or if other stresses are excessive, a stress-reduction program is indicated (exercises, relaxation programs, etc.).

Education/ Communication

- Teach the client and family to
  Develop an awareness of good body alignment
  Lift, push, and move with the least expenditure of energy and strain to muscle groups
  Push rather than pull
  Push or pull rather than lift
  Assemble work items so that the least amount of energy possible must be used to accomplish a task
  Carry objects close to the body
  Use assistance (e.g., another person or a device when possible)
  Engage in moderate exercise program to develop strength and flexibility
  Engage in stress-reduction measures, if appropriate

Evaluation of Health Promotion Activities

Quality Assurance/ Reassessment

- Periodically, observe the client/family member in the process of lifting, moving, and working to determine if principles of good body mechanics are being observed.

DOCUMENTATION

Charting for the Home Health Nurse
- Note the date and type of teaching performed.
- Note any special programs recommended for stress reduction or weight reduction and note progress.

Records Kept by the Client/Family
- Note any indication of muscle strain.
- Record progress in weight reduction and/or stress reduction.

Health Teaching Checklist

Name of Care Provider _____

Relationship to Client _____ Telephone # _____

Taught by _____ Date _____

	EXPLAINED	DEMONSTRATED
Good body alignment	_____	_____
Procedures for lifting, pushing, pulling	_____	_____
Measures for energy conservation	_____	

Product Availability

Casters that can be applied to heavy objects, dollies, and carts can be purchased at a hardware store. A mechanical lift or transfer board to assist in moving a person can be rented or purchased from a hospital-supply firm.

Selected Reference

Wolff L, Weitzel M, et al: Fundamentals of Nursing, 7th ed. Philadelphia, JB Lippincott, 1983

3   Low Back Pain Exercises

Background

The complaint of low back pain is a commonly occurring one. Most low back discomfort or pain reflects minor injury, overexertion, or the process of normal aging.

A healthy back is one that is straight, flexible, strong, and pain-free. It has good alignment and is supported by strong back and abdominal muscles.

The vertebrae and disks surrounding the spine have the largest and heaviest load to bear during exercise. The bones, disks, ligaments, and muscles of the back are heavily supplied with nerve endings. Low back pain occurs when the nerve endings are stimulated to send messages to the brain regarding pain. The back muscles, receiving the brain's message, try to protect the back. The result is that the muscles go into spasm and attempt to hold the back immobile and quiet.

In addition to the physical causes of low back pain, other factors are also involved: stress, fatigue, and the pressures of daily living.

The prevention of back strain is primarily controlled by posture and a daily exercise program designed to build strong, supporting, back muscles. It therefore requires persistence and daily motivation on the part of the client and family support if the exercise program is to be successful. These exercises should be performed under the guidance of a physician and/or a physical therapist.

Assessment of Self-Care Potential

Client/Family Assessment

- Assess the client's motivation to undertake and continue the exercise program.
- Assess the family's involvement, commitment, and support of the exercise program, since programs have been shown to be more likely to be continued if significant persons support and become involved in them.

Physical Assessment

- Note the client's weight in relation to height. Being overweight contributes to back pain.
- Assess the client's posture: the back should be straight and well aligned.
- Assess body mechanics in relation to lifting, pulling, and pushing.
- Assess the presence of excessive stress, fatigue, or work overload, each of which may be contributing to the back pain.

Environmental Assessment

- Determine if the home contains a space cleared of obstacles and large enough for the client and others participating to perform the exercises easily.
- Determine a time to be designed into the lifestyle for uninterrupted exercises (at least three 20- to 30-minute sessions weekly).

Planning Strategies

Potential Nursing Diagnoses

Mobility, impaired physical
Comfort, alteration in: pain

Expected Outcomes

Prevention of deformities
Relief of low back pain

Health Promotion Goals

- The client and family will
  Have a physical examination to determine the cause of back pain and to initiate medical treatment if necessary
  Become committed to consistent exercise
  Schedule the exercise program into their usual lifestyle
  Demonstrate the accurate performance of the recommended exercises

Equipment

All those performing the exercises should wear loose-fitting clothing and comfortable, low-heeled, laced shoes.

Interventions/Health Promotion

ACTION

1. Advise the client to have an initial physical examination and, if indicated, a physical therapist's evaluation.

2. Advise the client to use good body mechanics in standing, lifting, moving, and reaching.

RATIONALE/AMPLIFICATION

These evaluations will form the baseline data for designing the appropriate exercise program. An exercise prescription should result from the evaluations.

Good body mechanics will assist in preventing increases in pain or damage to the back.

Rest Positions That Relieve the Back and Ease Back Strain

1. Hold onto the back of a chair, in a squatting position with back held straight. Hold for 30 seconds. Build up to 2 to 5 minutes (Fig. 3-1).

These positions rest the back by straightening the spine and tilting the pelvis forward.

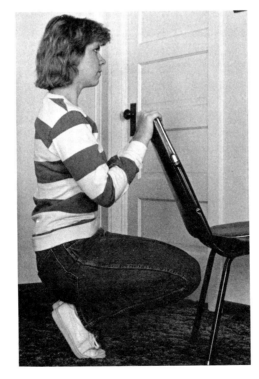

Figure 3.1

ACTION

RATIONALE/AMPLIFICATION

2. Sit on a chair of proper height to allow the feet to be flat on the floor. Bend forward and lower the head to the knees. Hold for 30 seconds. Build up to 2 to 5 minutes (Fig. 3-2).

This exercise can cause dizziness. The client may need a physician evaluation before beginning.

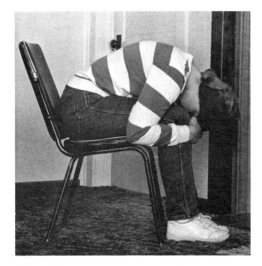

Figure 3.2

3. Lying supine on the floor, place legs on a chair or stool, remaining in place up to 15 minutes (Fig. 3-3).

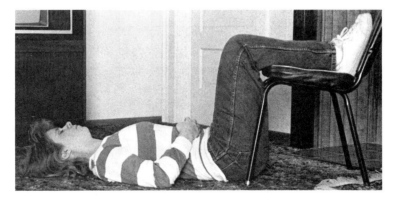

Figure 3.3

ACTION

RATIONALE/AMPLIFICATION

Active Exercises

1. Lie on the back with knees bent and hands clasped behind the neck. Place feet flat on the floor (Fig. 3-4). Take a deep breath and relax. Press the small of the back against the floor and tighten the stomach and buttock muscles (Fig. 3-5). This should cause the lower end of the pelvis to rotate forward and flatten the back against the floor. Hold for 5 seconds and relax.

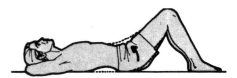

Figure 3.4

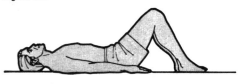

Figure 3.5

2. Lie on the back with knees bent, feet flat on the floor. Take a deep breath and relax. Grasp one knee with both hands and pull as close to the chest as possible (Fig. 3-6). Return to starting position. Straighten leg. Return to starting position. Repeat with alternate leg.

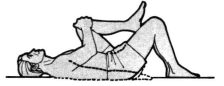

Figure 3.6

3. Lying on the back with legs bent and feet on the floor, take a deep breath and relax. Grasp *both* knees and pull them as close to the chest as possible (Fig. 3-7). Hold for 3 seconds, then return to starting position. Straighten legs and relax.

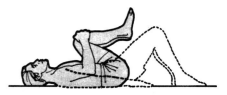

Figure 3.7

4. Lying on the back with knees bent and feet flat on the floor, take a deep breath and relax (Fig. 3-8). Draw one knee to chest (Fig. 3-9), then point leg upward as far as possible (Fig. 3-10). Return to starting position. Relax. Repeat with alternate leg. Note: this exercise is useful in stretching tight hamstring muscles, but it is not recommended for clients with sciatic pain associated with a herniated disk.

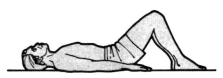

Figure 3.8

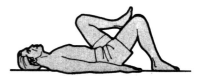

Figure 3.9

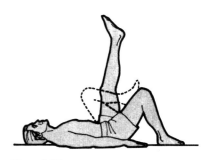

Figure 3.10

ACTION

RATIONALE/AMPLIFICATION

5. Lie on the stomach with hands clasped behind the back. Pull shoulders back and down by pushing hands downward toward feet, pinching shoulder blades together (Fig. 3-11), and lift head from floor. Take a deep breath. Hold for 2 seconds and relax.

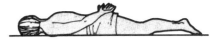

Figure 3.11

6. Stand erect. With one hand, grasp the thumb of the other hand behind the back, then pull downward toward the floor. Stand on toes and look at the ceiling while exerting the downward pull (Fig. 3-12). Hold a few seconds, and then relax. Repeat 10 times every two hours during the working day.

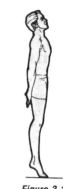

Figure 3.12

7. Stand with the back against a doorway. Place heels 4 inches away from the door frame. Take a deep breath and relax. Press the small of the back against the doorway. Tighten the stomach and buttock muscles, allowing the knees to bend slightly (Fig. 3-13). Press the neck up against the doorway. Press both hands against the opposite side of doorway and straighten both knees (Fig. 3-14). Hold for 2 seconds and relax.

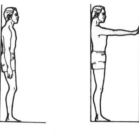

Figure 3.13   *Figure 3.14*

Advanced Exercises

1. Lie on the back with legs straight out, knees straight, and arms at the side. Take a deep breath and relax. Raise legs one at a time as high as is comfortable and lower to floor as slowly as possible (Fig. 3-15). Repeat five times for each leg.

These should not be started until pain-free and the other exercises have been done for several weeks. Physician or physical therapist consultation should precede beginning these exercises.

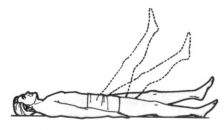

Figure 3.15

2. Hold onto a chair or a table. Squat in front of it, flexing head forward, bouncing up and down two or three times (Fig. 3-16), and then assuming an erect position.

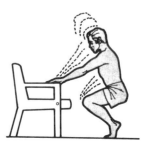

Figure 3.16

ACTION	*RATIONALE/AMPLIFICATION*
3. Lie on the back with knees bent and feet flat on the floor. Take a deep breath and relax. Pull up to a sitting position keeping knees bent (Fig. 3-17). Return to starting position and relax. Note: having someone hold the feet down facilitates the exercise.	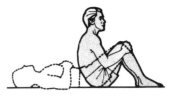 *Figure 3.17*

Related Care

1. Graduate exercises slowly.	As tolerance increases, quantity and quality of exercises can be increased.
2. Discontinue exercises that cause pain.	If pain occurs, consult the physician for advice before continuing exercises.

Referrals and Consultations

- Consult a physician or physical therapist for guidance on specific exercises and progression of the regimen. Pain, dizziness, and other unusual physiological responses should be reported.

Evaluation of Health Promotion Activities

Quality Assurance/ Reassessment

DOCUMENTATION

Charting for the Home Health Nurse
- Document the date, time, and type of exercises initiated.
- Chart the adherence to the exercise schedule.
- Note any resulting pain, documenting in client's terminology.
- Note and document accurate performance of exercise.

Records Kept by the Client/Family
Schedule of exercise program
Any pain or other concerns related to the exercise program

Health Teaching Checklist

Name of Care Provider _____

Relationship to Client _____ Telephone #_____

Taught by _____ Date _____

	EXPLAINED	DEMONSTRATED
Positions of rest	_____	_____
Exercises	_____	_____
Need to report pain or other concerns	_____	

Selected References

Brunner L, Suddarth D: Textbook of Medical–Surgical Nursing, 5th ed. Philadelphia, JB Lippincott, 1984
Back Owner's Manual: A Guide to Care of the Low Back. Patient Information Library. Daly City, CA, PAS Publishing, 1981

4　Postmastectomy Exercises

Background

The purpose of postmastectomy exercises is to strengthen the muscles of the arm and shoulder on the affected side. Exercises are usually begun within 24 hours after surgery and continued throughout the rehabilitation phase. The exercises are begun gradually and are progressed as the client gradually becomes more independent. The goal is to develop muscle use on the affected side to the preoperative state.

Assessment of Self-Care Potential

Client/Family Assessment

- Assess the client's and family's fears, concerns, and anxieties related to the pathological and psychological impact of the mastectomy.
- Assess the client's and family's acceptance of the client's altered body image.
- Determine if the client and family are committed to the client regaining independent functioning.
- Assess the role of the client within the family structure, along with her requirements for the use of the affected arm, such as for cooking, driving, typing, and so forth. Required role alterations of a temporary nature both in the home and in employment should be assessed.

Physical Assessment

- Test the involved arm, hand, and shoulder for strength as compared to that of the unaffected arm.
- Assess the level of granulation of the operative site. Assess the operative site also for drainage, redness, heat, or bleeding.
- Assess the level of pain present prior to, during, and following the performance of the exercises.
- Assess the affected arm for edema.

Environmental Assessment

- Locate an area in the home where there will be adequate space near a wall for the client to stand freely 18 inches from the wall and perform the exercises.

Planning Strategies

Potential Nursing Diagnoses

Mobility deficit, arm and shoulder
Alteration in comfort, pain
Body-image disturbance

Expected Outcomes

Return of strength and mobility in the affected arm and shoulder to preoperative levels
Relief of or decrease in pain
Client's and family's acceptance of the altered body image

Health Promotion Goals

- The client and family will
Progress from passive to totally independent exercise performance
Consistently perform prescribed exercises
Obtain and wear appropriately fitting prosthesis as recommended
Contact and attend postmastectomy support group meetings if available
Resolve body-image and sexual concerns related to the mastectomy

Interventions/Health Promotion

ACTION

1. Begin exercises slowly and within limits. Gradually increase scope and number of repetitions as strength returns.

2. *Wall-Climbing:* Stand facing a wall, with the toes as close to the wall as possible and the feet apart (Fig. 4-1). Place the palms on the wall at shoulder level with elbows slightly bent. Flex the fingers and work the hands up the wall until arms are fully extended. Work hands down to starting point. Increase scope each day, gradually bringing the feet closer to the wall.

RATIONALE/AMPLIFICATION

The purpose of the exercises is to achieve complete range-of-motion ability in the shoulder and arm of the affected side.

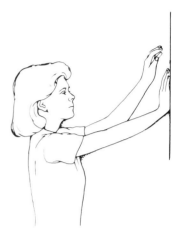

Figure 4.1
Wall-climbing exercise.

3. *Rope-Turning:* Stand facing a door. Tie a light rope to the door handle. Take the free end of the rope in the hand of the affected side. Place the other hand on the hip. With the affected arm extended and held away from the body, nearly parallel with the floor, turn the rope, making circles as wide as possible (Fig. 4-2). Perform circles slowly at first, gradually speeding the procedure.

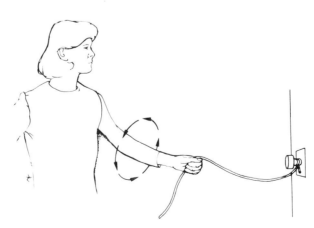

Figure 4.2
Rope-turning exercise.

ACTION   *RATIONALE/AMPLIFICATION*

4. *Rod- or Broom-Lifting:* Grasp broom handle or rod with both hands, held about 2 feet apart. With arms straight, raise broom handle above the head. Bend elbows, lowering the rod behind the head (Fig. 4-3). Reverse the procedure, raising rod above the head, and return to starting position.

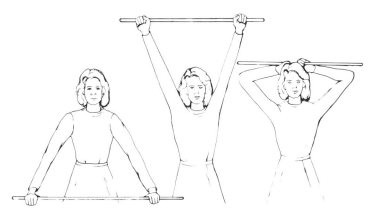

Figure 4.3
Rod-lifting exercise.

5. *Pulley:* Toss a light rope over a shower-curtain or doorway-curtain rod. Stand under the rod if possible. Grasp an end of the rope in each hand. Extend arms straight and away from the body. Pull left arm up by pulling down with right arm, then right arm up and left down in seesaw fashion (Fig. 4-4).

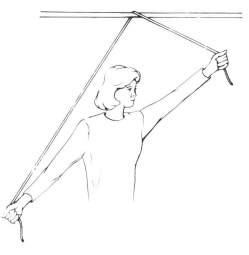

Figure 4.4
Pulley exercise.

ACTION	*RATIONALE/AMPLIFICATION*
6. Accomplish additional exercises of the affected arm by simple activities of daily living, for example, brushing hair using the affected arm, reaching for items on the floor and on shelves above the head with the affected arm, and vacuuming with the affected arm.	Any activity that will require movement and use of the affected arm will facilitate a return to preoperative strength of the arm.

Related Care

1. Encourage the client and family to verbalize feelings related to body-image alteration, the healing process, and the prognosis.	The alteration of body image often causes problems related to sexuality, self-concept, and wellness.
2. Initiate fittings for the prosthesis no later than two weeks following surgery.	A properly fitting prosthetic device assists in postmastectomy adjustment.
3. Wear an elastic sleeve over the affected arm, if recommended for edema.	The sleeve is a preventive measure against edema.

Education/ Communication

- Teach the client and family to
  Perform the exercises on a regular, consistent basis, increasing the repetitions and degree of the exercises as tolerance allows
  Discontinue the exercises if excessive pain or resistance occurs
  Maintain surveillance of the operative site for drainage, irritation, and pain
  Massage the scar, if directed, with the appropriate preparation
  Verbalize concerns and feelings with each other and the nurse
  Consistently wear the prosthetic device

Referrals and Consultations

- Consult the local affiliate of the American Cancer Society for literature and information regarding the existence of local self-help groups.
- Consult a social worker for assistance with problems of sexuality and/or self-image if needed.

Evaluation of Health Promotion Activities

Quality Assurance/ Reassessment

DOCUMENTATION

Charting for the Home Health Nurse
- Note the accuracy of exercise performance, with progression of range of motion and strength in performance.
- Assess the condition of the incision site: granulation, drainage, pain, edema of the arm.
- Consistently assess family concerns related to body image and sexuality.

Records Kept by the Client/Family
Questions and concerns
Any complications noted
Pain, resistance to exercises
Checklist of exercises performed

**Health Teaching
Checklist**

Name of Care Provider _____

Relationship to Client _____ Telephone #_____

Taught by _____ Date _____

	EXPLAINED	DEMONSTRATED
Exercises	_____	_____
Importance of involvement in self-help group	_____	
Purchase and wearing of prosthesis	_____	
Open communication with spouse and family regarding	_____	
Self-image alteration	_____	
Sexual adjustments	_____	

Product Availability

Prosthetic devices are available from a local prosthetist or through a physical therapist or the American Cancer Society.

Selected References

Brunner L, Suddarth D: Textbook of Medical–Surgical Nursing, 5th ed. Philadelphia, JB Lippincott, 1984
Help Yourself to Recovery. American Cancer Society

Circulation

5　Basic Life Support

Background

The techniques of basic life support (BLS) are similar whether resuscitating a child or an adult and whether there are one or more rescuers at the scene. Minor modifications allow a person to perform one-rescuer or two-rescuer cardiopulmonary resuscitation (CPR), child and infant CPR, and foreign body obstruction techniques. When health professionals arrive at the scene, they will proceed with advanced cardiac life support (ACLS) skills. The home health nurse should remain available to assist with procedures as requested or to relieve rescuers performing CPR. Family members will be able to assist the nurse until professional help arrives. The lay rescuer will be relieved of responsibility when no longer required.

Assessment of Self-Care Potential

Client/Family Assessment

- Assess whether family members are capable and willing to learn BLS techniques. Check whether BLS classes are available through community agencies or whether individual instruction will have to be given.
- Check whether special instructions on BLS will need to be given for tracheostomy or laryngectomy.
- If an apnea monitor will be used for monitoring an infant, determine whether a monitor can be rented. Check whether a third-party payor will reimburse the family.

Physical Assessment

- Determine if the client is at risk for sudden death or respiratory arrest.
- If the client is a neonate, determine if the infant is at risk for sudden infant death syndrome.

Environmental Assessment

- Assess the environment where a victim is found to determine if there is the possibility of a neck injury. Persons who are found unconscious near a fallen ladder or a diving board or in an automobile accident may have sustained neck injuries. Neck injuries require special precautions to prevent hyperextension of the neck and injury to the spinal cord. If the victim has been eating, suspect an airway obstruction.

Planning Strategies

Potential Nursing Diagnoses

Cardiac output, alteration in: decreased due to sudden death

Tissue perfusion, alteration in: decreased due to ineffective cardiac contractions

Injury, potential for sudden death due to...

Gas exchange, impaired due to respiratory arrest

Knowledge deficit, basic life support techniques

Expected Outcomes

Maintenance or restoration of adequate cardiac output

Maintenance of adequate tissue perfusion

Prevention of injury during resuscitation efforts

Prevention of brain damage due to anoxia

Increased knowledge of basic life support techniques

Health Promotion Goals

- The client and family will
  Demonstrate effective basic life support techniques

Interventions/Health Promotion

ACTION	*RATIONALE/AMPLIFICATION*
1. Determine whether the person is unresponsive. Gently shake the victim and shout "Are you OK?" Call for help, even if no one is in sight.	If the victim does not respond, calling for help may bring another person to the scene. This person can call for emergency medical service using a 911 emergency number, by calling the fire or police department to dispatch paramedics, or by following procedures specific to the community. Once professional help is on the way, the person can assist with basic life support.
2. Position the client supine on a firm surface.	Chest compressions will produce blood flow to the brain only if the body is in a vertical position. Use caution if a neck or back injury is suspected. Roll the person as a unit, without twisting the body, to prevent spinal cord injury.
3. Open the airway. *Head Tilt–Chin Lift Maneuver*	
• Place the fingers of one hand under the chin and lift the chin forward.	This supports the jaw and helps to tilt the head back.
• Use the other hand on the forehead to tilt the head back (Fig. 5-1).	Remove dentures only if they cannot be managed in place. Dentures make the mouth-to-mouth seal easier to accomplish.

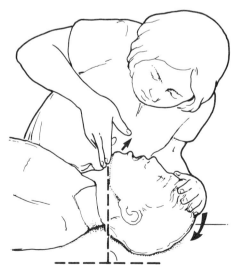

Figure 5.1
Head tilt–chin lift maneuver. Perpendicular line reflects proper neck extension. (© Reproduced with permission. Basic Life Support Instructors Manual. American Heart Association)

ACTION

Jaw-Thrust Maneuver
- Grasp the angles of the victim's lower jaw with one hand on each side. Lift the jaw while displacing the mandible forward and tilting the head back (Fig. 5-2).

RATIONALE/AMPLIFICATION

Use this maneuver if the airway cannot be opened by using the head tilt–chin lift maneuver.

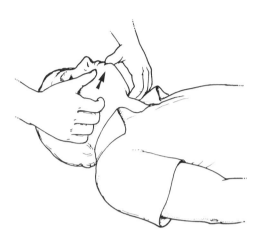

Figure 5.2
Jaw-thrust maneuver. (© Reproduced with permission. Basic Life Support Instructors Manual. American Heart Association)

4. Determine if the victim is breathing. Check for 3 to 5 seconds.

Breathlessness can be checked by looking for the chest to rise and fall, listening for air escaping during exhalation, and feeling the flow of exhaled air on the rescuer's cheek.

5. While maintaining the head tilt–chin lift, take a deep breath and seal the victim's lips with your lips. Pinch the victim's nostrils closed.
Blow air into the victim's mouth while watching for the chest to rise (Fig. 5-3). Give two quick breaths.

The head tilt–chin lift keeps the airway open. Pinching the nostrils stops air from escaping through the nose.

Mouth-to-nose breathing is an alternative. If this technique is used, hold the victim's mouth closed to prevent air from escaping.

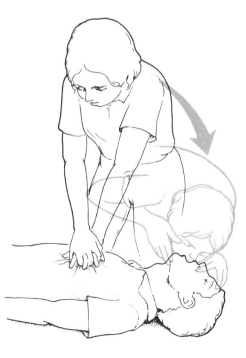

Figure 5.3
Mouth-to-mouth rescue breathing and chest compressions for one rescuer. Note proper position of rescuer: the rescuer's shoulders are directly over the victim's sternum, with elbows locked. (© Reproduced with permission. Basic Life Support Instructors Manual. American Heart Association)

ACTION	*RATIONALE/AMPLIFICATION*
6. If unable to ventilate the person, reposition the head and try again. If still unable to ventilate, perform foreign obstruction techniques (see Related Care, below).	Repositioning the head opens the airway. A closed airway is usually the reason that a person cannot be ventilated.
7. Check the carotid pulse while maintaining the head tilt.	Locate the carotid pulse on the side nearest the rescuer to prevent pressure on the trachea.
8. If there is a palpable pulse, initiate rescue breathing at the rate of 12 breaths/minute.	The rate of 12 breaths/minute is appropriate for one rescuer and an adult victim.
9. If there is no pulse, position your hands on the lower half of the victim's sternum and begin chest compressions at the rate of 80 to 100 per minute (see Fig. 5-3).	The correct hand position can be located by checking for the xiphoid process and placing the heel of the hand above the xiphoid process on the lower portion of the sternum. The sternum must be depressed 1½ to 2 inches (3.8 cm–5 cm) for the normal-sized adult. The compression is released to allow venous return to the heart. If the rescuer repeats the mnemonic "One-and, two-and," and so forth, this helps maintain the correct rate.
10. Open the airway and deliver two quick breaths. Locate the proper hand position and begin 15 more chest compressions (see Fig. 5-3).	The correct ratio is 2 breaths to 15 compressions for an adult, if one rescuer is involved.
11. If another person arrives to assist, request that that individual take over breathing or chest compressions. Exchange positions periodically to prevent fatigue.	The correct ratio for two rescuers is 1 breath to 5 chest compressions.
12. Periodically check to see if the pulse has returned. Check the carotid pulse while the other person does chest compressions and again after chest compressions are stopped. If the pulse returns, discontinue chest compressions. Continue rescue breathing unless the person starts breathing unassisted. Check both pulse and breathing periodically.	There should be a pulse for each chest compression. If the pulse is felt while no chest compressions are being performed, the pulse has returned.

Related Care

1. If a neck injury is suspected, use the jaw-thrust technique without the head tilt to open the airway.	Using the jaw thrust without the head tilt opens the airway without hyperextension of the neck, which can cause injury to the spinal cord.

ACTION

2. Use mouth-to-stoma breathing if the victim has a laryngectomy (Figs. 5-4 and 5-5) or tracheostomy.

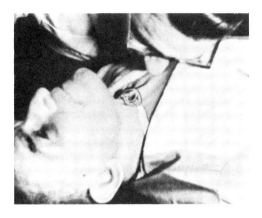

Figure 5.4
Mouth-to-stoma breathing. (Reprinted with permission of the American Cancer Society)

RATIONALE/AMPLIFICATION

A person with a laryngectomy breathes either entirely or partially through an opening (stoma) in the neck, as does the person with a tracheostomy. There may or may not be a tube in place. Tracheostomy tubes have a cuff. Inflate the cuff with air and a syringe to prevent air escaping around the tube. (See Technique 76, Tracheostomy Care.)

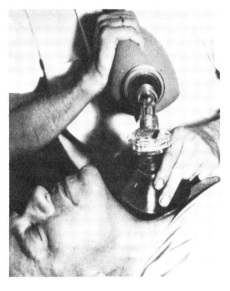

Figure 5.5
Adapting a facemask and Ambu bag to ventilate a laryngectomee. (Reprinted with permission of the American Cancer Society)

3. If an airway obstruction is suspected
   • Roll the person supine. Deliver abdominal or chest thrusts.

   • Sweep the mouth with the fingers to check for dislodged foreign material.
   • Attempt to ventilate the person if still not breathing. If the person still cannot be ventilated, repeat the maneuvers to dislodge the foreign body. When the person can be ventilated, give two breaths. Then check the carotid pulse (see Step 7, above).

Suspect obstruction of the airway with a foreign body if the person cannot be ventilated even after repositioning the head.
The thrusts are forceful in an attempt to relieve the obstruction.
Abdominal thrusts can be delivered while alongside or astride the person. Chest thrusts are appropriate for pregnant women or obese individuals.
Removing material that has been dislodged prevents it from being forced back into the airway during rescue breathing.

Age-Specific Modifications (Pediatric)

- A child can use the astride position (Fig. 5-6) to perform abdominal thrusts on an adult who is choking.

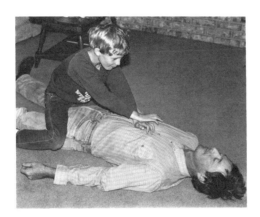

Figure 5.6
Administering an abdominal thrust using the astride position.

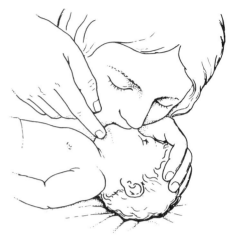

Figure 5.7
Rescue breathing with airtight seal for mouth and nose. (© Reproduced with permission. Basic Life Support Instructors Manual. American Heart Association)

- Seal both the mouth and nose to perform rescue breathing on a small infant (Fig. 5-7). Use small puffs of air to ventilate rather than a forceful breath that could cause damage to the lungs. For a child, ventilate only enough to cause the chest to rise. Breathe 20 times per minute for an infant and 15 times per minute for a child.
- Modify obstructed airway techniques for infants and children (Figs. 5-8, 5-9, and 5-10).

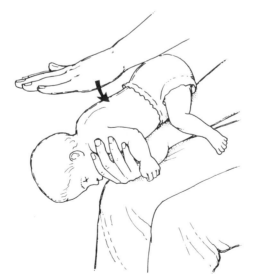

Figure 5.8
Back blows for management of foreign body airway obstruction in an infant. (© Reproduced with permission. Basic Life Support Instructors Manual. American Heart Association)

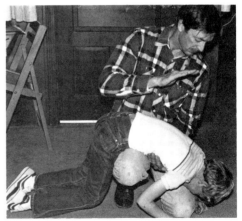

Figure 5.9
Back blows for management of foreign body airway obstruction in a child.

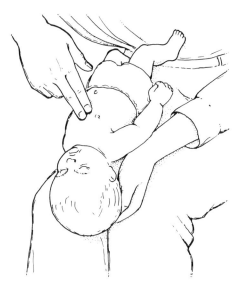

Figure 5.10
Chest thrust for management of foreign body airway obstruction in an infant. (© Reproduced with permission. Basic Life Support Instructors Manual. American Heart Association)

- For infants and small children, palpate to check for a brachial pulse rather than for a carotid pulse.
- Use two fingers to perform chest compressions on an infant (Fig. 5-11). Compress the midsternum between the nipples ½ to 1 inch (1.3 cm–2.5 cm). Use the heel of one hand for chest compressions in a child. Depress the sternum 1½ to 2 inches (2.5 cm–3.8 cm).

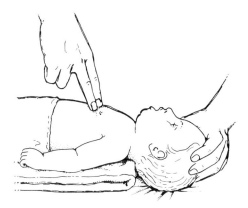

Figure 5.11
External chest compressions in an infant. (© Reproduced with permission. Basic Life Support Instructors Manual. American Heart Association)

- Perform chest compressions at a rate of 100 per minute for an infant and at a rate of 80 to 100 per minute for a child.
- Coordinate rescue breathing and chest compressions in a ratio of 1 breath to 5 chest compressions.

Education/ Communication

- Teach the family to
    Activate the emergency medical system immediately so that professional help will be dispatched. Ask a second person to phone for emergency assistance by calling 911, the police or fire department, or local emergency medical service.
    Remain with the victim and initiate BLS. Circulation must be established within 4 minutes to prevent brain damage.
    Count chest compressions aloud if a second rescuer is assisting (e.g., "one-one thousand, two-one thousand"). This assists the rescuer to maintain the proper rate and to pause briefly to enable the person doing rescue breathing to interpose breaths.
    Perform chest compressions on a firm surface with the victim supine

Reposition the head and continue BLS if air is entering the stomach. Realigning the airway is usually sufficient to prevent this. Check for swelling over the stomach, which indicates that air is entering the esophagus during rescue breathing.

Modify BLS techniques for infants or children

Discontinue BLS only if (1) you are exhausted and no help is available, (2) you are relieved by a qualified person, or (3) you are instructed to do so by a physician

Referrals and Consultations

• Refer the family to the American Red Cross, American Heart Association, local college continuing-education program, or local hospital for cardiopulmonary resuscitation training.

Evaluation of Health Promotion Activities

Quality Assurance/ Reassessment

• Check the family members' BLS skills yearly or refer them for yearly refresher course and practice.

DOCUMENTATION

Charting for the Home Health Nurse
• Record capabilities of family members to perform BLS.

• Assess client's risk for cardiac or respiratory arrest.

Health Teaching Checklist

Name of Care Provider _____

Relationship to Client _____ Telephone # _____

Taught by _____ Date _____

	EXPLAINED	DEMONSTRATED
BLS techniques	_____	_____
Specific modifications as required (e.g., neonatal resuscitation)	_____	_____
Activation of emergency medical system	_____	
Referral for yearly refresher course	_____	

Product Availability

Mannequins can be obtained for practice by contacting the American Heart Association, American Red Cross, a local college, or a community hospital.

Films and literature on basic life support are available from the American Heart Association and the American Red Cross. Films suitable for all audiences are available.

Selected References

Herrin TJ, Montgomery WH (eds): Instructors Manual for Basic Life Support. Dallas, American Heart Association, 1985

American Heart Association: Interim Teaching Guidelines for Revisions in Basic Life Support. Dallas, American Heart Association, 1986

6 Holter Monitor

Background

A Holter monitor is an electrocardiogram (ECG) recorder approximately the size of a small tape recorder. It is worn by the client during normal daily activities to record an ambulatory electrocardiogram (ECG). The heart action is recorded continuously for either 12 or 24 hours on tapes similar to those used in a tape recorder. This type of recording is useful to evaluate cardiac arrhythmias that occur intermittently and that have not been documented. Often arrhythmias occur during a specific daily activity.

The recorder is attached to the client by a technician. The client is instructed to record activity and symptoms in a diary, so that events can be correlated with the Holter tape (Fig. 6-1). The tape is scanned by a technician, using a computer that rapidly superimposes one ECG complex on another, so that an entire 24-hour recording can be scanned in less than 30 minutes. The home health nurse can teach the client and family about the Holter recording and help allay any anxiety experienced by the client.

PATIENT ACTIVITY DIARY

TIME	ACTIVITY	SYMPTOM
10 AM PM	START RECORDING	
10:30	driving to work on freeway	chest pounding
11:30	walking up stairs	chest pains
11:45	Took medication	
12:30	Ate lunch	relaxed
5	Argued with son	Chest pounding

Figure 6.1
Sample patient diary.

Assessment of Self-Care Potential

Client/Family Assessment
- Determine whether the client will be able to record activities in the diary or if a family member will have to assist.

Physical Assessment
- Determine the reason the client requires a Holter recording (e.g., blackouts, arrhythmias, palpitations, etc.).

Planning Strategies

Potential Nursing Diagnoses

Related to potential cardiac problem:

Cardiac output, alteration in: decreased

Self-concept, disturbance in: body image, related to the presence of the Holter monitor

Knowledge deficit: related to management of 12-hour or 24-hour Holter recording.

Expected Outcomes

Recording of a clean, artifact-free ambulatory ECG

Maintenance of adequate cardiac output

Acceptance of the Holter monitor as a diagnostic aid

Understanding of the goals, use, and maintenance of a Holter monitor

Health Promotion Goals

- The client and family will
  Continue with normal activities during the recording
  Protect the recorder from damage
  Record all events in the patient diary

Equipment

Holter recorder

Battery

Recording tape, new or cleanly erased

Snap leads

Hypoallergenic tape (1-inch)

Benzoin

Patient diary

Electrodes

Adhesive overlays (to secure electrodes)

Extension cable

Electrode-retainer clip

Belt or shoulder strap

4 × 4 gauze pads

70% Isopropyl alcohol

Felt-tip pen

Fine sandpaper (6/0 or 220 grit)

Razor

Empty take-up reel

Magnetic-tape head cleaner

Cotton-tipped swabs

Interventions/Health Promotion

ACTION	RATIONALE/AMPLIFICATION
1. Load tape into the recorder following the manufacturer's instructions. Record 3 to 5 minutes of calibration pulses at the beginning of the tape.	The calibration pulses enable the technician scanning the tape to determine that the recorder has been calibrated correctly.
2. Prepare the skin and apply electrodes: • Defat the skin with alcohol and 4 × 4s. Allow the skin to dry thoroughly.	Electrodes are the ECG pads that are attached to the skin and enable the heart rhythm to be recorded.
• Locate the bony sites for electrode application by palpation (Fig. 6-2).	Electrodes are placed over bone because Holter monitoring is an ambulatory ECG. The placement over bone and avoidance of adipose tissue decrease artifact on the tape.

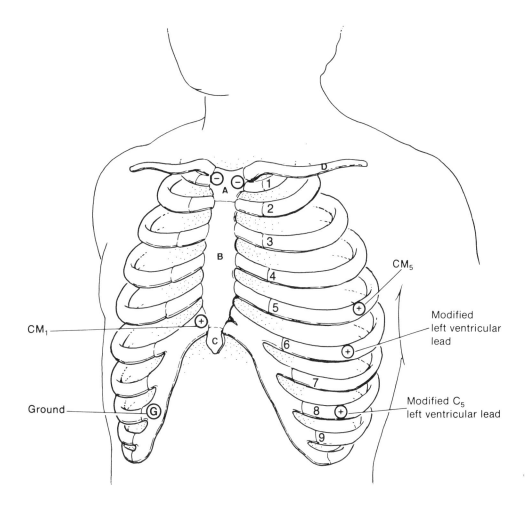

	ELECTRODE	PLACEMENT
Modified CM₅ left ventricular lead	Reference —	Right side of manubrial portion of sternum
	Exploring +	Left anterior axillary line, 5th rib
Modified CM₁ atrial and right ventricular lead	Reference —	Left side of manubrial portion of sternum
	Exploring +	2 cm right of xyphoid process, on lower rib margin
Ground	Ground (RL)	Right lower rib margin
Modified C₅ left ventricular lead	Reference —	Right side of manubrium
	Exploring +	Left 8th or 9th rib at anterior axillary line
Modified left ventricular lead	Reference —	Left side of manubrium
	Exploring +	Left 6th rib at anterior axillary line

Figure 6.2
Anatomical landmarks for applying electrodes. Select two leads if a 2-channel recorder is used. *Ref*, reference electrode; *Exp*, exploring electrode; *GND (RL)*, ground—right leg.

ACTION	*RATIONALE/AMPLIFICATION*
• Mark the electrode sites with a felt-tip pen.	
• Dry shave the hair from the electrode sites.	This should be done for men as well as women to improve electrode contact and decrease artifact on the tape.
• Gently abrade the skin, using fine sandpaper, until the skin is slightly pink.	This removes dead skin cells and decreases resistance, which enhances the ECG tracing.
• Using a cotton-tipped swab, apply benzoin to the skin that will be covered by the adhesive portion of the electrode.	This step is optional. Benzoin ensures adhesion of the electrode and protects the skin from irritation. Do not paint the skin under the center portion of the electrode where the gel will be in contact with the skin.
• Apply the disposable electrodes.	Check the electrodes to see that the gel is moist and has not dried while in storage.
• Remove the paper backing from the adhesive overlay and press the overlay over the electrode. Secure the overlay to the electrode and the surrounding skin.	This secures the electrode.

3. Connect the snap leads to the electrodes and the extension cable. Connect the extension cable to the recorder at the proper location.
4. Insert the battery into the recorder. Secure the recorder to the client's torso with the belt or shoulder strap (Fig. 6-3).

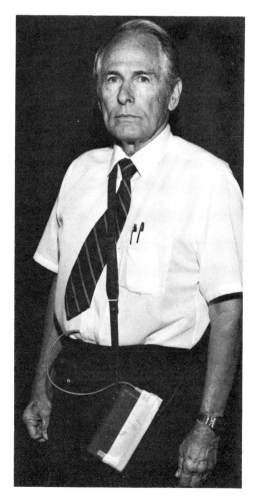

Figure 6.3
Holter monitor.

ACTION	*RATIONALE/AMPLIFICATION*

5. Following the manufacturer's instructions, test the client–electrode interface and the recorder before beginning the recording:
  • Connect the test cable to the scanner or ECG machine as directed by the instructions.
  • Obtain real-time write out from the ECG machine or scanner.
  • Observe the tracing for a minimum of 0.5-mV amplitude on at least one channel.
  • Gently tap each electrode with an index finger and observe the appropriate channel for artifact.
  • Replace the electrode if artifact is observed.
	Because the recording is not obtained in real time, problems with the recorder would not be observed until the tape is scanned 12 or 24 hours later. Testing the application of the recorder is important.
	
	If artifact is observed the electrode contact with the skin is not secure.

6. Secure the lead wires together with tape to reduce movement.	Movement produces artifact on the ECG tape.
7. Prepare the recorder to begin recording, and set the clock on the recorder.	
8. Enter the time when the recorder was started and the recorder serial number into the client's diary.	
9. Check that the recorder is functioning correctly: Is the clock reading the correct time? Is the tape being properly wound on the take-up reel? Is the tape still moving and the motor still operating? Is the pinch wheel still closed?	The events in the diary will be correlated with arrhythmias on the ECG tape.

Education/ Communication

• Explain to the client and family the reason for an extended recording in determining whether or not irregularities of the heartbeat are a problem. Most clients have had a resting ECG. The Holter recording can be likened to an ECG.

• Tell the client where to go to have the recorder removed at the end of the recording time.

• Teach the client how to record physical events or feelings in the diary. Communicate how important the diary will be in scanning the ECG tape.

• Show the client that the recorder can easily be concealed under a loose jacket, shirt, or blouse.

• Tell the client to participate in normal activities except for showering. Taking a sponge bath rather than a shower will protect the recorder from water. Reassure the client that the recorder is secure.

• Caution the client not to drop the recorder.

• Tell the client to reapply any electrode that becomes disconnected and to tape it in place with adhesive. The client should note the time of reapplying of electrodes in the diary.

- Tell the client and family to deal with episodes of chest pain as they have previously been instructed (e.g., nitroglycerin). The Holter recording will make no difference.

Referrals and Consultations

- Give the client and family a telephone number where assistance can be obtained in the event of problems with the recorder.

Evaluation of Health Promotion Activities

Quality Assurance/ Reassessment

- When the client returns to have the Holter monitor removed, discuss any problems that might have occurred that would decrease the quality of the recording.
- Determine that the client has a follow-up appointment with the cardiologist to evaluate the results of the recording.

DOCUMENTATION

Charting for the Home Health Nurse
- Document the application of the recorder and the time that the recording was commenced.
- Document the client's understanding of the reason for the recording and the importance of entering events into the diary.
- Note the position of the electrodes to document the lead that is being monitored.

Records Kept by the Client/Family
- Holter monitor diary

Health Teaching Checklist

Name of Care Provider _____

Relationship to Client _____ Telephone #_____

Taught by _____ Date _____

	EXPLAINED	DEMONSTRATED
Purpose of Holter recording	_____	
Recording symptoms in diary	_____	_____
Importance of carrying out normal daily activities	_____	
Importance of protecting recording from water or damage	_____	
Replacing electrodes if disconnected	_____	_____
Telephone number to contact technician or home health nurse if problems develop with the recorder	_____	
Where to report to have the recorder removed at the end of the recording period	_____	

7 Permanent Pacemaker

Background

People who have permanent dysfunction of the normal cardiac conduction system and whose condition cannot be controlled with drugs may be candidates for the insertion of a permanent artificial pacemaker. One of the most common reasons that a permanent pacemaker is inserted is complete heart block following trauma, surgery, or myocardial infarction. Other problems include severe bradycardia, sick sinus syndrome, Stokes-Adams attacks, and certain rapid dysrhythmias. (In the event of a rapid rhythm such as atrial tachycardia, the rate of the pacemaker can be turned higher than the client's rate and take over pacing. Then the rate can be gradually lowered to a normal rate.) More commonly, pacemakers are inserted for people with heart rates too slow to maintain an adequate cardiac output. The client will show symptoms of fainting, dizziness, and fluid accumulation, as indicated by swollen ankles, for example.

A permanent pacemaker system consists of a power source (called the *pulse generator*), electrodes that deliver an electrical impulse to the myocardium, and leads that connect the generator and electrodes. Pacemaker activity (firing) is indicated on the electrocardiogram (ECG) by a pacemaker spike or artifact (Figs. 7-1 and 7-2).

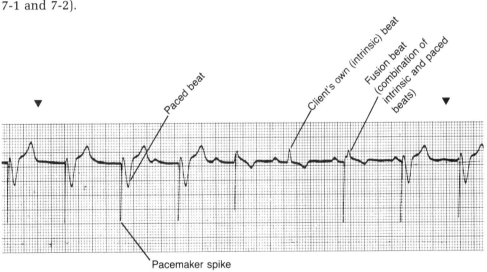

Figure 7.1
Demand ventricular pacemaker. The pacemaker spike will be followed by a ventricular complex wider than normal.

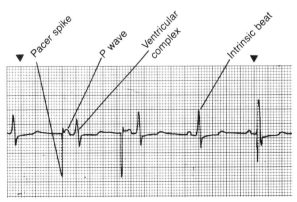

Figure 7.2
Atrial pacemaker. The pacer spike will be followed by a P wave.

The most common type, a *transvenous* or *endocardial* pacemaker, is placed in the operating room or x-ray department under local anesthesia. The generator is sutured in a subcutaneous pocket on the right shoulder, leaving a flat bulge (Fig. 7-3). The leads are threaded through the venous system and stabilized in the right side of the heart. Less commonly, an *epicardial* pacemaker is inserted during chest surgery under general anesthesia, and the electrodes are sutured directly onto the left ventricle. The generator can also be positioned in the abdominal subcutaneous tissue or on the left shoulder if the client prefers; for example, placing the generator in a pocket on the left shoulder would enable a person who likes hunting to continue with this sport without the recoil of the gun affecting the pacemaker.

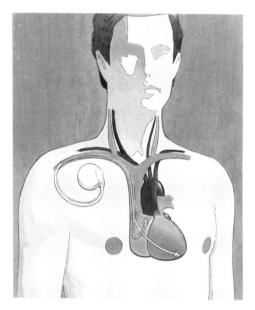

Figure 7.3
Transvenous AV synchronous pacemaker. The electrodes are implanted in both the atrium and ventricle. (Copyright © 1985, by Medtronic, Inc.)

Pacemaker Terminology

Atrial pacemaker: The electrode is inserted in the atrium to overcome problems with the sinus node. On the ECG the pacer spike will precede the P wave (see Fig. 7-2).

Ventricular pacemaker: The electrode is inserted in the ventricle because of conduction problems in the atrioventricular (AV) node or ventricle. The pacer spike will be followed by a wide QRS complex on the ECG. P waves may or may not be present (see Fig. 7-1).

AV synchronous pacemaker: Electrodes are inserted into both the atrium and the ventricle to mimic the normal conduction between the two chambers (see Fig. 7-3).

Fixed rate (asynchronous) pacemaker: The pacemaker is set at a predetermined rate and fires regardless of the client's rate. This type of pacemaker does not have a mechanism to sense the heart's normal beats, and it is not inserted very often.

Demand pacemaker: The pacemaker will not fire unless the client's rate drops below a predetermined rate, usually about 72 beats per minute. This type of pacemaker contains both sensing and firing components.

Hysteresis pacemaker: This pacemaker allows some leeway before it starts to fire at the preset rate. For example, if the rate is set at 70 beats per minute, the pacemaker may not fire until the rate reaches 60. This prevents the pacemaker from firing when the heart normally slows down (e.g., during rest).

Programmable pacemaker: The generator settings (e.g., rate) can be altered by signals from an external pacemaker programmer. This is a noninvasive procedure. Pacemakers that are not programmable have the parameters set during manufacture.

Capture: When a pacemaker spike is followed by contraction of the heart, it is said to capture the heart.

Assessment of Self-Care Potential

Client/Family Assessment

- Determine the level of knowledge of the client and family related to the implanted pacemaker.
- Assess the ability and willingness of the client or family member to check pacemaker function.
- Determine the amount of assistance that will be required from the home health nurse.
- Assess whether the client's altered body image has been accepted by both the client and family members.
- Determine whether insurance counseling has been provided and whether the family will be able to meet the expenses of pacemaker insertion and maintenance. Third-party payors including Medicare, Veterans Administration, and private insurance companies may cover the costs of the pacemaker. If this is not available, assess the availability of community aid.
- Assist the client and family to determine whether a telephone pacemaker follow-up clinic will be useful. This depends on how far the client must travel to the cardiologist's office and whether travel is a problem. Assist the client and family to determine which company will best meet the client's needs.

Physical Assessment

- Perform a complete physical assessment. Emphasize cardiovascular and pacemaker assessment on subsequent visits. Determine whether the client has experienced any injuries caused by falls prior to pacemaker insertion.
- Assess for the return of pre-pacemaker symptoms (e.g., dizziness, falls, shortness of breath, or swollen ankles).
- Check whether the client has experienced any chest pain.
- Assess personal cleanliness. The client will be discharged from the hospital without a dressing on the suture line of the pacemaker pocket.

Environmental Assessment

- Assess the location of a telephone and whether it will be feasible to use it for telephone pacemaker checks.

Planning Strategies

Potential Nursing Diagnoses

Cardiac output, alteration in: decreased due to conduction disturbance in cardiac tissue

Tissue perfusion, alteration in: low cardiac output due to inability to maintain effective heartbeat

Health maintenance, alteration in: permanent pacemaker implantation

Knowledge deficit, learning need related to implanted heart pacemaker

Anxiety, due to pacemaker insertion or impending pacemaker generator replacement

Expected Outcomes

Maintenance of adequate cardiac output by supplementing the client's normal (intrinsic) rhythm with paced beats

Maintenance of tissue perfusion

Relief of symptoms of conduction disorder

Knowledge of the management of the implanted pacemaker

Decreased anxiety due to increased knowledge of pacemaker system

Health Promotion Goals

• The client and family will

Perform pacemaker function checks daily and telephone checks as directed

Inspect the subcutaneous pocket for signs of infection or tissue breakdown

Understand that the pacemaker will deliver an electrical signal to the myocardium to stimulate the heart to beat

Realize that a pacemaker does not cure heart problems or repair damaged tissue

Be prepared for surgery to replace the generator or other parts of the pacing system should this become necessary. The life of the generator will depend on the type of generator and the amount of use.

Keep regular appointments with the cardiologist

Continue their present lifestyle with minimal changes

Equipment

For daily pulse checks:
    Watch with second hand or stopwatch
    Pacemaker magnet (optional)

For periodic telephone clinic checks:
    Any telephone
    ECG transmitter
    Electrodes: finger, bracelet, chest, or underarm
    Pacemaker magnet

For radio pulse checks:
    Small transistor radio
    Magnet (unless pacemaker is fixed rate)

For telephone transmitter checks:
    Transmitter
    Electrodes

Interventions/Health Promotion

ACTION	*RATIONALE/AMPLIFICATION*
1. Teach the client to check pulse rate daily on awakening each morning (see Technique 42, Vital Signs). Use a watch with a second hand and take the pulse for one full minute.	Check the pulse while seated on the side of the bed and before ambulating. A gradual decrease in pulse rate over a period of time will alert the cardiologist to schedule the client for generator replacement. If the pacemaker is functioning correctly, the heart rate, whether from the pacemaker or normal heartbeats, should not be below

ACTION

RATIONALE/AMPLIFICATION

the preset rate. When the voltage in a lithium battery drops to a certain point, the pacemaker automatically decreases the rate of stimulation by 5 to 10 beats per minute.

2. If requested by the cardiologist, place a magnet over the pacemaker generator before taking the pulse.

The magnet places the pacemaker in the fixed-rate mode, so that the pulse rate will reflect pacemaker function. Expect a slight decrease in the rate when the magnet is placed over the generator. There is a slight risk of triggering ventricular arrhythmias when the pacemaker is in the asynchronous mode. Use this pulse check when other family members are present.

3. Perform a telephone pacemaker check as required:

When a specially designed transmitter is used, the heart's sounds are converted to electronic signals that can be transmitted over the telephone. A device at the other end records the client's ECG (Fig. 7-4). This form of checkup is helpful for the elderly or for people who have to travel long distances to a pacemaker clinic. Telephone monitoring may not be covered by third-party payors. Check to be sure.

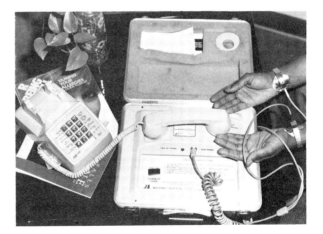

Figure 7.4
Monitoring a permanent pacemaker using wrist electrodes. The electrocardiogram is recorded at a remote facility by telephone. (Copyright © 1985, by Medtronic, Inc.)

• When the pacemaker clinic calls, place the electrodes on the skin.

Most services have a 24-hour set-up where a client can call if problems develop with the pacemaker.

• Turn on the ECG transmitter.

Reassure the client that telephone checks in no way use power from the pacemaker generator.

ACTION	RATIONALE/AMPLIFICATION
• Place the mouthpiece of the telephone over the transmitter's audio output (this usually makes a beeping sound).	
• The ECG is automatically transmitted.	
• If requested by the technician, place the magnet over the generator. The client may lie down and place the magnet over the generator if unable to hold it.	This enables evaluation of the pacemaker. If there are any problems with the pacemaker, the technician will alert the client to seek medical attention.
4. Use the radio test to determine the rate of pacemaker stimulation:	This will not work on all pacemakers. Check with the physician to see if it is suitable.
• Turn on the transistor radio and tune it to 55 or 550 AM.	
• Lie down and place the magnet over the generator.	For a fixed-rate pacemaker, place the radio directly over the generator. The magnet will not be required.
• Listen for clicks on the radio.	These clicks correspond to the rate of stimulation.
• Check the pulse at the same time. Each click should correspond with a heartbeat.	This checks that the pacemaker leads are intact. If they are not, the click indicating pacemaker stimulation will not be followed by a heartbeat, indicated by a pulse. If the client feels the pulse without the click, this means that the heart is beating without the aid of the pacemaker.
• Contact the cardiologist if the pulse rate with the magnet decreases by 5 or more beats per minute.	Generator replacement may be necessary.
Alternative:	
• Use the telephone transmitter to count the pulse.	
• Turn on the transmitter and connect the electrodes to the body in the same manner that is used for telephone transmission.	
• Count the beeps.	The drawback to this method is that there is no way to differentiate between natural and paced heartbeats.

Education/ Communication

• Teach the client and family to

Expect minimal incisional discomfort following pacemaker insertion. This can be relieved by acetaminophen or a similar oral pain medication. Chest pain may occur just the same as before the pacemaker insertion. Follow the physician's instructions for treatment of chest pain.

Stay on bed rest, with the head no higher than 30 degrees, for 48 to 72 hours after pacemaker insertion to prevent dislodging the electrode. After 72 hours, enough tissue will have formed around the electrode to secure it to the endocardium.

Report any signs of infection of the subcutaneous pocket (e.g., redness, drainage, or an unusual amount of pain)

Limit vigorous movement of the arms for 6 weeks following surgery to prevent electrode displacement. Resume all previous activities after 6 weeks. Discourage contact sports that could result in chest trauma. Swim, bathe, and shower as desired once the wound has healed. The generator will be watertight.

Check the pacemaker function daily by taking the pulse. Do not be concerned if the rate changes slightly from day to day. The pacemaker might be required more on some days than others. The rate should not drop below the preset pacemaker rate.

Avoid *close exposure* to sources of electromagnetic interference (EMI) (e.g., heliarc welding equipment, radar installations, malfunctioning electrical appliances or tools, dental treatment devices such as drills and ultrasonic cleaners, internal combustion engines, and microwave ovens with faulty shielding). These can affect pacemaker function. Certain radio frequencies used by ham radio operators and citizen's band radio can affect pacemaker function. The most common frequencies that affect pacemaker function are 3.5 MHz and 28.5 MHz. Internal combustion engines, such as snowmobile engines, car engines, or lawnmower engines, are safe unless the person leans up against them. Hospital devices such as diathermy or electrocautery can affect pacemaker function.

Electronic metal detectors used by airport security personnel or libraries will not affect pacemaker function but will set off the alarm. Living near a radar installation such as an airport will not affect pacemaker function. If any device interferes with pacemaker function, as indicated by dizziness or fainting, move away from the source.

Check the information received when the pacemaker was inserted to determine whether the pacemaker meets the standards established by the Association for the Advancement of Medical Instrumentation (AAMI). Most pacemakers meet these standards, and the client can be reasonably sure the EMI will not affect pacemaker function.

Wear a Medic-Alert bracelet or neck chain. Carry a card that has details of the type of pacemaker.

Be prepared for battery replacement at a future date. The leads do not necessarily have to be replaced at the same time. Mercury–zinc batteries last 3 to 5 years, lithium batteries last 7 to 15 years, and nuclear pacemakers last 15 to 20 years.

- Teach the client that
Sexual activity can be resumed in 6 weeks
The pulse generator can be easily covered by wearing appropriate clothing. Tight clothing that might put pressure on the incision should be avoided (e.g., tight bra straps).

Age-Specific Modifications (Pediatric)

- Reassure the family and client that
As the child matures and the normal heart rate slows, the pacemaker can be programmed externally to fire at a slower rate
The cardiologist will be able to determine when new leads will be required to adapt the system to the growth of the child. When the pacemaker is inserted, the excess lead is coiled in a loop. Periodic x-ray films will show how much the coil has diminished because of the child's growth.
The normal activities and falls of childhood will not cause problems with the pacemaker. Extremely violent activities should be discouraged.

Referrals and Consultations

- Refer the client to the cardiologist for pacemaker problems determined by telephone evaluation or suspected because of return of pre-pacemaker symptoms.

- Obtain a physician consultation if signs of infection of the pocket are present, such as redness, drainage, excessive pain, or elevated temperature.
- Refer the client to the American Heart Association for teaching materials about pacemakers and for cookbooks containing low-cholesterol and low-sodium recipes.
- Refer the family to the American Red Cross, American Heart Association, or local hospital for cardiopulmonary resuscitation (CPR) training should the client develop heart problems.
- Refer the client to the home health nurse or cardiologist for suture removal when the pocket has healed, about 5 days to 7 days after pacemaker insertion.
- Refer the client to self-help pacemaker groups:
International Association of Pacemaker Patients, Inc.
PO Box 54305
Atlanta, GA 30308
This is a nonprofit group that promotes communication among pacemaker recipients. They also publish a magazine, *Pulse*, for people with pacemakers.

Pacemakers Unlimited, Inc.
PO Box 5481
Fort Lauderdale, FL 33310
This is an international nonprofit group started in 1976 by a group of pacemaker recipients and their families. The group aids pacemaker recipients before and after surgery.

Mended Hearts, Inc.
721 Huntington Avenue
Boston, MA 02115
This group does not limit itself to people with pacemakers, but includes all people who have had heart surgery. The group members usually organize visits to clients who are anticipating surgery.

Local hospital groups
Many hospitals have local pacemaker clubs where clients can interact with other pacemaker recipients. Starting or joining such a group may be helpful.

- Refer the client to pacemaker monitoring agencies (if appropriate):
Cardiac Data Corp.
1280 Blue Hills Avenue
Bloomfield, CT 06002
or
1705 Walnut Street
Philadelphia, PA 19103
or
4500 Biscayne
Suite 220
Miami, FL 33137

Cardiac Monitoring, Inc.
10384 Riverside Drive
Palm Beach Gardens, FL 33401

Cardiocare
Division of Medtronic, Inc.
425 East 61st Street
New York, NY 10021

Cardiopace
3181 SW Sam Jackson Park Road
Portland, OR 97201

Dart Medical
500 Hogsback Road
PO Box 212
Mason, MI 48854

Instromedix
10950 SW 5th Avenue
Beaverton, OR 97005

Intermedics, Inc.
PO Box 617
Freeport, TX 77541

MedAlert
1 Penn Plaza
New York, NY 10001

MedPace Analysis, Inc.
1166 East 86th Street
Brooklyn, NY 11236

Pacemaker Diagnostic Clinic
4020 Newberry Road
Gainesville, FL 32607

Pacesetter
12884 Bradley Avenue
Sylmer, CA 91342

United Medical Corp.
Cardio Data Systems
56 Haddon Avenue
PO Box 117
Haddonfield, NJ 08033

Veterans Administration

- In addition, local hospitals or physicians may have telephone pacemaker follow-up clinics.

Evaluation of Health Promotion Activities

Quality Assurance/ Reassessment

- Check the client for the return of symptoms experienced before the pacemaker was inserted (e.g., dizziness, swollen ankles, or shortness of breath). This might indicate pacemaker malfunction.
- Check a 12-lead ECG as necessary.
- Monitor reports of pacemaker telephone evaluation for indications of pacemaker malfunction. The urgency of obtaining medical attention will be determined by the degree that the client is pacemaker-dependent:

  Loss of sensing is caused by lead displacement in the heart. There will be no pacer spikes on the ECG although the client's heart rate falls below the preset rate of the pacemaker. This could also occur if there is a malfunction in the sensing apparatus in the pulse generator.

  Loss of capture may have occurred if the client shows symptoms of pre-pacemaker condition. The ECG will show either no pacer spikes although the client's heart rate is lower than the preset pacemaker rate or the pacemaker spikes are not followed by a cardiac contraction (QRS). Loss of capture can occur if the leads are displaced or by a pacemaker impulse (MA) that is not strong enough.

  Perforation occurs if the electrode lead penetrates the ventricular wall. This will be indicated on the ECG by the absence of pacemaker spikes even though the client's heart rate is less than the pacemaker rate. The client might experience hiccups if the electrode happens to be in the vicinity of the diaphragm. The client will exhibit pre-pacemaker symptoms.

DOCUMENTATION

Charting for the Home Health Nurse
- Determine the following:

  The client's or family's understanding of the reason for and function of the pacemaker

  The client's or family's ability to perform daily pacemaker checks and periodic telephone checks

  The client's or family's ability to pay for pacemaker insertion and maintenance

  The condition of the pacemaker pocket

  Relief of the client's pre-pacemaker symptoms

  Psychological responses of the client and family regarding lifestyle or body-image changes

  Client's or family's understanding of the time period before generator replacement will be likely

  Alterations in activities of daily living (ADL) that may be necessary, including activity limitations if any

  Safety precautions such as avoidance of EMI

Records Kept by the Client/Family
Daily pulse checks
Record of adverse symptoms such as dizziness and the corresponding activity

Health Teaching Checklist

Name of Care Provider _____

Relationship to Client _____ Telephone #_____

Taught by _____ Date _____

	EXPLAINED	DEMONSTRATED
Reason for pacemaker insertion	_____	
Function of the pacemaker	_____	_____
Specific type of pacemaker inserted	_____	
Time that replacement will likely be required	_____	
Lifestyle changes (if any)	_____	
Activity	_____	
Precautions such as avoidance of EMI	_____	
Follow-up appointments	_____	
Daily pacemaker checks	_____	_____
Telephone surveillance (if appropriate)	_____	_____
Basic life support (CPR)	_____	_____
Emergency telephone numbers	_____	
Insurance coverage/other third-party payor	_____	

Product Availability

Paperback book aimed at clients and their families: *Understanding Pacemakers*, by D. Sonnenburg, M. Birnbaum, and E. A. Naclerio (1982), available from
Michael Kesend Publishing, Ltd.
1025 5th Avenue, New York, NY 10028
$12.95

Selected References

Hudak CM, Lohr T, Gallo BM: Critical Care Nursing, 3rd ed. Philadelphia, JB Lippincott, 1982

Slusarczyk SM, Hicks FD: Helping your patient to live with a permanent pacemaker. Nursing '83 13(4):58–63, 1983

Sonnenburg D, Birnbaum M, Naclerio EA: Understanding Pacemakers. New York, Michael Kesend Publishing, 1982

Elimination

8 Assistive Devices for Elimination

Background

The bedpan and urinal are devices used to collect feces and urine. They are used in the home primarily for clients who are unable to ambulate to other toileting facilities.

Bedpans and urinals are constructed of either stainless steel or plastic. They are of two types:

Fracture pans that are shallow at the upper end (the end that fits under the sacrum) and deeper at the other end

The usual bedpans that are approximately two inches deep on all sides

Assessment of Self-Care Potential

Client/Family Assessment

- Assess the family to determine if a family member is willing and capable of providing the assistance necessary in helping the client with the bedpan/urinal.
- Assess the family to determine if there is a family member who feels comfortable assisting the client and with whom the client feels comfortable.

Physical Assessment

- Assess the client to determine which assistive device is the one of choice (a bedside commode or a bedpan). Criteria for assessment include client independence and strength.
- Assess the client to determine the level of assistance required in the use of the devices and to determine the feasibility of installing an over-bed trapeze to allow the client to assist in the transfer from bed to bedpan or bedside commode.
- Assess the client for skin breakdown caused by improper cleaning, pressure, or urinary incontinence.

Environmental Assessment

- Assess the availability of privacy and freedom from interruption for the client while using the elimination devices.
- Assess the bedroom area to determine if a call light or bell is within the client's reach for summoning assistance while using the devices.

Planning Strategies

Potential Nursing Diagnoses

Alteration in elimination
    Alteration in bowel elimination, constipation
    Alteration in bowel elimination, diarrhea or incontinence
    Urinary elimination pattern, alteration in

Skin integrity, impaired

Self-esteem disturbance

Expected Outcomes

Prevention of bowel or urinary elimination alterations by establishment of a routine at scheduled times or at client request

Prevention of skin breakdown

Maintenance or resumption of client functioning with maximum possible independence and preservation of self-esteem

Health Promotion Goals

- The client and family will
  Assist the client with use of the bedpan, urinal, or bedside commode, using safe body mechanics
  Install an over-bed trapeze if necessary to assist the client with transfer to assistive devices
  Properly clean elimination devices and control odor effectively
  Resolve any feelings of guilt or embarrassment

Equipment

Indicated assistive device (bedpan, urinal, or bedside commode)

A method of elevating the head of the bed during use of the bedpan

Toilet tissue placed within easy reach

Bell, call light, or other device for summoning assistance

Washcloth, soap and water, and towel

Aerosol air freshener if needed

Bedpan or urinal cover

Over-bed trapeze if needed to assist with lifting of hips

Interventions/Health Promotion

ACTION	RATIONALE/AMPLIFICATION
Bedpan	
1. Position the client with the upper body in a raised position (Fig. 8-1).	Elimination is enhanced with the body in a normal physiological position. If the client is to be bedfast for a lengthy period of time, a hospital bed can be rented. If this is not feasible, an elevation device can be constructed using plywood that is then padded. If neither of these options is feasible, prop the upper body up with pillows.

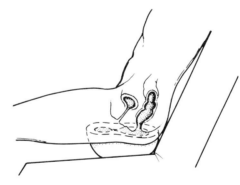

Figure 8.1
Proper positioning on the bedpan. If a hospital bed is not available for elevation of the upper body, prop the patient's upper body with pillows or construct an elevating device using padded plywood.

ACTION	RATIONALE/AMPLIFICATION
2. If the bedpan is a stainless-steel one, run warm water over it to warm it. Dry and powder the bedpan.	The warm water will reduce the cold feeling of the metal. Powder reduces friction, making it easier to insert the bedpan under the client.
3. Instruct the client to raise the hips for easier insertion of the bedpan.	If unable to raise hips, an over-bed trapeze to assist the client in lifting the hips can be installed.
4. If unable to raise hips and if arm strength is insufficient to use an over-bed trapeze effectively, turn the client to one side. Place the	If this method is used, do not elevate the head of the bed until the client is placed on the bedpan to promote ease in turning.

ACTION

RATIONALE/AMPLIFICATION

bedpan against the client's hips in proper position and turn the client back onto the bedpan.

5. Place toilet tissue and summoning device within easy reach of the client.

Privacy is provided to the extent that it is safe.

6. Remove the bedpan in the same manner that it was inserted.

Cover the bedpan as it is removed.

7. Clean the perineal and rectal areas with soap and water and dry well.

Improper cleansing predisposes to skin irritation and skin breakdown. Encourage the client to perform as much of the cleaning procedure as possible.

Urinal

1. If the client is unable to place the urinal, place it gently with a minimum of exposure.

Encourage independent use of the urinal.

2. Place calling device within easy reach.

Provide privacy and freedom from interruption.

Bedside Commode

1. Place the bedside commode parallel with and on side of the bed (Fig. 8-2). Lock the wheels.

The sitting position permits a more normal physiological position, as well as a feeling of independent functioning.

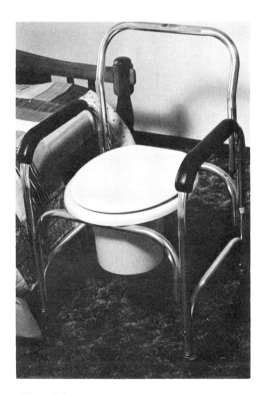

Figure 8.2
Bedside commode properly placed.

ACTION	*RATIONALE/AMPLIFICATION*
2. Assist the client to sit on the commode. Place toilet tissue and calling device within easy reach.	Provide privacy and freedom from interruption.

Related Care

1. Offer the client a wet washcloth, soap, and a towel following each use of the bedpan or urinal.	Handwashing is an effective method of preventing contamination.
2. Rinse bedpans, urinals, and bedside commode inserts with cold water. Follow by washing with soap and water.	Soak with vinegar and water (1¼ cups vinegar to 1 gallon of water) for odor control.
3. Assess perineal area, sacral area, and other pressure areas daily for irritation and skin breakdown.	Friction, pressure, and inadequate cleansing predispose to skin breakdown.
4. Include adequate amounts of bulk, fiber, and liquids in the diet.	These assist in preventing constipation.

Age-Specific Modifications

1. Use smaller pediatric-size bedpan for children.	Adaptations in size improve client ability to perform eliminative functions.
2. For a toddler, a potty-chair can be used rather than a bedside commode.	

Education/ Communication

- Teach the client and family to
  Position the client properly on the bedpan. Focus on body alignment and normal physiological positioning.
  Safely assist the client with the bedpan (refer to Technique 2, Body Mechanics). This is especially important if the client is an adult with a high level of physical dependence.
  Cleanse anal and perineal areas following urination and defecation to prevent skin irritation and skin breakdown
  Use cleansing and odor control measures for bedpan, urinal, or insert of bedside commode
  Assess perineal area and sacral area daily for skin breakdown

Evaluation of Health Promotion Activities

Quality Assurance/ Reassessment

- Observe the placement of the bedpan and/or urinal and evaluate for good body alignment of the client and good body mechanics of the assistant.
- Observe if needed items are left within easy reach of the client (bell or other summoning device and toilet tissue).
- Evaluate the sacral area for irritation or indications of beginning pressure sores.
- Evaluate the perineal and rectal areas for chafing, redness, or other signs of irritation.

DOCUMENTATION

Charting for the Home Health Nurse
- Document the ability of the client/family to perform the procedure accurately.
- Note any occurrences of diarrhea, constipation, impaction, signs of skin irritation and/or breakdown, or signs of urinary tract infection.

Records Kept by the Client/Family

Questions and concerns

Presence of blood in the urine or feces; pain on urination or defecation; urinary frequency, diarrhea, or constipation

Perineal/sacral skin irritation/breakdown

Health Teaching Checklist

Name of Care Provider _____

Relationship to Client _____ Telephone #_____

Taught by _____ Date _____

	EXPLAINED	DEMONSTRATED
Positioning of client	_____	_____
Assistance in use of device	_____	_____
Appropriate cleansing of skin and handwashing following urination and defecation	_____	_____
Cleansing and odor control measures for bedpan, urinal, or insert of bedside commode	_____	_____
Daily assessment of perineal skin and sacral area	_____	_____

Product Availability

The bedside commode is available for rental or purchase through hospital-supply firms. Bedpans and urinals are available by purchase through hospital-supply firms and some pharmacies. An over-bed trapeze can be rented or purchased, also from hospital-supply firms.

9   Bladder Training Program (Incontinence)

Background

The term *urinary incontinence* refers to the inability of the external urinary sphincter to control the urinary flow from the bladder. The condition may be temporary or permanent. Two classes of urinary incontinence exist. Stress incontinence occurs with laughing, coughing, exercise, or any activity causing an increase in intra-abdominal pressure. Urge incontinence, on the other hand, occurs when the client's urge to void is so immediate that there is not sufficient time to get to toileting facilities. This is commonly caused by lower urinary tract infections or bladder spasms.

A bladder training program consisting of exercises of the sphincter can be initiated to reduce the frequency of urinary incontinence. The program is a lengthy one. Motivation, persistence, and family support are essential to the success of the program.

Assessment of Self-Care Potential

Client/Family Assessment

- Assess family support of the program. Determine family/client attitudes toward incontinence, because these are basic to developing support for the client's progress.
- If the client has, additionally, a mobility deficit, assess the willingness and capability of a family member to provide the needed assistance.

Physical Assessment

- Assess the times and situations associated with incontinence (e.g., when laughing, exercising, coughing, or sneezing).
- Assess potential causes of incontinence (e.g., enlarged prostate gland, spinal cord injury, loss of consciousness, medication interaction, medications that interfere with sphincter control, or bladder infection or spasms).
- Palpate the abdomen for tenderness, pain, or masses. Palpate the renal area for tenderness, pain, or masses. Note if incontinence is accompanied by pain or hematuria.

Environmental Assessment

- Determine if toilet, bedpan, portable commode, or other urinary device is easily accessible.
- Determine if means to provide privacy during urinary attempts are available.

Planning Strategies

Potential Nursing Diagnoses

Urinary elimination, impairment of: incontinence

Self-esteem disturbance

Expected Outcomes

Restoration of normal urinary elimination pattern

Restoration of maintenance of client's self-confidence

Health Promotion Goals
- The client and family will
  Promote fluid intake to an adequate level
  Prevent skin breakdown and/or irritation
  Alleviate client embarrassment regarding the procedure
  Initiate and adhere to the prescribed sphincter exercise program
  Reduce the frequency of incontinence

Equipment

Toilet, bedpan, portable commode, or other urinary device

Underclothing with disposable liners or waterproof pants worn with sanitary pads (e.g., Proctor & Gamble's ATTENDS)

Interventions/Health Promotion

ACTION	RATIONALE/AMPLIFICATION
1. If drug therapy is contributing to the incontinence, notify the client's physician.	Another drug with similar effects but without the side-effects leading to incontinence may be ordered.
2. If weakened pelvic musculature is related to the incontinence, initiate pelvic-floor exercises. • Tighten the anal sphincter for a count of 5 and relax. • Tighten urinary and pelvic musculature for a count of 5 and relax. • Perform several times each hour, lengthening the duration of muscle contraction each day.	Pelvic-floor exercises will strengthen the sphincter and thus reduce urinary incontinence due to weakness of the sphincter. Persistent performance of the exercises is essential to the reduction of incontinence.
3. Assist the client to establish a regular voiding schedule; for example, every 1 to 2 hours, whether or not the urge to void is felt.	The consistent, frequent stretching and relaxing of the musculature caused by voiding attempts assist in strengthening the sphincter.
4. Initiate increased fluid intake to at least 2000 ml daily. Encourage the client to avoid carbonated drinks and citrus juices. Initiate a pattern of fluid intake 30 minutes prior to voiding times. Encourage the client to avoid liquids at bedtime.	Adequate fluid intake assists in successfully establishing a voiding schedule. Citrus juices and carbonated drinks are alkalizing and thus are irritating to the bladder.
5. Encourage an increase in physical activity.	Muscle tone and circulation are increased with activity, thus improving urinary retention.
6. Encourage client to arrange family schedule to ensure easy access to toilet or bedpan at the scheduled times or as needed.	Ready availability of urinary devices prevents accidental incontinence.

ACTION	*RATIONALE/AMPLIFICATION*
7. Apply pads to the bed and encourage the wearing of waterproof clothing if desired. Advise the client to change these often and wash the skin where it is in contact with urine frequently with soap and water.	Particularly in social situations, these protective devices assist in reducing embarrassment. Frequent changing and cleansing of skin reduces chances of skin irritation and breakdown due to urinary acidity.

**Education/
Communication**

- Teach the family and client to
  Perform the exercises appropriately and consistently, several times hourly
  Have toileting needs available and easily accessible to client at scheduled voiding times
  Refer to waterproof clothing needs in those terms rather than as "diapers"
  Engage in desired social activities, with proper protection
  Wash perineal skin often with soap and water
  Change undergarments frequently
  Ingest at least 2000 ml of fluids daily; avoid fluids at bedtime; avoid citrus juices, carbonated drinks, and caffeinated drinks; take fluids 30 minutes prior to scheduled voiding times
  Increase physical exercise within physical limitations
  Notify the nurse or physican if hematuria or painful urination occurs
  Notify the nurse if skin irritation or breakdown occurs due to exposure to urine

Evaluation of Health Promotion Activities

**Quality Assurance/
Reassessment**

- Evaluate the client for alterations in frequency of urinary incontinence.
- Assess the perineal area for chafing and/or breakdown due to constant presence of urine on the skin.
- Observe the client for improvement in self-esteem.
- Evaluate the client's willingness to participate in desired social activities and/or functions of usual lifestyle.

DOCUMENTATION

Charting for the Home Health Nurse
- Record the frequency of urinary incontinence and associated events.
- Document any alterations in frequency or pattern of incontinence.
- Note the client/family attitude to the recommended exercises and indications of consistent performance of the exercises.

Records Kept by the Client/Family
The frequency and associated events of urinary incontinence are noted; this can be done in a notebook or tablet.

Successes and failures of voiding at the scheduled times are documented.

Adherence to pelvic-floor exercises is noted, as well as maintenance of physical activity recommendations and fluid intake.

**Health Teaching
Checklist**

Name of Care Provider _____

Relationship to Client _____ Telephone #_____

Taught by _____ Date _____

	EXPLAINED	DEMONSTRATED
Pelvic-floor exercises	_____	_____
Fluid intake	_____	
Voiding schedule	_____	
Increased physical exercise	_____	

Product Availability

Waterproof underclothing is available from hospital-supply firms and drug stores (one example is Proctor & Gamble's ATTENDS). A portable commode, if needed, can be rented or purchased from a hospital-supply firm. If additional protective devices are desired while the client is incontinent, external collection devices (for males; Fig. 9-1) are available (e.g., condom catheters, urinary sheaths, or dribble sheaths).

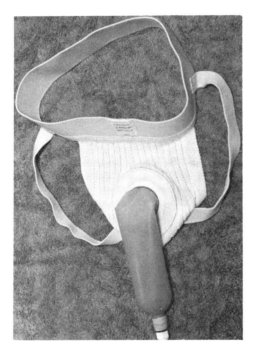

Figure 9.1
An example of an external protective device
that can be used for male incontinence.

10 Bowel Training

Background

Bowel incontinence results from the inability to control the anal sphincter muscle in relation to the urge to defecate. This, in turn, is often related to an impairment of the sphincter itself or to the neural mechanism controlling it. Many clients can be assisted to regain bowel control through a systematic program of bowel training exercises performed regularly and consistently.

Assessment of Self-Care Potential

Client/Family Assessment

- Assess family support and cooperation, which are necessary to a successful program.
- Assess meal preparation to ensure inclusion of fiber and client intake of foods containing fiber since fiber adds bulk, weight, and form to the stool and improves evacuation of the rectum and colon.
- Assess availability of opportunity for privacy and adequate time in the bathroom at the designated time for bowel movement.

Physical Assessment

- Inspect the anal area for presence of hemorrhoids.
- Perform rectal–digital examination to detect masses and/or tenderness in the rectal anterior and posterior walls.
- Assess current level of exercise, since adequate exercise supports bowel elimination.

Environmental Assessment

- Assess the bathroom area. Determine if the bathroom is situated in such a manner that the commode is accessible to the client when needed. In addition, determine if the client can walk to the bathroom or if a wheelchair or portable commode must be used. If assistance is required to go to the bathroom, assess whether a family member will be available and is willing to assist the client at the specified times to go to the bathroom.
- Assess the bathroom accessories. Determine if the height of the commode is sufficient for the client to sit comfortably on it with both feet on a solid surface such as a footstool or the floor. If a mobility disability is present, determine if the commode must be equipped with stable armrests to assist in sitting and rising from the commode.
- Assess the need for a mechanism for calling for assistance if the client has a mobility deficit. Determine how this can be placed within easy reach of the client during use of the commode, such as by using a light string or a bell.
- If the client is unable to go to the bathroom, or if sufficient time and privacy are not available as needed for the program, assess the need to rent or purchase a portable commode. Determine if there is adequate room in the bedroom for this equipment while still maintaining privacy and time for the accomplishment of the training program.

Planning Strategies

Potential Nursing Diagnoses

Bowel elimination, alteration in: incontinence

Self-concept, disturbance in self-esteem

Expected Outcomes
Achievement of fecal continence to the maximum level possible within the physical limitations present

Alterations of dietary habits as necessary

Maintenance of exercise program

Health Promotion Goals
- The client and family will
  Verbalize feelings regarding fecal incontinence and the bowel training program
  Drink warm fluids early in the morning to stimulate peristalsis
  Administer a laxative, stool softener, or enema as ordered
  Alter diet to include fiber and adequate fluid intake if indicated
  Replace medications contributing to bowel incontinence
  Establish regular times for bowel evacuation
  Provide availability and accessibility without interruption at the specified times each day
  Initiate and support an exercise program within the client's physical limitations
  Assume proper positioning while on the toilet

Equipment
Commode of proper height (if too high, a footstool can be placed in front of the commode to alter the sitting height)

Portable commode (rented or purchased) if needed

Oral stool softeners or laxative suppository

Interventions/Health Promotion

ACTION	*RATIONALE/AMPLIFICATION*
1. Designate with the client the time of day most suitable for bowel evacuation, such as after breakfast.	After breakfast the gastrocolic reflex is stimulated and defecation may be induced more easily than at other times of the day.
2. Instruct the client to drink a cup of warm liquid in the early morning.	Warm liquid stimulates peristalsis, thus increasing the probability of bowel evacuation.
3. Administer an oral stool softener or a laxative suppository approximately 30 minutes prior to the scheduled defecation time.	Stool softeners and suppositories stimulate the rectal mucosa to initiate a bowel evacuation.
4. At the specified time, arrange with the family to have the bathroom or portable commode available for the client's use.	Privacy and freedom from interruption are essential to the success of the program.
5. Advise the client to assume a sitting position on the commode, leaning forward at the hips, applying manual pressure on the lower abdomen, and bearing down to a normal degree (avoid straining, which will produce or aggravate hemorrhoids).	Pressure on the large colon is increased by this position, increasing the probability of bowel evacuation.

ACTION	RATIONALE/AMPLIFICATION
6. Put a summoning device (bell or light cord) and toilet tissue within easy reach of the client. Provide privacy and freedom from interruption. A time limit of 25 minutes is usually adequate for each sitting.	Some clients find that reading during this time assists with relaxation.

Related Care

1. Initiate needed dietary alterations to increase fiber, roughage, and adequate fluid intake.	Fiber increases the bulk, weight, and form of the stool, thus assisting in bowel evacuation.
2. Evaluate medications currently being taken for effect on bowel habits.	Medications can usually be altered to another form that is equally effective.
3. Initiate an exercise program within the physical and social limitations of the client.	Exercise stimulates regular bowel habits, thus increasing the probability of success of the program.
4. Demonstrate respectful behaviors toward the client. Assume an encouraging attitude toward the client/family.	Bowel incontinence is usually embarrassing. The program is lengthy and thus often discouraging both to the client and the family.
5. Encourage the client/family to provide rewards for themselves when successes are achieved.	Positive reinforcement increases the probability of success.
6. Advise the client of the availability of specially designed underwear with disposable liners to provide security in social situations.	Do not refer to these items as "diapers" but as underclothing.
7. Advise the client/family of the need to keep the area surrounding the anus clean and dry, washing with soap and water as frequently as is necessary.	Keeping the area clean and dry prevents tissue irritation and breakdown.

**Education/
Communication**

• Teach the client and family to
  Make recommended dietary alterations to include adequate fluid intake and adequate fiber and bulk. Foods that are individually constipating should be avoided. Foods that are individually gas-forming should be avoided. Warm liquid taken early in the morning should be encouraged.
  Perform the procedure correctly, with emphasis on regularity and consistency. Adequate time should be allowed for scheduled bowel movements, with provisions for privacy and freedom from interruption.

Evaluation of Health Promotion Activities

**Quality Assurance/
Reassessment**

• Document the progress in achieving bowel control.

• Assess the initiation and adherence to the bowel training program.

• Occasionally schedule a home visit to coincide with a meal to assess the dietary patterns. A periodic food-intake diary to be kept by the client can also assist in assessing food patterns.

DOCUMENTATION

Charting for the Home Health Nurse
- Note client/family adherence to steps of designated program.
- Assess client/family commitment to the program.
- Record progress of retraining development.
- Record client/family adherence to dietary, exercise, and fluid intake recommendations.

Records Kept by the Client/Family
Outcomes of the program, both successes and failures
Questions and concerns
Occurrences of constipation/diarrhea

Health Teaching Checklist

Name of Care Provider _____

Relationship to Client _____ Telephone #_____

Taught by _____ Date _____

	EXPLAINED	DEMONSTRATED
Nutritional changes needed	_____	_____
Exercise program	_____	_____
Time of day for bowel movement	_____	
Use of stool softener or suppository	_____	
Proper positioning on commode	_____	_____
Need for privacy	_____	
Need for adequate uninterrupted time for scheduled bowel movements	_____	

Product Availability

A portable commode can be rented or purchased from a medical equipment store. Underclothing containing disposable liners can be purchased from pharmacies, hospital-supply firms, or from a hospital itself (one example is Proctor & Gamble's ATTENDS).

Selected Reference

Nursing Photobook: Helping Geriatric Patients. Springhouse, PA, Springhouse Corporation, 1983

11 Digital Removal of Fecal Impaction

Background

The term *fecal impaction* refers to the accumulation of a mass of hardened feces in the rectum, caused by prolonged constipation. Symptoms of fecal impaction include seepage of liquid around the impacted mass, constipation, frequent but nonproductive urges to defecate, and sometimes rectal pain. Clients often describe a general feeling of malaise, distended abdomen, and sometimes nausea and vomiting.

The development of an impaction is related to many factors, including poor nutrition, low fluid intake, poor elimination habits, inadequate bulk in the diet, lack of exercise, weakened muscle tone, and stress.

Prevention is the goal. However, therapeutic measures are sometimes necessary to remove the impaction. If enemas do not relieve the impaction, digital removal is indicated. By this process the fecal mass is digitally broken into small parts, dislodged from the rectal mucosa, and removed.

Assessment of Self-Care Potential

Client/Family Assessment

- Determine if the client wants a family member to be in attendance during the procedure, since it is often uncomfortable, tiring, embarrassing, and sometimes painful.

Physical Assessment

- Assess the client's usual pattern of defecation, including frequency, quantity, and time of day.
- Assess the client's current bowel status, including amount of time since last defecation and quality of last bowel movement.
- Auscultate abdomen to determine presence of bowel sounds. Unusually intense and frequent bowel sounds indicate enteritis or an obstruction of the small intestine.
- Palpate the abdomen for pain, tenderness, and/or masses.
- Examine for presence of hemorrhoids. If present, the procedure must be performed so as not to cause unnecessary pain.
- Assess lifestyle contributors to constipation:
  Insufficient exercise
  Inadequate fluid intake
  Current stressors in life
  Low intake of bulk and fiber; irregular meals
  Medications currently being taken

Environmental Assessment

- Assess the environment to determine if privacy and freedom from interruption can be provided during the procedure.
- Determine if toileting facilities are readily available and accessible.

Planning Strategies

Potential Nursing Diagnoses

Alteration in bowel elimination, constipation

Comfort, alteration in

Expected Outcomes
Removal of impaction with minimal discomfort

Establishment of normal bowel elimination patterns

Health Promotion Goals
- The client and family will
Experience a minimum of discomfort, exhaustion, embarrassment, and pain
Be ensured of privacy during the procedure
Learn and initiate methods of preventing a recurrence of the impaction
Have the impaction removed

Equipment
Oil retention enema

Cleansing enema set-up

Rubber gloves and lubricating jelly

Draping sheets

Bedpan, bedside commode, or other toileting device

Waterproof bedpad

Interventions/Health Promotion

ACTION	RATIONALE/AMPLIFICATION
1. Ensure that privacy and freedom from interruption can be guaranteed. Have the client assume a side-lying position, back to the nurse and within easy reach of the nurse.	Privacy is essential to the comfort and dignity of the client.
2. Place a waterproof pad under the client's hips. Drape the client. Place the bedpan within easy reach of the nurse.	Proper draping provides warmth and comfort for the client.
3. Explain the procedure to the client.	Knowing what will happen reduces anxiety.
4. Double glove, using clean technique. Lubricate the index finger with water-soluble lubricant.	Lubricant reduces friction, thereby reducing discomfort during the procedure.
5. Insert the index finger gently into rectum (Fig. 11-1). Rotate the finger toward the umbilicus, gently loosening and dislodging the fecal	Take care to avoid aggressive removal of fecal material to avoid damage to the rectal mucosa. Examine the glove periodically for the presence of blood.

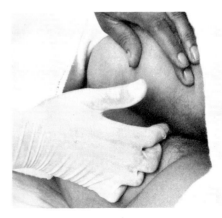

Figure 11.1
Inserting the lubricated finger into the rectum for removal of fecal impaction.

ACTION	*RATIONALE/AMPLIFICATION*
material and breaking it into smaller pieces (Fig. 11-2). Remove the fecal material from the rectum and place it in the bedpan for disposal.	
6. Continually assess the client for signs of exhaustion and/or pain. If either occurs, discontinue the procedure until the client indicates readiness to resume.	The procedure is usually very tiring due to manipulation of the rectum, discomfort, and embarrassment.
7. Remove as much fecal material as possible. Clean the client. Change linens if necessary. Remove bedpan and clean. Assist the client to the bathroom for toileting if desired. Encourage the client to rest following the procedure.	Manipulation of the rectum creates an urge to defecate.
8. Wash hands. Record procedure.	Handwashing and cleaning of soiled equipment are essential to prevent cross-contamination.

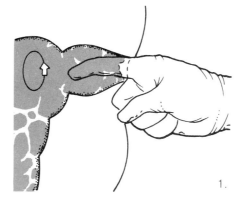 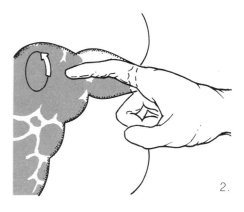

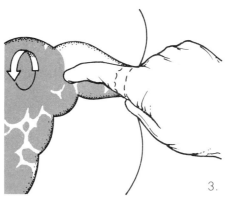 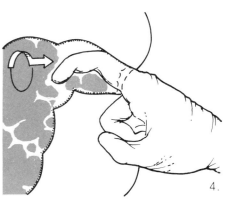

Figure 11.2
Schematic drawing of digital removal of fecal impaction.

ACTION	RATIONALE/AMPLIFICATION
Related Care	
1. Administer an oil retention enema prior to digital removal of the impaction.	The oil retention enema softens the fecal mass to facilitate removal.
2. Administer a cleansing enema following the removal of the impaction.	Do not administer if the client is overly tired.
3. Advise the client to make dietary changes as needed. Tell him to avoid fiber laxatives.	Increase in bulk and fiber and regularity of meals help prevent constipation. Add bran and prunes to the diet, if needed.
4. Advise the client to increase exercise level if indicated.	Exercise within physical limitations prevents constipation.
5. If the client is under undue stress, find means of stress reduction.	Measures such as exercise programs, hobbies, and counseling are among those that assist persons to reduce stress.
6. Increase fluid intake if indicated.	Inadequate fluids frequently increase constipation.

Education/ Communication

- Teach the client and family to
  Take measures to establish a regular pattern of bowel functioning
  With physician consultation, make dietary alterations as indicated to include bulk, fiber, and adequate fluid intake. Advise the client to add commercially available bulk and fiber supplements.
  Increase daily level of exercise within physical limitations
  Find means of stress reduction

Referrals and Consultations

- Notify the client's physician if there is evidence of bleeding during the procedure or if there is excessive pain or presence of masses in the abdomen.

Evaluation of Health Promotion Activities

Quality Assurance/ Reassessment

- During each visit, assess the client for incidents of constipation.
- Evaluate the client's progress in relation to alteration in dietary habits, increase in fluid intake, adequate exercise within physical limitations, and initiation of stress-reduction measures (if indicated).

DOCUMENTATION

Charting for the Home Health Nurse
- Document the performance of the procedure to include results, client toleration, presence of pain or tenderness, notation of hemorrhoids or other observed lesions, any complications, and preventive measures taught.

Records Kept by the Client/Family
A record should be kept of frequency of bowel movements. Client questions and concerns should be written for communication to the nurse or physician.

Health Teaching Checklist

Name of Care Provider _____

Relationship to Client _____ Telephone # _____

Taught by _____ Date _____

	EXPLAINED	DEMONSTRATED
Need to establish regular bowel pattern	_____	
Dietary alterations recommended	_____	
Available bulk/fiber supplements	_____	
Recommended exercise program	_____	_____
Recommended stress-reduction measures	_____	

Product Availability

Fiber and bulk supplements are available in grocery stores or pharmacies without prescription.

12　Enema Administration

Background

The administration of an enema involves the introduction of solution into the rectum and sigmoid colon, with the solution returning by natural or artificial means. An enema is used for any of the following purposes:

To remove fecal material or gases from the lower bowel

To stimulate peristalsis in the lower bowel

To soothe and treat irritation of the rectal and colon mucosa

To decrease body temperature

To treat local hemorrhage

To introduce medication into the gastrointestinal system

Assessment of Self-Care Potential

Client/Family Assessment

- Assess the client/family to determine if a family member is capable and willing to administer the enema correctly and if the client feels comfortable having the family member perform the procedure in the nurse's absence.
- Assess the capability and willingness of the client to self-administer the enema if the enema prescribed is a self-administrative type.

Physical Assessment

- Auscultate the abdomen for the presence of bowel sounds. Unusually intense and frequent bowel sounds indicate enteritis or an obstruction of the small intestine.
- Palpate the abdomen for pain and/or masses. If pain is present in the right lower quadrant, or if rebound tenderness is present, notify a physician before proceeding.

Environmental Assessment

- Assess the home for a place where the enema can be given with uninterrupted privacy for the duration of the procedure.
- Determine if the room where the enema is to be given has a bed and has some provision for warmth during the procedure.
- Determine if the bathroom (or bedside commode or bedpan) is readily available and accessible.

Planning Strategies

Potential Nursing Diagnoses

Alteration in bowel elimination, constipation

Anxiety, mild

Expected Outcomes

Establishment and maintenance of regular bowel function

Achievement of the therapeutic purpose for which the enema is being given

Relief of anxiety and restoration of a sense of well-being

Health Promotion Goals

- The client and family will
  Experience the minimum amount of discomfort and embarrassment related to the procedure

Introduce the indicated amount of the correct solution into the client's
   rectum
Prepare the enema solution at the proper temperature
Retain the solution for the required length of time before expelling the
   solution
Record the results of the enema
Notify the nurse of any complications, such as abdominal pain or resistance
   to the introduction of the enema tubing

Equipment

Enema set-up (disposable or reusable) or commercial self-administrative enema
   (e.g., Fleet)

Thermometer by means of which to determine solution temperature of 100°F to
   110°F

Linen for protection of bed and for covering of client to provide warmth and
   dignity

Bedpan, bedside commode, or easily accessible bathroom

Solution as ordered. Types of solution commonly ordered are the following:
Liquid soap: 1 teaspoon to 1000 ml of water

Saline: 1 teaspoon to 1000 ml of water

Sodium bicarbonate: 1 to 2 teaspoons to 1000 ml of water

Olive oil: 2 to 5 ounces warmed to 100°F

Paraldehyde: dosage ordered in 2 ounces of water

Glycerin and water: 3 ounces glycerin in 4 ounces of water

Commercially prepared solutions: give according to manufacturer's directions.
   (Cleansing, oil, and carminative enemas are available in self-administrative
   and self-contained units.)

Rectal tubing

Water-soluble lubricant

Interventions/Health Promotion

ACTION	*RATIONALE/AMPLIFICATION*
1. Wash hands and assemble equipment. Don gloves, if desired, using clean technique.	Having all equipment available and ready to use prevents needless interruption of the procedure. Handwashing reduces the probability of cross-contamination.
2. Prepare the solution with emphasis on proper amount and proper temperature. The tubing is clamped off.	The solution must be of the proper temperature because heat stimulates the nerve plexuses of the intestinal mucosa and thus enhances the action of the enema.
3. Lubricate the tip of the enema tubing generously with a water-soluble lubricant.	Lubricant reduces friction, thus inhibiting potential for damage of rectal mucosa.
4. Position the client on the left side, lying flat in bed with the right leg flexed.	The descending colon is on the left side. Lying on the left side will aid gravity flow of the solution. If the client is unable to retain the enema solution, alter the position to a supine position on the bedpan, with the right knee flexed more than the left.

ACTION

5. Expel the air from the tubing by filling the tubing with the solution and closing the clamp.

6. Slowly insert the enema tube into the rectum for 4 to 5 inches as the client takes a deep breath (Figs. 12-1 and 12-2). Do not force if resistance is encountered; instead, withdraw the tubing approximately 1 inch and allow the solution to flow as the tubing is advanced again. If resistance is again encountered, discontinue the enema and consult the client's physician.

RATIONALE/AMPLIFICATION

Air introduced into the colon may overly distend the walls of the colon, causing unnecessary discomfort.

The anal canal is approximately 1 to 1½ inches long in the adult. Slow introduction of a well-lubricated tube reduces spasm of the intestinal wall.

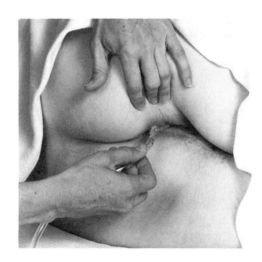

Figure 12.1
Inserting the enema tubing into the rectum at an angle pointing toward the umbilicus.

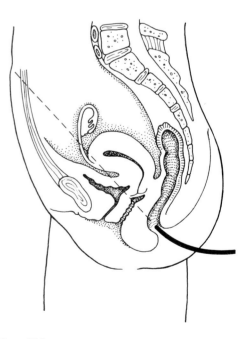

Figure 12.2
Lateral view of the correct angle of insertion of the enema tubing. (The tubing is inserted 2–3 inches.)

ACTION	RATIONALE/AMPLIFICATION
7. Allow the solution to flow by gravity. The maximum elevation of the enema container for an adult is 18 to 24 inches. If the client experiences cramping in the process of the procedure, lower the container, clamp the tubing, and wait for a minute. Then resume the procedure.	Distention and irritation of the intestinal wall often produce strong peristaltic action. This can be reduced by lowering the pressure of the administration.
8. When almost all of the solution has been introduced into the colon, clamp the tubing and withdraw the tubing from the client's rectum.	This will prevent entry of air into the colon.
9. Instruct the client to retain the solution.	Nonretention evacuative-type solutions should be retained for 5 to 10 minutes. Retention solutions should be retained according to the physician's prescription or the manufacturer's directions.
10. Assist the client to the bathroom or portable commode and provide privacy and safety measures that will best enhance evacuation.	If the client is left alone, some type of call system should be within easy reach to summon assistance. If the client requires, proper restraints and supportive devices are applied to assist in safety.
11. If the enema is not expelled in 1 hour, position the client on the right side near the edge of the bed. Insert the enema tubing into the rectum and place the enema container at a level lower than the client's body, allowing the solution to return.	Allowing the solution to return by gravity is a trauma-free method of obtaining the return of the solution.
12. Assist the client to bathe, shower, or wash. Clean equipment and replace.	A client's sense of well-being is enhanced if in a clean and fresh condition.
13. Advise the client/family to notify the nurse if the solution does not return or if excessive pain or bleeding is present.	Any of these could indicate the presence of complications for which further treatment may be indicated.

Related Care

ACTION	RATIONALE/AMPLIFICATION
1. Do not give enemas or laxatives on a regular basis.	Regular use creates dependence on these assistive measures and can cause a loss of muscle tone and inability to have an unassisted bowel evacuation.
2. If ordered, give a laxative in conjunction with the enema.	The action of a laxative is usually less severe than that of an enema. If given when constipation is not severe, a laxative may prevent the need for an enema.

ACTION	RATIONALE/AMPLIFICATION
Major types of laxatives include Bulk-forming laxatives (e.g., Metamucil)	These expand in water, forming a gelatinous mass, thereby increasing bulk. They are the safest type of laxative for stool evacuation. Their action is slow and gentle.
Emollient laxatives (e.g., Dulcolax)	These soften the stool by allowing water to enter the fecal mass, thus softening the stool and increasing the mass. They are indicated for clients with hemorrhoids or clients who are post-myocardial infarction.
Lubricant laxatives (e.g., glycerin)	These reduce friction and soften feces. Primary indication is for persons who should avoid straining with bowel movement.
Saline laxatives (e.g., milk of magnesia)	These draw water into the intestine through an osmotic effect, thus increasing the bulk. Action is rapid, usually within 3 hours.
Stimulants (e.g., Senokot)	These act directly on intestinal smooth muscle, increasing peristalsis. Cramping and bowel action usually occur within 6 to 8 hours.

Age-Specific Modifications

ACTION	RATIONALE/AMPLIFICATION
1. Alter the quantity of solution according to client's age.	Adult: 750 to 1000 ml School-age child: 500 to 1000 ml Toddler to preschooler: 500 ml Infant: 250 ml or less
2. Alter the temperature of the solution according to client's age.	Cooling enemas, all ages: 95°F Other enemas, adult: 105°F to 110°F; children: 100°F
3. Alter size of tubing and depth of insertion according to client's age.	For an infant or small child, a size 12 to 16 French catheter is used. For a small child, the tubing is inserted only 2 to 3 inches.
4. Familiarize a child with the equipment and teach the child mouth breathing prior to beginning the procedure.	Mouth breathing relaxes the sphincter and permits easier insertion of the enema tubing. Distraction from the procedure may also assist the child to relax.

Education/ Communication

- Teach the client and family to
  Perform the procedure accurately. Place emphasis on age-specific modifications as well as on the need to hold the enema solution container no more than 18 to 24 inches above the client's body.
  Report any complications prior to initiation of the procedure. If complications such as bleeding occur while in the process of administration, the enema must be discontinued.
  Attempt other means of initiating bowel evacuation, such as dietary alterations and exercise, to preclude dependence on assistive measures

Evaluation of Health Promotion Activities

Quality Assurance/ Reassessment

- Make a home visit at the time the family member is to perform the procedure to observe the technique.
- Assess the client/family member's knowledge of complications that would preclude the administration or continuation of the procedure.

DOCUMENTATION

Charting for the Home Health Nurse

Type of enema administered

Person administering the enema

Results of enema

Any reported complications

Date of enema administration

Records Kept by the Client/Family

Date enema given

Type and amount of enema solution

Results of enema administration

Any difficulties or problems encountered

Health Teaching Checklist

Name of Care Provider _____

Relationship to Client _____ Telephone #_____

Taught by _____ Date _____

	EXPLAINED	DEMONSTRATED
Handwashing	_____	_____
Assembly of equipment	_____	_____
Enema administration	_____	_____
Recording of results	_____	_____

Product Availability

Commercially prepared enemas are available through local drug stores and some supermarkets. Enema equipment can be purchased through any hospital-supply firm. Some therapeutic solutions might require a prescription.

Selected Reference

Wolff L, Weitzel MH, Zornow RA, Zsohar H: Fundamentals of Nursing, 7th ed. Philadelphia, JB Lippincott, 1983

13 Hemodialysis Shunt Care

Background

Hemodialysis

Dialysis is the process by which water and waste products are removed from the body in the presence of acute or chronic kidney failure. During dialysis, solutes and water equilibrate across a semipermeable membrane. This can be done either through peritoneal dialysis or hemodialysis. During peritoneal dialysis, the peritoneum is the semipermeable membrane used for dialysis. Hemodialysis requires the use of an external (extracorporeal) artificial kidney, where the dialysis takes place through a semipermeable membrane immersed in a special bath.

Clients on a chronic dialysis program usually dialyze two or three times per week. The treatment sessions last from 3½ to 4½ hours each. To prevent clotting in the extracorporeal system, either regional or systemic anticoagulation is required. Regional heparinization involves the anticoagulation of the blood only while it is in the artificial kidney; the heparin is neutralized before the blood is returned to the client. Systemic heparinization requires a standard anticoagulant regimen.

Weight (fluid) loss during hemodialysis is based on the principle of ultrafiltration. The amount of positive or negative pressure applied to the membrane of the kidney can be altered depending on the amount of fluid to be removed. Pretreatment laboratory work usually includes a blood urea nitrogen (BUN), serum creatinine, and electrolytes. Post-treatment laboratory tests should be delayed for up to 6 hours after the treatment to allow for equilibration of the electrolytes in the intracellular, interstitial, and intravascular fluid spaces. The client will be instructed in an individualized home dialysis protocol for laboratory work. Extracorporeal blood flow increases the chance of hypotension, angina, and arrhythmias. It is essential that the home dialysis team have a hemodialysis nurse and physician readily available by telephone in the event of problems.

Vascular Access for Hemodialysis

For effective hemodialysis, blood must flow through the kidney at 200 ml to 300 ml per minute. The small blood vessels used for intravenous (IV) therapy are not large enough to supply blood at this rate. For chronic dialysis, an external arteriovenous shunt or an internal arteriovenous fistula will be required.

The arteriovenous shunt is an external connection of an artery and a vein using synthetic tubing. The shunt is placed surgically and an external loop of tubing is joined by a removable connector. The connector is removed and the limbs of the shunt are connected to the artificial kidney during dialysis. A straight connector or a T connector can be used to connect the shunt limbs (Fig. 13-1). A T connector permits vascular access between dialysis treatments without additional venipunctures.

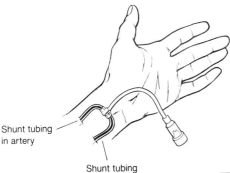

Figure 13.1
External arteriovenous hemodialysis shunt with T connector.

Shunt tubing in artery

Shunt tubing in vein

The advantage of the arteriovenous shunt is that it can be readily inserted, requiring generally less than 1 hour for surgical placement, and thereafter it can be used immediately for dialysis. There are several problems associated with an external shunt, including preventing infection and clotting and preventing accidental dislodgement of the shunt (decannulation). Even when the shunt is covered with an elastic bandage between dialysis treatments, many clients have body-image problems associated with it.

An arteriovenous fistula is the internal surgical anastomosis of an artery and a vein that results in the direct flow of arterial blood into a vein. The vein distends and becomes tougher and thicker as the fistula matures. Needles are inserted into the fistula to connect the client to the artificial kidney for hemodialysis (Fig. 13-2). The needles are removed at the conclusion of the treatment. There is much less chance of infection with the fistula, and there is less chance of clotting of the fistula because there is no synthetic material involved. Clients have fewer problems with body image changes because, unlike the arteriovenous shunt, the fistula is not readily apparent to the observer. The main disadvantage of the fistula is that it requires up to 8 weeks to mature. Also, improper cannulation for dialysis can cause problems such as clotting or infection. While the fistula is maturing, the client will require another means of vascular access, usually an external shunt.

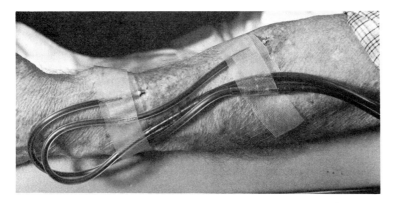

Figure 13.2
Needle placement in arteriovenous fistula during hemodialysis.

To decrease the costs of long-term chronic dialysis, and to improve the quality of life for persons with chronic renal failure, selected clients may be enrolled in a home dialysis program. Concentrated training is provided to the client and a partner who assists with the dialysis treatment. Although the program is always supervised by nurses and technicians specially trained in hemodialysis, the home health nurse may be involved in caring for other health needs of the person who is on a home dialysis program. The nurse may be able to offer assistance if the client has problems caring for the external hemodialysis shunt.

Assessment of Self-Care Potential

Client/Family Assessment

- Determine the willingness and the ability of family members to assist the client in assuming self-care activities.
- Determine whether the client will be dialyzed at a dialysis center as an outpatient or in a home hemodialysis program.
- Check whether the client and family have received insurance counseling. (See Technique 18, Peritoneal Dialysis.)
- Assist the client to choose an appropriate vendor for the artificial kidney and dialysis supplies.

- Determine whether the client is on a waiting list for a kidney transplant. Determine if third-party payment is available for a kidney transplant.

Physical Assessment

- Determine the reason the client requires hemodialysis (e.g., chronic renal failure, awaiting maturation of arteriovenous fistula [weeks to months], or awaiting a kidney transplant).
- Check the shunt every 4 hours for patency:
  Absence of a bruit or thrill in the shunt (using a stethoscope)
  Absence of pulsation in the shunt
  Evidence that blood in the shunt is darkened or separated into serum and cells
  Kinking of shunt tubing
  Dressing applied too tightly
  Decreased temperature of shunt tubing
- Check the shunt every 4 hours to prevent bleeding:
  Presence of blood on the elastic bandage
  Loose shunt connector
  Tension on the shunt tubing
  Alligator clamps clipped to the elastic bandage
- Check for evidence of infection:
  Redness, tenderness, drainage at the shunt insertion site (Check during dressing changes.)
  Skin erosion at the insertion site
  Elevated white cell count
  Elevated temperature
  Chills, fever
- Assess for fluid volume excess (hypervolemia):
  Body weight
  Shortness of breath
  Presence of third heart sound (S_3 gallop), indicating heart failure
  Neck vein distention
  Periorbital, presacral, or ankle edema
  Intake in excess of output
  Hypertension (systolic and diastolic)
- Assess for hyperkalemia:
  Profound skeletal muscle weakness
  Intestinal cramping
  Voice changes (e.g., hoarseness)
  Increased serum potassium
  ECG changes if ECG is available (peaked T wave, prolonged QRS interval, prolonged PR interval, absent P waves, ventricular ectopy)
- Check for evidence of metabolic acidosis:
  Drowsiness or disorientation
  Decreased pH
  Asterixis, myoclonus, or seizures
- Check for evidence of uremia:
  Gastrointestinal disturbances
  Hiccups
  Muscle cramps
  Pruritus
  Anorexia and weight loss
  Fatigue, lethargy
  Behavioral changes
  Bleeding tendencies, occult blood in stool
  Elevated serum creatinine

• Check for bleeding tendencies if the client is on systemic anticoagulants.

Environmental Assessment

• Check that appropriate facilities are available in the home if the client is on a home dialysis program. Adequate space will be required for storing the artificial kidney machine. A water supply will be required for mixing dialysate. In areas where hard water is a problem, deionization of water may be required. A free-flowing drain will be required to drain the dialysate.

• Check that standard hygiene practices are followed in the home. Dialysis must be carried out in clean surroundings. Aseptic technique is required for shunt care.

Planning Strategies

Potential Nursing Diagnoses

Urinary elimination, alteration in, due to renal failure

Fluid volume, alteration in, excess due to diminished urinary output

Infection or hemorrhage, potential for, due to indwelling vascular access

Knowledge deficit, hemodialysis shunt care

Self-concept, disturbance in: body-image changes due to presence of hemodialysis shunt

Expected Outcomes

Maintenance of adequate renal function

Intact hemodialysis shunt promoting effective fluid and waste removal during hemodialysis

Prevention of infection and bleeding; maintenance of shunt patency

Increased knowledge of shunt care

Acceptance of body-image changes

Health Promotion Goals

• The client and family will
Perform self-care activities related to hemodialysis shunt care
Adapt activities of daily living to incorporate hemodialysis and shunt care
Accept body-image changes related to the hemodialysis shunt

Equipment

For shunt dressing:
Stethoscope
Nontraumatic shunt clamps
Elastic bandage
Sterile 4 × 4s (including 2 precut 4 × 4s)
Alcohol swab sticks or prep pads
Iodophor swab sticks
Iodophor ointment

For declotting a shunt:
Dressing supplies
Sterile towels
Sterile gloves
Sterile shunt clamps
Sterile 10-ml syringes, 2
Sterile shunt connector or T connector

Interventions/Health Promotion

ACTION	*RATIONALE/AMPLIFICATION*
1. Wash hands thoroughly. Remove the soiled elastic bandage and dressings from the shunt.	Retrieve the shunt clamps connected to the bandage.
2. Open sterile supplies onto a clean, dry nightstand or TV tray.	The inside of the packages can be used as a sterile field.
3. Clean around the insertion sites with an alcohol swab stick or alcohol prep pad, taking care not to touch the site or shunt tubing.	Use a separate swab stick or prep pad for each insertion site to prevent the spread of infection from one site to another. One side of the shunt may be infected and the other not.
4. Repeat the cleaning procedure with an iodophor swab stick. Apply iodophor ointment to the insertion sites.	Take care not to touch the tube opening to anything or the tube will be contaminated.
5. Place a precut sterile 4 × 4 around each insertion site. Place a 4 × 4 beneath the shunt tubing. Cover with 4 × 4s and tape the dressing in place.	A 4 × 4 beneath the tubing protects the skin, and is more comfortable for the client. Avoid circular wrapping of the arm with tape because this can interfere with circulation and may cause the shunt to clot.
6. Cover the dressing with the elastic bandage. Cover the entire shunt with the bandage, but cover in such a way that the client can check the shunt tubing for patency or bleeding. Clip two shunt clamps to the dressing.	The shunt clamps are used to clamp both sides of the shunt if it is accidentally disconnected.
7. Discard soiled dressings. Wash hands thoroughly.	Thorough handwashing is mandatory when there is the possibility of exposure to infections that are transmitted by blood.

Related Care

1. Launder the elastic bandage for re-use.	
2. Use a shunt T connector for heparin administration if ordered.	
3. Do not draw blood from a maturing fistula.	Entering the fistula carries the chance of introducing infection or causing clotting.
4. Do not take blood pressure reading on the arm with the external shunt.	Interrupting blood flow can encourage clotting of the shunt.
5. Attempt to declot a clotted shunt: • Assist the client to a comfortable position with the shunt arm extended on a table.	

ACTION	RATIONALE/AMPLIFICATION
• Wash hands thoroughly and remove the elastic bandage and dressings. Use sterile towels to create a sterile field around the shunt. Open sterile supplies onto the sterile field.	Sterile technique is necessary to prevent infection because the shunt will be disconnected to declot.
• Put on sterile gloves.	
• Clean the shunt connector and adjacent tubing with iodophor swabs. Place a sterile shunt clamp on each limb of the shunt.	Cleaning the shunt with iodophor is necessary to prevent infection of the shunt and possible systemic infection. The limbs of the shunt are clamped to prevent bleeding from the shunt. Although the shunt is not patent, one side of the shunt may not be clotted. The venous limb of the shunt tends to clot before the arterial side.
• Separate the shunt tubing. Attach a sterile 10-ml syringe to one limb of the shunt. While holding the syringe in one hand, remove the shunt clamp with the other. Aspirate gently. Reapply the clamp.	Gentle suction with the syringe can remove a newly formed clot and re-establish patency. Pressure with the syringe can force a clot into the circulation, causing an embolus.
• Repeat the procedure for the other limb of the shunt using a second syringe.	
• Reconnect the shunt using a sterile shunt connector or T connector.	Always use a new connector. If the old connector has been damaged in any way it could cause clotting. The old connector may be contaminated and cause infection.
• Evaluate the shunt for patency. If it is not patent, contact the physician for embolectomy using a Fogarty catheter.	
• Redress the shunt.	

Education/ Communication

• Teach the client and family to

Dress the shunt 3 times a week in conjunction with dialysis treatments and if the dressing becomes wet or soiled. Use aseptic technique during dressing changes to prevent infection.

Check the shunt every 4 hours for patency and leakage

Notify health-care professionals of a maturing fistula. The vessel cannot be used for drawing blood. Blood pressures should not be taken on the arm that has the external shunt to prevent clotting.

Refrain from strenuous activities that can damage the shunt. Avoid getting the shunt and elastic bandage wet to prevent infection. Cover the bandage with plastic wrap while bathing to prevent inadvertent wetting from splashing. Keep the shunt arm out of the shower.

Keep a set of nontraumatic alligator clamps clipped to the elastic bandage for clamping the shunt if bleeding occurs. Other clamps can damage the shunt.

Seek emergency medical attention if accidental decannulation occurs. Apply manual pressure to the bleeding site using dressing folded in four.

Seek medical attention or notify the home health nurse as soon as possible if the shunt has clotted

Maintain fluid and dietary restrictions between dialysis treatments
Weigh the client before and after dialysis. Check blood pressure before and
after dialysis and as instructed during dialysis.

Referrals and Consultations

- Refer the client to emergency medical attention in the event of accidental decannulation.
- Instruct the client to contact the home health nurse or seek medical attention as soon as possible for a clotted shunt.

Evaluation of Health Promotion Activities

Quality Assurance/ Reassessment

- Check the client's body weight to estimate fluid gain between dialysis sessions. Check body weight before and after dialysis to determine the amount of fluid removed.
- Check shunt for evidence of bleeding, infection, or clotting.
- Obtain a culture if drainage is present at the shunt insertion sites.
- Check blood pressure. Hypertension can indicate fluid retention.
- Check for signs of fluid overload, uremia, or hyperkalemia.

DOCUMENTATION

Charting for the Home Health Nurse
Condition of the external shunt

Condition of the new fistula if using a shunt while the fistula matures

Physical assessment

Body weight and blood pressure

Compliance with dietary restrictions

Laboratory work flowsheet

Specific records related to the dialysis treatment will be maintained by the home dialysis personnel.

Records Kept by the Client/Family
Predialysis and postdialysis body weight

Vital signs and temperature

Fluid intake

Condition of the shunt

Problems during dialysis

Health Teaching Checklist

Name of Care Provider _____

Relationship to Client _____ Telephone #_____

Taught by _____ Date _____

	EXPLAINED	DEMONSTRATED
Shunt care	_____	_____
Patency checks	_____	_____
Alterations in activity (if necessary)	_____	
Fluid and dietary restrictions	_____	
Emergency procedures (decannulation, clotting)	_____	_____

Product Availability

Dressing supplies are available at drug stores and large grocery stores. Shunt clamps are available through medical-supply companies.

Selected References

Baer CL: Dialysis therapy. In Kinney MR, Dear CB, Packa DR, Voorman DMN (eds): AACN's Clinical Reference for Critical Care Nursing. New York, McGraw-Hill, 1981

Chambers JK, Mekstroth S: Acute hemodialysis. In Persons CB (ed): Critical Care Procedures and Protocols: The Nursing Process. Philadelphia, JB Lippincott, 1987

Grant MM: Renal-urinary disturbances. In Jones DA, Dunbar CF, Jiroreec MM (eds): Medical–Surgical Nursing: A Conceptual Approach. New York, McGraw-Hill, 1982

Lancaster LE (ed): The Patient With End Stage Renal Disease. New York, John Wiley & Sons, 1984

14   Care of the Indwelling Catheter

Background

Indwelling catheters are tubes that are inserted directly into the bladder through the urethra or through an artificial opening in the abdominal wall. The indwelling catheter is made of rubber, Teflon, or Silex. Generally these catheters are held in place by an inflated balloon that wedges against the side of the bladder wall at the site of insertion to secure the catheter in the bladder.

Assessment of Self-Care Potential

Client/Family Assessment

- Assess the client and family members who are to assist with the care to determine if they are willing and capable of performing the required procedure.
- Assess the client/assisting family member for fine motor skills adequate to insert the catheter properly, using sterile technique.
- Assess the visual acuity for ability to determine color changes in the urine as well as to assess for skin breakdown.

Physical Assessment

- Assess the perineal skin daily for irritation or breakdown.
- Assess the mucous membranes for irritation, redness, drainage, and bleeding.
- A sample of urine should be assessed daily to detect color change, cloudiness, presence of blood, and/or mucous threads or particles.
- A urine specimen should be analyzed by a laboratory technician periodically, at times directed by the physician, or when pain, bleeding, or change in urine indicates.

Environmental Assessment

- Assess the environment for a place where the drainage tubing and urinary drainage receptacle can be cleansed and hung to dry.
- Assess the client's bed for a way to apply a hook from which to hang the drainage bag while the client sleeps.

Planning Strategies

Potential Nursing Diagnoses

Urinary elimination pattern, altered

Skin integrity, potential skin breakdown

Body-image disturbance, potential

Expected Outcomes

Maintenance of adequate urine elimination

Maintenance of indwelling catheter without bladder infection, skin breakdown, or renal calculi

Continuation or resumption of usual pattern of daily living with a high level of independent functioning

Health Promotion Goals

- The client and family will
  Demonstrate proper cleaning technique of the drainage system
  Maintain an odor-free status
  Demonstrate appropriate technique for emptying the drainage system

If using a leg-attached receptacle, demonstrate proper technique when changing from one drainage system to another

Demonstrate cleansing technique of the catheter insertion site

Equipment

White vinegar

Povidone-iodine swabs

Pan large enough to cleanse tubing and bag

Urine specimen containers as needed

Funnel or 50-ml syringe

Clean towel

Pan to boil equipment

Additional equipment if leg-attached system is used
Rubber or plastic leg-attached drainage apparatus (reusable or disposable) to include drainage tubing and bag with antireflux valve

Additional equipment for closed drainage system
Presterilized, disposable drainage system containing collection bag, tubing, and clamp with antireflux valve

Interventions/Health Promotion

ACTION	RATIONALE/AMPLIFICATION
1. Change the catheter on a set schedule.	The frequency for changing the catheter depends on the material of which the catheter is made as well as on whether or not the catheter becomes obstructed or is otherwise defective. Changing the catheter on a set schedule, prior to the development of obstruction or defect, will help prevent complications.
2. Secure the catheter in such a manner that stress or pulling on the catheter is prevented.	Stress on the catheter can cause bladder trauma and extreme discomfort.
3. For males, anchor the tubing so as to eliminate pressure and irritation at the penoscrotal angle (Fig. 14-1).	Allowing some slack contributes to preventing stress on the catheter and the bladder wall.

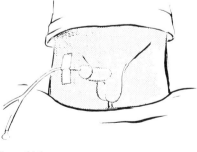

Figure 14.1
Proper taping of the catheter in males reduces pressure on the bladder as well as on the penoscrotal angle.

ACTION	*RATIONALE/AMPLIFICATION*
For females, secure the drainage tube with nonallergenic tape to the inner thigh just below the vagina, leaving some slack in the tubing.	
4. Hang the tubing in such a manner that kinking and loops are prevented. Place the urinary receptacle in a position so that it is always below the level of the bladder whether the client is sitting, lying, or standing. Empty the urinary receptacle as needed, at least every 8 hours. Empty the leg bag more frequently.	Proper positioning of the tubing prevents the urine from pooling and standing in the tubing, which encourages bacterial growth in the urine.
5. Wash the area around the insertion site with soap and water at least twice daily. Wash the anal area with soap and water after each bowel movement.	Consistent cleanliness reduces the probability of irritation from the acidity of the urine.
6. Force fluids daily.	Adequate fluid intake reduces the risk of renal calculi and assists in odor control.

Care of the Closed Drainage System

1. Do not interrupt the closed drainage system.	Interruption encourages introduction of bacteria into the urinary system.
2. Empty the drainage system according to the manufacturer's directions. Unclamp the drainage tube, being careful not to touch the tip. Cleanse the tip with povidone-iodine, if available, or with soap and water. Drain the urine into the toilet or other suitable container. Wash the end of the tube with povidone-iodine or soap and water. Reapply the clamping device and replace according to the manufacturer's directions.	Cleansing the end of the tubing before and after draining the bag will offer additional protection against contamination of the system.

Care of the Leg-Attached Drainage Bag

1. Do not interrupt the drainage system unnecessarily.	Even though the leg-attached bag is used during the day, the closed drainage bag is used during sleep. This allows for hanging of the drainage bag below the level of the bladder while the client is lying down. In addition, since the closed drainage bag is larger, it does not require emptying as frequently as the bag that is worn on the leg.
2. Procedure for emptying is identical to that for the closed drainage system (above).	Empty every 4 to 6 hours.

ACTION	*RATIONALE/AMPLIFICATION*
Changing From Leg-Attached Bag to Closed Drainage System (Nighttime)	
1. Empty leg-attached bag according to manufacturer's directions.	Emptying the bag prior to disconnecting reduces the possibility of contamination.
2. Clamp the catheter near its end and cleanse with povidone-iodine.	The system is interrupted. Therefore, means must be taken to ensure a clean system following reestablishment of the system.
3. Connect the closed drainage system and unclamp the catheter.	
Care of the Leg-Attached and/or Closed Drainage Bags	
1. After disconnecting the drainage apparatus, rinse with warm, soapy water. Rinse with vinegar-and-water solution (1½ cups white vinegar to 2 quarts water). Soak for 2 hours.	Warm, soapy water cleanses the system. Vinegar and water are used for odor control. Commercial preparations are also available for odor control that do not affect the color or longevity of the tubing.
2. Allow hot water to run through the tubing and allow tubing to air dry.	
Irrigation of the Catheter	
1. Place the barrel of a sterile 50-ml syringe in the distal end of the catheter after cleansing the distal end of the catheter with povodine-iodine or soap and water.	A disposable or a reusable glass syringe can be used. If neither is feasible, a metal funnel can be used. Both the glass syringe and the funnel can be sterilized by boiling for 5 minutes.
2. Pour the irrigating solution into the syringe barrel or the funnel. Allow solution to flow by gravity. Remove the barrel or funnel and allow the solution to return by gravity flow.	Allowing gravity flow prevents the use of excessive force or pressure while introducing or withdrawing the irrigating solution. If pressure or suction is necessary, the nurse or physician should be contacted for further direction.
Maintaining Cleanliness of the Meatus	
1. *Female:* Separate labia minora with thumb and forefinger. Clean with soap-saturated cotton balls, from the meatus downward and outward, using a clean cotton ball for each stroke (Fig. 14-2). Rinse in the same manner, using clean, warm water.	Secretions, menstrual flow, and feces soiling the catheter cause a prime colonization site for bacteria.
2. *Male:* Raise the penis and retract the foreskin. Clean the meatus with one cotton ball. Using another cotton ball, clean the catheter in a circular motion from the insertion site outward (Fig. 14-3).	The mucous membrane should be kept clean to prevent infection resulting from infective exudate and excretions.
3. *Both males and females:* Clean the catheter insertion site at least twice daily and following each bowel movement.	Consistent cleanliness is the best preventive measure against infection and irritation.

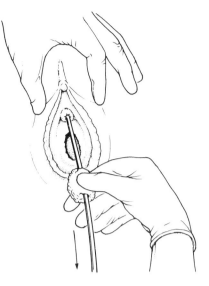

Figure 14.2
Cleansing the meatus and catheter in a female.

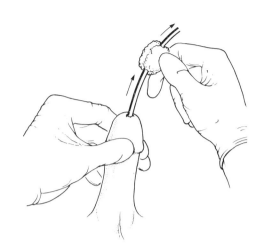

Figure 14.3
Cleansing the meatus and catheter in a male.

ACTION	RATIONALE/AMPLIFICATION
Related Care	
1. Inspect urine daily by holding up specimen to observe in a well-lighted area (at a window, for example).	Inspect for changes in color and clarity and for presence of blood.
2. If the client is allergic to tape, use the top of a nylon stocking to secure the catheter to the thigh.	A slip knot on one side of the stocking secures the catheter in place, yet has enough "give" to provide ease to the catheter.
3. See Technique 15, Insertion and Removal of a Foley Catheter.	

Education/ Communication

- Teach the client and family to
  Irrigate the catheter, using gravity flow
  Clean drainage tubing and drainage bag/bottle
  Observe the urine twice daily for color changes, presence of mucus or blood, and cloudiness
  Collect urine specimen for analysis if any changes are observed
  Clean perineal area/penis with soap and water twice daily
  Wash rectal area with soap and water after each bowel movement
  Maintain flow of drainage tubing to prevent kinks, loops, and a position of the drainage receptacle below the level of the bladder
  Maintain odor control by use of vinegar-and-water solution for washing equipment
  Secure catheter/drainage tubing to thigh in such a manner as to prevent stress and pull on the bladder
  Notify the nurse if
    The irrigating solution does not return by gravity
    The urine changes color
    The urine is cloudy or contains blood or mucous threads
    The catheter is inadvertently removed
    Pain is experienced in the bladder area or at the insertion site
    There is no urinary drainage for more than a 1-hour period

Referrals and Consultations

Referral to a urologist may be needed if pain or discoloration of the urine occurs.

Evaluation of Health Promotion Activities

Quality Assurance/ Reassessment

- Make periodic home visits to evaluate quality of care of the catheter and cleanliness of the insertion site.
- Periodically collect urine samples for laboratory analysis (once monthly or more often if indicated).
- Observe a family member or the client irrigate the catheter.
- Inspect the urinary drainage system to determine proper placement in relation to the bladder.
- Inspect the areas where the drainage tubing is taped to the skin to determine the presence of skin irritation or breakdown.

DOCUMENTATION

Charting for the Home Health Nurse
The condition of the insertion site, the quality and quantity of urinary output, and the skin condition at the taping site should be examined and recorded at each visit.

Records Kept by the Client/Family
Questions and concerns
Perineal/sacral skin irritation/breakdown
Presence of blood in the urine; pain on urination

Health Teaching Checklist

Name of Care Provider _____

Relationship to Client _____ Telephone #_____

Taught by _____ Date _____

	EXPLAINED	DEMONSTRATED
Cleaning of Equipment	_____	_____
Proper positioning of devices	_____	_____
Irrigation of catheter	_____	_____
Odor control	_____	_____

Product Availability

All items needed are available from a hospital-supply firm.

Selected Reference

Kniep-Hardy M, Votova K, Stubbings MJ: Managing indwelling catheters in the home. Geriatric Nursing, September/October, 1985, pp 280–285

15 Insertion and Removal of a Foley Catheter

Background

A Foley catheter is an indwelling or retention catheter. It is held in place at the outlet of the bladder by means of a balloon filled with sterile water that is injected into a lumen at the end of the catheter. The catheter is selected for size, graded according to a French scale (the larger the number, the larger the lumen); for capacity of the balloon (indicating the number of milliliters to be injected into the lumen, 5 ml, 10 ml); and for composition (Silex, Teflon-lined, or rubber).

Assessment of Self-Care Potential

Client/Family Assessment

- Assess the client/family for willingness and ability to observe the catheter for urinary flow and to notify the nurse immediately in the event of obstruction or other observed complication.

Physical Assessment

- Take vital signs prior to insertion of the catheter.
- Assess fluid intake.
- Inspect the abdomen for a greatly distended bladder, which can be observed as an enlargement just above the symphysis pubis.
- Percuss the bladder. Unless filled with urine, the bladder can be neither palpated or percussed. A full bladder produces a dull sound; an empty one produces a resonant sound.
- Palpate the bladder. If distended or full, it can be palpated as a firm, smooth mass.
- Assess the urethral orifice. In males, it is situated at the tip of the penis. In females, it lies between the clitoris and the vaginal orifice. Normally it lies in the midline (Fig. 15-1). Variations in both male and female structures can occur and should be noted prior to attempting catheterization.
- Inspect the perineal area for odors, drainage, inflammation, tumors, ulcers, or chancres. The presence of any of these should be documented carefully.

Environmental Assessment

- Assess the bed, chair, wheelchair, or walker used by the client to determine if a hook or other device can be attached for hanging the closed drainage bag. The bag must not be placed on the floor because of the possibility of contamination. It should at all times be hung below the level of the bladder.

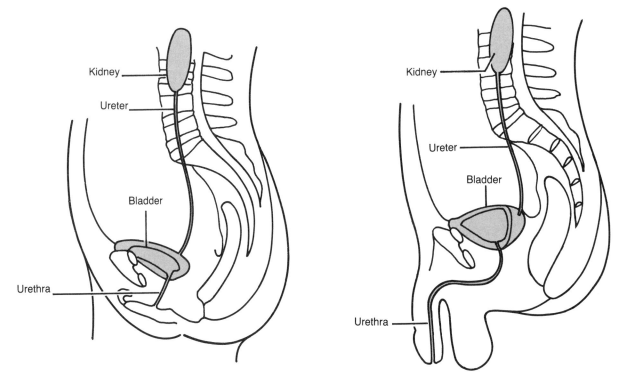

Figure 15.1
Schematic lateral illustrations of female (*left*) and male (*right*) urinary tracts.

Planning Strategies

Potential Nursing Diagnoses

Urinary elimination pattern, altered

Alteration in comfort, pain

Expected Outcomes

Restoration of adequate urine elimination by artificial means

Maintenance of the catheter without complication or excessive discomfort

No significant alteration in client/family's lifestyle

Health Promotion Goals

- The client and family will
  Be relieved of discomfort due to bladder distention/urinary retention
  Keep the drainage bag and tubing hung at a level lower than the bladder
  Respect the need for privacy for the client in the process of catheterization or catheter removal

Equipment

Appropriate catheter (number 16 or 18 French with 5-ml balloon for adults unless a larger size is ordered)

Adequate lighting source

Appropriate draping to provide for modesty and dignity

Gloves

Fenestrated drape to place over perineum

Cotton balls or gauze squares to apply the antiseptic

Water-soluble lubricant to lubricate the tip of the catheter

A urine specimen container

Hypoallergenic tape

Drapes to protect the bed and provide sterile field

An antiseptic cleansing solution to clean labia and urinary meatus

Forceps to apply the antiseptic

A 10-ml syringe filled with sterile solution for injection into the balloon

A receptacle for urine collection

A drainage bag with tubing

Interventions/Health Promotion

ACTION	*RATIONALE/AMPLIFICATION*
1. Explain the procedure to the client.	Knowing what to expect will assist in reducing anxiety.
2. Provide for privacy, modesty, and dignity, and arrange to be free of interruption during the procedure.	Any measures that will assist in preventing embarrassment or loss of dignity will contribute to the comfort and ease of the procedure.
3. Position the client in such a manner as to relax the abdominal and perineal muscles during insertion of the catheter.	The female is placed recumbent with knees flexed; the male is placed supine. Pillows can be used to support the knees and elevate the female buttocks, thus providing better visualization.
4. Place a light source in such a manner as to provide good visualization, yet so it does not burn the client.	If a gooseneck or similar lamp is unavailable, a flashlight can be used.
5. Wash the perineal area with soap and water prior to beginning the procedure.	

Catheterization of Female Clients

1. Using sterile technique, open the catheterization tray at the bedside. Don the sterile gloves aseptically and place the tray between the client's thighs.	If the client is overly anxious or is unable to follow directions, provide assistance to prevent movement of the legs onto the sterile field.
2. Drape the client with the sterile drapes provided, cautiously protecting the sterility of the gloves. The first drape is inserted under the buttocks, with the edges cuffed over the gloves, thus preventing contamination of the gloves.	All steps of preparation must be done completely prior to the initiation of the procedure to prevent having to interrupt the procedure.
3. The fenestrated drape is placed over the perineum.	This will adequately expose the perineal area.
4. Thigh drapes are placed over the thighs.	Draping the thigh farthest away first will allow the draping of both thighs without contamination.
5. Pick up the catheter and check the balloon for leaks by injecting 5-ml of sterile solution into the lumen and then withdrawing the solution if there are no leaks.	If the balloon is defective, the catheter cannot be retained in place.

ACTION

RATIONALE/AMPLIFICATION

6. Lubricate the tip of the catheter liberally with the lubricating jelly provided.

Lubrication reduces friction, thus minimizing the mechanical injury to tissue while inserting the catheter.

7. Place the urine specimen container within easy reach on the sterile field, with lid removed.

8. Cleanse the perineum: Two fingers of the nondominant hand are used to separate the labia majora. Cleanse the labia majora on each side, using cotton balls saturated with the antiseptic solution. Each cotton ball is used only once. The movement for cleansing is downward from the pubic area to the anus (Fig. 15-2).

The area is thus cleansed from the area of least contamination to that of greatest contamination.

The cotton balls are held with the forceps by the dominant hand.

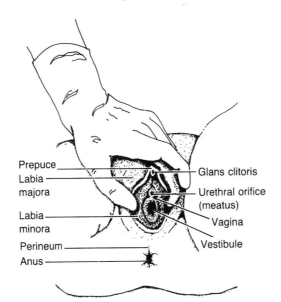

Figure 15.2

9. Separate the labia minora with the thumb and another clean finger of the nondominant hand, using the same procedure as above to cleanse the area surrounding the urinary meatus, retracting the tissue sufficiently to visualize the meatus. *Important*: once the meatus is cleansed, the labia must not be allowed to close over it.

The hand that has touched the client's skin is considered contaminated. It therefore is used to expose the meatus, freeing the other hand to accomplish the sterile catheterization.

10. Place the distal end of the catheter into the urine receptacle. Grasp the proximal end of the catheter with the sterile forceps, approximately 2 to 3 inches.

The female urethra is approximately 1.5 inches long. The catheter is held far enough from the tip to allow for full insertion into the bladder.

ACTION

RATIONALE/AMPLIFICATION

11. The catheter is inserted into the meatus approximately 2 inches or until urine flows (Fig. 15-3).

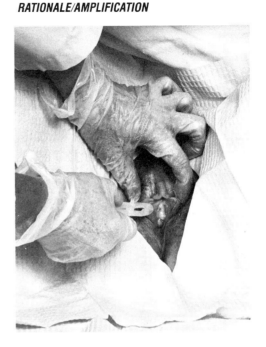

Figure 15.3

12. If resistance is encountered, ask the client to breathe deeply. Attempt to complete insertion during expiration. If resistance is still encountered, discontinue attempts and consult the physician.

Forceful pressure can cause damage to the tissues.

13. When urine returns, grasp the catheter with the contaminated hand, holding the catheter in place.

14. Collect the urine specimen. Empty the bladder (stopping after 700 ml has been drained).

Removing large quantities of urine rapidly can produce hypovolemic shock.

15. Inject the premeasured sterile solution into the lumen connected to the balloon. If the client expresses that she feels pain, withdraw the solution, insert the catheter further, and inject the sterile solution again. Withdraw the catheter slightly until resistance is felt.

If pain is indicated when the solution is injected, the tip of the catheter may be located in the urethra. Inserting it further will place it well into the bladder.

16. Connect the catheter to the drainage tubing, hanging the bag below the level of the bladder. Tape the tubing to the client's inner thigh, just below the perineum.

Securing with tape prevents pull on the bladder.

17. Remove and discard equipment. Make client comfortable. Deliver urine specimen for analysis.

ACTION	*RATIONALE/AMPLIFICATION*

Catheterization of Male Clients

1. Assist the client to assume a supine position, knees slightly bent and legs slightly apart.

   This allows relaxation of abdominal and perineal muscles, easing the process of catheter insertion.

2. The penis and perineal area are washed with soap and water and dried.

3. Drape the client so that the penis is exposed.

   Proper draping protects modesty and ensures warmth.

4. Open the catheter kit, using aseptic technique. Place equipment within easy reach at the bedside.

   If a bedside table is not available, a chair can be placed at the bedside for work space.

5. Put on gloves. Pour antiseptic solution over cotton balls.

6. Inject 5 ml of the sterile solution into the lumen leading to the inflatable balloon. If no leaks are found, remove the solution.

   The balloon is examined for leaks.

7. Lubricate the distal end of the catheter with the sterile lubricating jelly provided.

   Lubrication reduces friction, thus reducing trauma to the urethra during catheter insertion.

8. Drape the client with the sterile drapes provided.

   Cover the thighs with one drape. Place the fenestrated drape over the abdomen and guide the penis through the precut opening.

9. Hold the penis in the nondominant hand during the remainder of the procedure.

   That hand is now considered contaminated.

10. If the client is uncircumcised, pull back the foreskin with the contaminated hand.

11. With the uncontaminated hand, grasp a cotton ball with the forceps and clean the meatus with the cotton ball. Repeat with each cotton ball.

    Use a circular motion, starting at the meatus and ending at the corona.

12. Hold the penis at a 90-degree angle to the thighs. Grasp the catheter with the uncontaminated hand or sterile forceps, 7 to 10 inches from the tip (Fig. 15-4). Gently insert into the meatus. Lower the penis to a 60-degree angle.

    This angle permits easier insertion of the catheter.

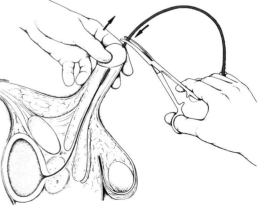

Figure 15.4
Technique of male catheter insertion.

ACTION

    Note: a few inches into the urethra, some resistance will be encountered. Ask the client to exhale, then inhale. Advance the catheter during the inhalation phase.

13. If the catheter bends inside the penis or springs back when released, increase the traction on the penis and gently attempt to insert.

14. When urine returns, hold the catheter in place with the contaminated hand. Collect the urine specimen. Empty the bladder (up to 700 ml at a time).

15. Inject 5 ml of sterile solution into the lumen of the balloon. Withdraw the catheter slightly until resistance is encountered.

16. Connect the catheter to the drainage tubing, hanging the bag below the level of the bladder. Tape the catheter to the client's lower abdomen.

17. Remove and discard equipment. Assist client to become comfortable. Deliver urine specimen for analysis.

RATIONALE/AMPLIFICATION

If the insertion cannot be accomplished with gentle pressure, the physician should be notified.

This problem is often encountered at the external sphincter.

Emptying the bladder too suddenly can result in hypovolemic shock.

The balloon will be inflated just inside the outlet of the bladder, thus securing the catheter.

Taping the catheter prevents traction on the bladder (Figs. 15-5 and 15-6).

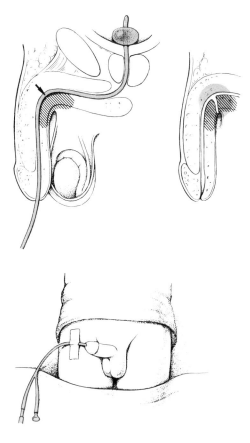

Figure 15.5
Illustration of compression of the penoscrotal angle resulting from the straightening of the catheter, producing pressure that can cause soreness, abscesses, and fistula formation. This can be prevented by proper taping of the catheter (see Fig. 15.6).

Figure 15.6
Illustration of the proper taping of the catheter to eliminate the penoscrotal angle and thus prevent abscess formation and fistula formation.

ACTION	RATIONALE/AMPLIFICATION
Removing the Foley Catheter	
1. Assemble equipment: clean examining gloves, sterile needle, 5-ml syringe to collect withdrawn solution.	Having all required equipment available prevents unnecessary interruptions.
2. Attach needle to syringe. Swab the inflation site with antiseptic solution. Insert needle and withdraw solution.	
3. Pinch the catheter near its tip and withdraw gently.	Pinching the catheter prevents urine from entering the meatus during withdrawal of the catheter.

Age-Specific Modifications

The catheter size should be adapted if the client is a child.

Education/ Communication

- Teach the client and family to
  Maintain proper positioning of the urine collection device (below the level of the bladder)
  Maintain positioning of the catheter, tubing, and collection device to prevent pull on the bladder
  Maintain the collection tubing without kinks
  Apply the tape to secure the catheter properly (to the thigh or lower abdomen)
  Remove the catheter in the event of complications
  Observe for catheter obstruction, hematuria, changing character of urine

Referrals and Consultations

- Consult a urologist if excessive resistance or bleeding is encountered in the process of catheterization.

Evaluation of Health Promotion Activities

Quality Assurance/ Reassessment

- Evaluate the placement of the collection device relative to the tubing and bladder. It should always be below the level of the bladder. The tubing should not be kinked and should not produce unnecessary pull on the bladder.
- Observe a return demonstration of removing the catheter.
- Evaluate the character of the urine periodically by taking a urine sample to the laboratory for analysis.
- Evaluate the daily fluid intake to ensure it is adequate.

DOCUMENTATION

Charting for the Home Health Nurse
- Note the date and time of catheterization.
- Document client toleration of the procedure, the quantity of urine return, and character of urine return.
- Note any complications encountered during the procedure.

Records Kept by the Client/Family
Any changes in the character of the urine

Marked decrease in urine volume

Any difficulties encountered with the catheter

Questions and concerns

Health Teaching Checklist

Name of Care Provider _____

Relationship to Client _____ Telephone # _____

Taught by _____ Date _____

	EXPLAINED	DEMONSTRATED
Positioning of bag and tubing	_____	_____
Assessing for catheter obstruction and changes in urine character	_____	_____
Removal of catheter	_____	_____

Product Availability

All needed supplies are available at hospital-supply or medical-supply firms. Prescriptions are required for purchase of catheters.

Selected Reference

Wolff L, Weitzel MH, Zornow RA, Zsohar H: Fundamentals of Nursing, 7th ed. Philadelphia, JB Lippincott, 1983

16 Intermittent Self-Catheterization

Background

Intermittent self-catheterization refers to the introduction of a catheter into the bladder at a set schedule by either the client or a person assisting the client. Since the client determines the timing of the procedure, catheterization can take place prior to the bladder becoming distended, thus reducing the traumatic effect of an overly distended bladder. In addition, since the catheter is not an indwelling one, irritation to the urethra and bladder is reduced. By controlling urinary functions, the client exercises a higher level of independence in basic living functions.

Assessment of Self-Care Potential

Client/Family Assessment

- Assess the willingness and capability of a family member to assist the client with the procedure until the client gains independence in its performance, as well as in the event of an emergency.
- Assess the fine motor movement and visual acuity of the person assisting with the procedure.

Physical Assessment

- Assess the client's anal sphincter muscle tone. The absence of anal sphincter tone is an indicator of inadequate bladder capacity since both the vesicle neck and the anal sphincter share the same neuronal pathway.
- Determine if the bladder capacity is at least 500 ml. A smaller capacity requires catheterizations too frequently.

Environmental Assessment

- Determine that adequate lighting exists in the area to be used for the procedure.
- Determine that privacy and freedom from interruption can be provided the client during the procedure.

Planning Strategies

Potential Nursing Diagnoses

Urinary elimination, impairment of: incontinence

Skin integrity, potential skin breakdown

Expected Outcomes

Development of new levels of independence in urinary control

Prevention of skin breakdown

Incorporation of self-catheterization on an intermittent schedule into the client/family lifestyle

Health Promotion Goals

- The client and family will
  Obtain required catheterization equipment. If finances do not permit the purchase of the equipment, social worker assistance will be obtained.
  Properly clean and store the catheterization equipment
  Adhere to the recommended catheterization schedule
  Demonstrate the ability to adapt the performance of the procedure to environments other than the home as needed

Prepare a travel kit to take needed supplies when away from home

Initiate and continue recommended dietary alterations

Equipment

Straight rubber catheters (minimum of one day's supply, wrapped in aluminum foil)

Clean washcloth

Soap and water

Water-soluble lubricant

Plastic bag to be used as receptacle for used catheters

Container for draining urine if toilet is not available

A hand-held mirror for a female in the early stages of learning the procedure

Interventions/Health Promotion

ACTION	RATIONALE/AMPLIFICATION
Female Self-Catheterization	
1. Wash hands and assemble equipment.	The procedure must be kept as free of infection-inducing bacteria as possible. Handwashing is a primary means of preventing infection. All needed equipment must be readily available so that the procedure is not interrupted unnecessarily. Note: the importance of catheterizing at the scheduled time cannot be over-emphasized. Therefore, even if some supplies are not presently available due to some unforeseen incident (soap, for instance), the catheterization should still be performed at the scheduled time. The bladder's natural resistance to bacteria will assist in inhibiting infection.
2. Attempt to urinate.	Do this by applying moderate pressure on the lower abdomen and/or by stroking the thighs. Running water might also induce urination.
3. Assume a sitting position on a bed or chair or on a toilet.	If using a bed or chair, protect the surface with plastic covered with a towel.
4. Separate the vaginal folds with one hand. With the other hand, use downward strokes while washing with the washcloth and soap and water.	Downward strokes proceed from the less-contaminated area to the more-contaminated area, thus reducing the possibility of introducing rectal bacteria into the urinary tract.
5. Lubricate the end of the catheter with water-soluble lubricant.	This will reduce friction, thus reducing damage to the urethra.
6. Keeping the vaginal folds separated with one hand, insert the catheter with the other hand about 3 inches or until the urine begins to flow.	Holding the catheter like a pencil in the dominant hand as it is inserted will aid in the procedure.

ACTION	*RATIONALE/AMPLIFICATION*
7. Press down with abdominal muscles.	This maneuver will aid in emptying the bladder.
8. Allow all urine to drain. Remove the catheter by pinching it off and holding the tip upward above the rest of the catheter.	This prevents urine from draining into the urethra.
9. Rinse the catheter in cold water. Wash with warm soapy water. Place into plastic bag provided for used catheters.	Proper cleansing of catheters prolongs their effective use.

Male Self-Catheterization

1. Wash hands and assemble equipment.	The procedure must be kept as free of infection-inducing bacteria as possible. Handwashing is a primary means of preventing infection. All needed equipment must be readily available so that the procedure is not interrupted unnecessarily. Note: the importance of catheterizing at the scheduled time cannot be over-emphasized. Therefore, even if some supplies are not presently available due to some unforeseen incident (soap, for instance), the catheterization should still be performed at the scheduled time. The bladder's natural resistance to bacteria will assist in inhibiting infection.
2. Attempt to urinate.	Do this by applying moderate pressure on the lower abdomen and/or by stroking the thighs. Running water also induces urination for some persons.
3. Assume a sitting position on a bed, chair, or toilet.	If using a bed or chair, protect the surface with plastic covered with a towel.
4. If uncircumcised, retract the foreskin and keep it retracted for the entire procedure. Wash the tip of the penis thoroughly with the washcloth and soap and water.	Proper cleansing is necessary to prevent spread of bacteria.
5. Lubricate the first 7 inches to 10 inches of the catheter.	Lubricant reduces friction, thus reducing damage to the urethra.
6. Hold the penis with one hand at a right angle to the body. With the other hand, grasp the catheter like a pencil and insert 7 inches to 10 inches into the penis or until urine begins to flow. Then insert it 1 inch further.	Proper positioning of the penis is important to prevent unnecessary pressure and possible damage to structures.
7. Apply moderate pressure on abdominal muscles.	This maneuver aids in emptying the bladder.

ACTION	***RATIONALE/AMPLIFICATION***
8. When urine stops flowing, pinch the catheter off and remove. Pull the foreskin back into position.	This prevents leakage of urine into the urethra.
9. Rinse the catheter in cold water. Wash with warm soapy water. Place into plastic bag provided for used catheters.	Proper cleansing of catheters prolongs their effective use.

Related Care

1. Medications are commonly prescribed in conjunction with intermittent self-catheterization.	The most commonly prescribed medications are Methenamine mandelate (Mandelamine): acidifies urine, thus preventing infection Ascorbic acid: maintains urine acidity Bethanechol chloride (Urecholine): acts on parasympathetic nerves, assisting in bladder contraction Propantheline (Pro-Banthine): acts on postganglionic nerve endings to relax bladder muscles, thus promoting retention of urine Oxybutynin chloride (Ditropan): assists in retention of urine, much as probantheline Phenoxybenzamine (Dibenzyline): relaxes urethral sphincter, increasing urine flow
2. Initially schedule the procedure every 6 hours.	Instruct the client to attempt to void prior to catheterization. The urine is measured; if less than 200 ml is obtained, the schedule can be increased to every 8 hours or more.
3. Monitor fluid intake.	From 1500 ml to 2000 ml should be taken daily.
4. Avoid calcium-rich and phosphorus-rich foods.	Avoid eating more than 1 milk product daily. Avoidance of these foods will reduce the chance of kidney stone formation.
5. Maintain good skin care.	If left on the skin without washing frequently, the acidity of urine will cause skin breakdown. Wash the skin frequently with soap and water and pat dry.
6. Ask the male client if he wishes to wear an external urinary collection device until the schedule for catheterization is effective.	This will eliminate soiling the clothing.
7. Ask the female client if she wishes to wear underclothing with disposable liners until the catheterization schedule is effective.	This will eliminate soiling the clothing.

ACTION	*RATIONALE/AMPLIFICATION*
Care of the Catheters	
1. Purchase a new supply of catheters as needed.	Purchase them monthly or when the ones being used become brittle. Purchase at least one day's supply of catheters.
2. Use each catheter only once after it has been washed.	Following use, place the catheter in a plastic bag provided for used catheters, to be washed later.
3. Soak the catheters in soapy water and rinse with clear water. Boil for 20 minutes in a pan of water.	Drain the catheters and store in a folder of aluminum foil or in a freshly laundered towel.

Age-Specific Modifications

This procedure has been shown to be effective for children also. Generally, the age guidelines are that intermittent self-catheterization can be performed by anyone old enough to follow and remember directions accurately.

Education/ Communication

• Teach the family and client to
  Perform the procedure accurately
  Understand the importance of following the established time schedule exactly
  Clean equipment thoroughly
  Maintain adequate fluid intake of 1500 ml to 2000 ml daily
  Adhere to recommended dietary alterations
  Follow medical regimen accurately
  Notify the nurse if pain is experienced during catheterization; if blood, mucus, or visible particles are seen in the urine; if the urine has an uncharacteristic odor; or if the urine decreases significantly in volume.

Evaluation of Health Promotion Activities

Quality Assurance/ Reassessment

• Following the successful return demonstration of the procedure, periodically observe the procedure to ensure ongoing accurate performance.
• Periodically collect a urine sample for laboratory analysis.
• Assess the frequency of incontinence to determine if it is reducing.

DOCUMENTATION

Charting for the Home Health Nurse
Return demonstration of catheterization procedure

Adherence to recommended schedule of catheterization

Quality of urine

Quantity of urine

Daily intake and output

Status of urinary control by means of catheterizations

Condition of skin

Client satisfaction with procedures

Records Kept by the Client/Family
Questions and concerns regarding the procedure

Any pain or resistance felt in the process of catheterization

The presence of blood, mucous threads, or visible particles in the urine

Any uncharacteristic odor of the urine

Any indication of skin breakdown due to urine
Any significant change in urinary volume
Success in preventing urinary incontinence

**Health Teaching
Checklist**

Name of Care Provider _____

Relationship to Client _____ Telephone #_____

Taught by _____ Date _____

	EXPLAINED	DEMONSTRATED
Catheterization procedure	_____	_____
Importance of maintaining the schedule	_____	
Cleaning equipment	_____	_____
Dietary recommendations	_____	
Recognition of complications: need to notify nurse	_____	
Elements of record keeping	_____	_____
Medication schedule	_____	_____

Product Availability

The catheters are available through hospital-supply or medical-supply firms. A prescription will be needed to purchase the catheters. The external urinary collection device (male) and underwear with liners can also be purchased from a medical-supply firm. All other needed supplies are available in the home.

Selected Reference

Wolff L, Weitzel MH, Zornow RA, Zsohar H: Fundamentals of Nursing, 7th ed. Philadelphia, JB Lippincott, 1983

17 Ostomy Care

Background

The term *ostomy* refers to a surgical diversion of waste products through an artificially created opening on the abdominal surface. The term *stoma* refers to the artificially created opening into the bowel system. Ostomy care relates to care of the stoma and peristoma, irrigation procedures if ordered, cleansing of equipment, and odor control. In addition, the client and family often require assistance with body-image adaptations.

Assessment of Self-Care Potential

Client/Family Assessment

- Assess the stage of acceptance of the ostomy:
  Determine if the client can look at the stoma.
  Assess the ability of the client/family to speak realistically of the ostomy.
- Determine if at least one family member is willing and able to assist with ostomy care until the client can perform it independently. In addition, another family member will be needed to assist the client in the event of an emergency for backup.
- Assess the presence of role/relational difficulties arising from adaptations required by the ostomy (sexual and/or social).

Physical Assessment

- Assess the condition of the skin surrounding the orifice. Drainage from the ostomy causes skin excoriation.
- Assess the current and preoperative patterns of elimination.
- Assess the color of the stoma. It should be bright red. If deep red or bluish, a circulatory problem may be present.

Environmental Assessment

- Determine if bathroom privacy and freedom from interruption can be provided at the scheduled time of ostomy care.
- Determine if there is a towel rack or other device from which to hang the irrigation device (if irrigating). It should be shoulder height to the client.
- Assess the adequacy of lighting in the bathroom. Lighting should be sufficient to allow the procedures to be performed accurately, the skin surrounding the stoma to be assessed, and appropriate cleansing to be done.

Planning Strategies

Potential Nursing Diagnoses

Alteration in elimination

Skin integrity, potential impairment of

Body image disturbance

Expected Outcomes

Reestablishment of acceptable elimination pattern

Prevention of skin breakdown

Acceptance of alteration of body image and resumption of independent activities of daily living

Health Promotion Goals

- The client and family will
  Obtain needed equipment
  Perform skin care properly
  Perform irrigation procedure (if prescribed)
  Measure and properly fit the stoma bag according to the size of stoma opening
  Initiate and maintain contact with an ostomy support group or former ostomy client. If appropriate, the client/family will attend "I Can Cope" group sessions
  Initiate and maintain recommended dietary alterations
  Assemble a travel kit to be kept in the car and in the luggage if traveling by commercial means

Equipment

Irrigation appliance (if indicated): disposable or reusable, enema or bulb-type irrigation devices

Commode or other toileting device (portable commode, bedpan)

Stand, hook, or towel rack to hold irrigating solution (while procedure is being done) at shoulder height to client. (A wire coat hanger can be bent to hang on towel rack and hold bag on its hook.)

Clean dressing and pouch

Water-soluble lubricant

Glove

Benzoin/Karaya paste/stoma adhesive as recommended

Interventions/Health Promotion

ACTION	RATIONALE/AMPLIFICATION
Changing Pouch and Applying Dressing	
1. Wash hands and assemble equipment.	In addition to the equipment listed, scissors will be required if the skin barrier or pouch has to be enlarged to provide a good fit.
2. Remove the used pouch, using warm water to loosen the seal.	The skin surrounding the stoma is highly sensitive. Constant irritation by abrasive removal of the pouch causes skin breakdown. Loosening the seal with warm water reduces the trauma. The frequency of changing the pouch and emptying it depends on the type of ostomy: iliostomies require more frequent emptying and changing. Frequent emptying and changing also assist in providing odor control.

ACTION

RATIONALE/AMPLIFICATION

3. Wash the peristomal area gently but thoroughly with warm water and mild soap. Follow with thorough rinsing. Pat area dry (Fig. 17-1).

Cleanliness is the greatest deterrent to tissue breakdown.

4. Hold a piece of gauze over the stoma to absorb drainage. Apply the skin barrier/seal of choice (benzoin, Karaya paste, stoma adhesive).

The gauze prevents irritating drainage from seeping onto the cleansed peristomal skin. Seepage also prevents a good seal from taking place.

5. Remove the paper backing from the foam pad on the faceplate of the pouch. Fit the faceplate over the stoma and gently press in place, being careful to avoid wrinkles. (Figs. 17-2 to 17-4).

Wrinkles prevent proper sealing and provide places where the drainage is in contact with the skin, thus promoting skin breakdown and irritation.

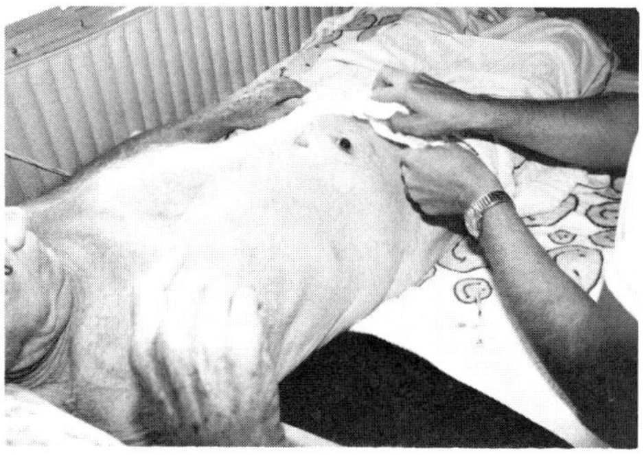

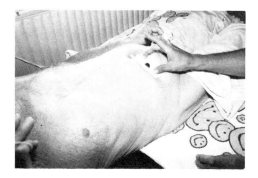

Figure 17.1
Cleansing and gently drying the periostomy area.

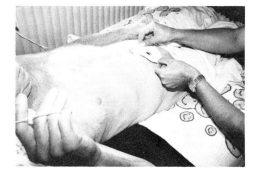

Figure 17.2
Applying the faceplate (shield), making sure the hole fits the ostomy.

Figure 17.3
Press gently to remove any wrinkles.

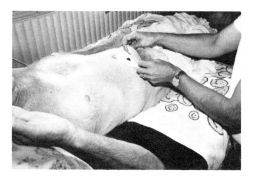

Figure 17.4
Apply the pouch.

ACTION   **RATIONALE/AMPLIFICATION**

Enema Type of Irrigation

1. Wash hands. Assemble and con-
    veniently arrange equipment (Fig.
    17-5).

The prescribed solution is warmed to
105°F. Adjust the amount of solution
to the needs of the individual client,
sometimes up to 1500 ml. Solution
that is too warm causes injury to the
mucous lining; solution that is too
cool causes cramping.

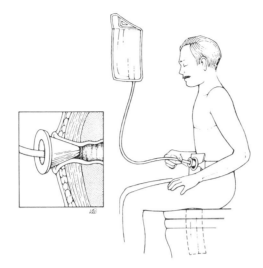

Figure 17.5

2. Hang solution at shoulder height
    to the client.

If a can is used, a stand can be
located conveniently near. If the solution is in a collapsible bag, it can be
suspended from a towel rack using a
bent coathanger, or a hook at the
proper height can be installed.

3. Fill the tubing with solution.
    Close the flow clamp tightly.
    Place a stoma guard below the
    flow clamp.

This prevents large amounts of air
from entering the intestine from the
tubing.

4. Have the client assume a sitting
    position on the commode. Re-
    move dressing and used pouch
    and dispose of them (if reusable,
    place in receptacle provided).

If the client cannot sit on the commode, a sitting position on a chair in
front of the commode, on a bedside
commode, or in front of a bedpan can
substitute.

5. Attach the irrigation appliance
    according to the manufacturer's
    directions.

The most commonly used irrigation
device consists of a plastic bag with
openings at both top and bottom. It is
attached around the client's waist by
means of a belt. A gasket on one side
fits around the stoma. The irrigating
tube is inserted into the stoma through
the upper bag opening. The lower
opening is hung into the commode for
drainage purposes.

6. Lubricate the end of the tubing
    with a water-soluble lubricant.

This reduces friction.

ACTION	RATIONALE/AMPLIFICATION
7. Insert the irrigating tubing through the stoma guard and into the stoma, 6 to 8 inches. Do not use force if resistance is encountered. If resistance is felt, pull the tube out slightly, release some fluid, and attempt to insert again. If resistance is still met, stop the procedure and notify the nurse.	Excessive force could result in perforation of the bowel.
8. Open the clamp and allow the solution to flow by gravity into the colon. The solution should remain in the colon for 5 to 15 minutes.	If cramping occurs, lower the pressure by lowering the solution container and advise the client to rest a short while.
9. Remove the tubing from the stoma. Clamp the top opening of the irrigating appliance.	The solution usually is evacuated in 30 minutes.
10. Clean the stoma and surrounding skin. Pat dry. Apply adhesive and the pouch (see Changing Pouch and Applying Dressing, above). Clean equipment and replace it.	Keeping the peristomal skin clean and dry prevents skin irritation and promotes a feeling of well-being.

Bulb Method of Irrigation

ACTION	RATIONALE/AMPLIFICATION
1. Wash hands and assemble equipment.	Use a 250-ml soft bulb syringe with the hard tip cut off and a number 24 French catheter attached. No more than 24 ounces of warm water is used.
2. Direct the client to sit on the commode and tuck the bag into the commode. Squeeze the bulb to insert the water.	Leave the bag in place for 15 minutes to drain.
3. Cover the stoma with a piece of gauze or other substance desired.	This method of irrigation stimulates fecal return rather than washing the feces out. Since no water is trapped in the colon, there is usually no spillage during the day (Fig. 17-6).

Dilating the Stoma

ACTION	RATIONALE/AMPLIFICATION
1. Don a glove or a finger cot.	Lubricate well with water-soluble lubricant.
2. Insert finger into stoma.	Insert gently and slowly to avoid pain and anxiety.

Related Care

ACTION	RATIONALE/AMPLIFICATION
1. To clean the pouch and belt, wash the irrigating bag, belt, and pouch in soapy water, soak in solution that is one part vinegar and one part water, rinse well, air dry, and dust with cornstarch.	Advise the client to obtain a second belt and pouch so one can be drying and airing while the other is being worn.

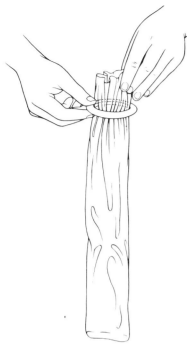

1. Insert one end of drainage sheath through the plastic ring.

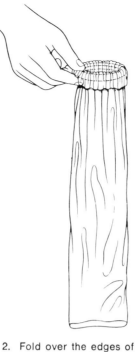

2. Fold over the edges of the sheath and roll around ring securely and evenly.

3. The ring with sheath is placed over the stoma, and the belt clips hooked onto the ring. This holds the appliance securely over the opening.

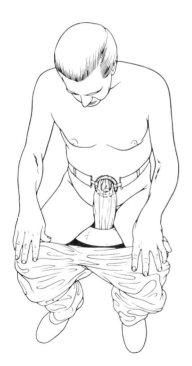

4. After cutting a small hole in the sheath above and to one side of the stoma, the sheath is tucked between the legs so that it leads directly into the toilet.

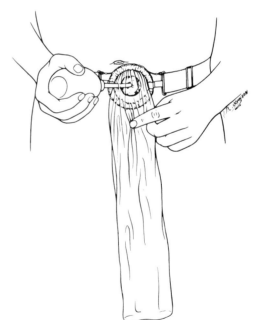

5. Moisten the tip of the syringe with a standard lubricating jelly. Insert the lubricated syringe tip through the hole of the drainage sheath and gently into the stoma about 7.5–12.5 cm. (3–5 inches).

Figure 17.6
Irrigating the colostomy using the bulb method. (Postel AH, Grier WRN, Localio SA: Training the Patient in the Bulb Syringe Method of Colostomy Irrigation. New York, New York University Medical Center)

ACTION	*RATIONALE/AMPLIFICATION*
Dietary Alterations	
1. *Colostomy:* avoid baked beans, onions, asparagus, vegetables in the cabbage family, eggs, fish, and alcohol.	Each of these foods causes increased fecal odor. Add new foods one at a time to determine their effect.
2. *Iliostomy:* avoid high-fiber foods and hard-to-digest foods such as celery, popcorn, corn on the cob, and coconut. Fluids may be a problem in the summer, since they are lost through the iliostomy as well as through other routes. Drinking Gatorade can assist in maintaining electrolyte balance. If discharge is too watery, restrict fibrous foods; if too dry, increase salt intake.	These alterations will reduce flatus and indigestion and will assist in maintaining electrolyte balance.
3. *Urinary diversions:* Monitor diet to avoid diarrhea or constipation.	Some recommend ingestion of cranberry juice on a daily basis to reduce odor.
Other Concerns	
1. *Sexual implications:* There are no sexual restrictions on a physiological basis. However, couples frequently have sexual difficulties related to body-image difficulties.	The client and partner may wish to explore alternative positions and methods of intercourse. If desired, counseling of both partners should be initiated by referral to a counselor or social worker. In addition, two publications effectively address the problem: *Sex, Pregnancy and the Female Ostomate* and *Sex and the Male Ostomate.* Both are available through the United Ostomy Association (call the local American Cancer Society for the address).
2. *Travel:* develop a travel kit containing all needed supplies for irrigation and dressing change.	These are available commercially or can be made personally. If traveling on a plane, hand-carry the kit to prevent loss. Keep one kit in the car for short trips or unexpected delays on short trips.
3. *Clothing:* wear comfortable clothing. Avoid tight clothing.	Modern appliances, deodorants, and accessories effectively conceal the presence of an ostomy.
4. *Sports:* Continue all sports except rough contact sports.	Swimming is allowed. Many swimming suits can be worn without notice.

ACTION	*RATIONALE/AMPLIFICATION*
5. *Skin care:* Karaya is available in powder form, rings, or disks. Place these directly on excoriated skin or use as a measure to prevent skin irritation around the stoma. For a covering over the stoma, a variety of items can be used, for example, facial tissue covered with petrolatum, plastic wrap, or disposable patches.	If the skin is wrinkled in the peristomal area, hypoallergenic skin shields (*i.e.,* Stomahesive, Hollihesive) can be used instead of Karaya washers. Both Stomahesive and Hollihesive adhere well to weeping skin and allow healing to take place. Always use hypoallergenic tape.
6. *Odor control:* liquids (Nilodor, Deodrops) and tablets (charcoal, chlorophyl, aspirin) can be inserted into the pouch after each emptying to prevent odors.	In the event of an emergency, underarm aerosol deodorants can be used to clear odors from a room. Since antibiotics cause strong odors that cling to the appliance, advise the client to use an old pouch while on antibiotics.

Age-Specific Modifications

Irrigation tubings, quantity of solution, and other equipment are adapted for children, as directed by the physician or ostomy therapist.

Education/ Communication

- Teach the client and family to
  Change the ostomy dressing. Focus on consistency of dressing change. Stress the importance of keeping drainage off the skin and prevention of skin irritation and breakdown. Advise them to notify the nurse if skin breakdown occurs.
  Irrigate the ostomy.* Regularity of irrigation will assist in establishing normal bowel evacuation. Discuss with the family the timing for irrigation that will fit into their usual lifestyle so another adjustment will not be necessary when the client resumes work, school, and other such activities.
  Make necessary dietary alterations. Some experimentation will be necessary to determine which foods cause gas and increased fecal odor. Advise the family to observe for any changes as each new food is added.
  Be concerned with clothing and grooming. Clothing and grooming should conform to the former lifestyle. Good grooming contributes to a feeling of well-being and should not be altered because of the ostomy.
  Become active in a local ostomy self-help group
  Assemble travel kits for long and short trips. Emergencies or unexpected delays may occur on these trips. If the equipment is available in the travel kit to care for the ostomy, embarrassment and inconvenience will be reduced.
  Return to former lifestyle. Social engagements, sports (except rough contact sports), and sexual activity should not have to be altered.

Referrals and Consultations

- Consult an ostomy therapist for assistance with complications.
- Refer to the local ostomy support group.
- If sexual problems or body-image problems persist, refer to a counsellor or social worker.

* If directed, for iliostomy or colostomy.

Evaluation of Health Promotion Activities

Quality Assurance/ Reassessment

- Observe peristomal skin and mucous membrane to determine that they are intact and healthy.
- Weigh client periodically to detect any weight changes.
- Determine quality of appetite.
- Evaluate client/family acceptance of body image alterations.
- Evaluate process of achieving regular bowel elimination.
- Determine if dietary alterations are adhered to.
- Observe if activities of usual lifestyle have been resumed within the existing limitations.

DOCUMENTATION

Charting for the Home Health Nurse
- Document the quality of peristomal skin.
- Note the abilities of client/family in relation to dressing change and irrigation. Also note client progress in developing regular bowel habits.
- Note progress in resuming former lifestyle.
- Describe indications of client attitude toward body-image changes and family attitudes.
- Document any indications of complications.

Records Kept by the Client/Family
Questions and concerns

Progress in establishing regular bowel habits (color, consistency, amount, and frequency of stools)

Presence of pain, drainage, bleeding, excessive flatus

Skin irritation or breakdown in the peristomal area

Health Teaching Checklist

Name of Care Provider _____

Relationship to Client _____ Telephone #_____

Taught by _____ Date _____

	EXPLAINED	DEMONSTRATED
Dressing change	_____	_____
Irrigation procedure	_____	_____
Assessment of skin integrity	_____	_____
Reporting of complications	_____	
Assembly of travel kit	_____	
Resumption of lifestyle	_____	

Product Availability

Informational literature is available from the local cancer society and The United Ostomy Association, Inc., Department N81, PO Box 4000, Princeton, NJ 90057.
     All other products are available through local medical equipment sales firms or pharmacies.

Selected References

American Cancer Society Publications: Sex and the Male Ostomate, and Sex and Pregnancy in the Female Ostomate

Mahoney J: What you should know about ostomies. Nursing '78 8(5):78–84, 1978

Wilpizeski M: Helping the ostomate return to normal life. Nursing '81 11(3):62–66, 1981

18 Peritoneal Dialysis

Background

Because of recent advances in techniques and the movement toward home health care, home peritoneal dialysis is available, as an alternative to hemodialysis, to a growing number of clients in the treatment of chronic renal failure. It is safer and less expensive than hemodialysis and does not require the extensive training period that is necessary to manage hemodialysis on an outpatient basis.

Soft, pliable, cuffed peritoneal catheters have reduced the risk of peritonitis, making long-term peritoneal dialysis possible. The Tenckhoff Silastic catheter in use today has two bonded cuffs; one cuff rests on the fascia covering the peritoneal membrane and the other in the subcutaneous tissue (Fig. 18-1). Tissue overgrowth prevents bacterial invasion along the catheter tunnel and provides an anchor for the catheter. The peritoneal catheter is placed surgically under local or general anesthesia. Optimal catheter position is in the left lower quadrant between the bowel loops and the anterior abdominal wall (Fig. 18-2).

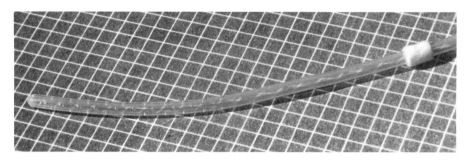

Figure 18.1
Tenckhoff cuffed peritoneal catheter. (Courtesy of Davol Inc., Cranston, Rhode Island)

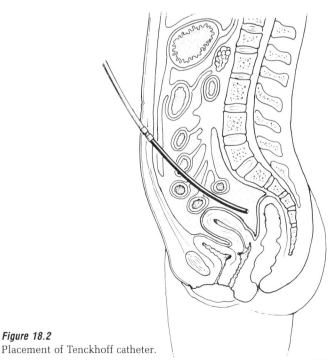

Figure 18.2
Placement of Tenckhoff catheter.

Candidates for Peritoneal Dialysis

Peritoneal dialysis may be performed by the client with or without assistance, an advantage over hemodialysis. If the peritoneal surface is intact, peritoneal dialysis is an option. Blood flow to the peritoneum must be adequate to remove excess metabolic products. The process is slower than hemodialysis and is therefore considered more physiologically normal. It may be appropriate for a client with cardiovascular problems or a pediatric client. It is also used for people who no longer have a vascular access or shunt site for hemodialysis.

Dialysate Composition

During dialysis, substances in the bloodstream and in the dialysate equilibrate across the peritoneum, which is a semipermeable membrane. Flow rate, temperature, pH, and osmolality of the dialysate alter the effectiveness of dialysis. To increase waste removal, the rate of exchange is increased rather than the amount of fluid infused with each cycle. Warming the dialysate to body temperature improves metabolic end-product clearance and minimizes loss of body heat. Generally, the pH of the dialysate does not affect clearance, but acid dialysate may cause pain on inflow.

Adding dextrose to the dialysate increases osmolality; an increase in solute clearance occurs because of the osmotic pull of the dextrose. Fluid removal can be accelerated by increasing the dextrose concentration. However, using dextrose concentrations greater than 4.25% can result in hypernatremia, rapid fluid loss, and hypovolemic shock. Because dextrose is absorbed by the body from the dialysate, blood glucose can increase. The diabetic client must be assessed for increased insulin coverage. Nondiabetics require insulin only if symptoms of hyperglycemia occur.

Dietary Modifications

Dietary restrictions for the person on peritoneal dialysis are much less rigid than those for persons on hemodialysis. Protein is lost across the peritoneal membrane and is further depleted if infection is present. Adequate protein intake becomes a problem, particularly if the person has an aversion to meat, as do many people with renal failure. It is seldom necessary to restrict dietary potassium; the dialysate is potassium-free, encouraging potassium loss into the dialysate. Dietary restriction of sodium and fluid depends on blood pressure and fluid weight gains.

Dialysis Modalities

MANUAL DIALYSIS

To accomplish dialysis manually, containers of dialysate are heated in water to body temperature and hung to allow gravity flow into the peritoneal cavity. The inflow of 2 liters of dialysate takes approximately 10 to 20 minutes. Dwell time for each exchange is determined by the person's needs and is generally about 10 to 25 minutes. The inflow bag is then placed below the level of the client's abdomen to facilitate outflow of the dialysate by gravity.

CONTINUOUS AMBULATORY PERITONEAL DIALYSIS

For continuous ambulatory peritoneal dialysis (CAPD), exchanges are controlled by gravity flow, using disposable solution bags and tubing. Upon completion of inflow, the bag and tubing are folded and secured to the client's torso in a pouch or pocket and used later for the outflow, which takes about 20 minutes. Dwell time is between 4 and 6 hours. Four exchanges are completed each day, with the last exchange of the day allowed to dwell overnight. CAPD allows the client freedom from a dialysis center and is easily managed in the home setting.

CONTINUOUS CYCLED PERITONEAL DIALYSIS

For continuous cycled peritoneal dialysis (CCPD), three to five exchanges are performed automatically at night using automated equipment (cycler) to regulate dialysate flow (Fig. 18-3). The abdomen is left full during the day. The cycler eliminates many of the problems associated with manual dialysis. The dialysate is automatically warmed. Several bags of dialysate can be hung at once, decreasing the number of entries into the system. Inflow and outflow of dialysate are managed automatically. An alarm system alerts the client to inflow or outflow difficulties.

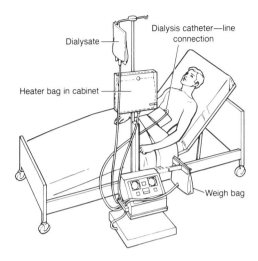

Figure 18.3
Automatic cycling equipment for peritoneal dialysis.

Assessment of Self-Care Potential

Client/Family Assessment

- Determine whether insurance counseling has been provided. Individuals requiring chronic dialysis are classified with other end-stage renal problems and are eligible for Part B Medicare funds for home dialysis. Determine whether hospitalization insurance will pay for treatment in the hospital prior to Medicare eligibility. Part B Medicare will pick up 80% of the cost after a 3-month waiting period. Check whether the 20% that is not covered will be reimbursed by private health insurance. If the client does not qualify for private insurance, investigate other funding sources (e.g., state kidney disease program, private kidney disease fund, or Medicaid). If the client is a veteran, determine eligibility for payment through the Veterans Administration.

- Determine the family's cultural background and budget. These factors can assist the dietitian in planning menus to include dietary modifications (e.g., sodium, potassium, or fluid restrictions and assurance of adequate protein intake).

- Determine what type of exchange system has been prescribed for the client (manual, CAPD, or CCPD). Assess whether the client and family are willing and able to assume management of dialysis at home. Determine the knowledge level of the family and client and the amount of intervention that will be required of the home health nurse.

- Assist the client to determine the vendor that best suits the client's needs.

Physical Assessment

- Assess the client for symptoms of infection (e.g., abdominal pain on inflow, cloudy dialysate return, low-grade fever, general malaise, and loss of appetite). Check for rebound tenderness, which indicates peritonitis.

- Assess the client for complications of peritoneal dialysis:
  Inflow pain resulting from intraperitoneal irritation, cold dialysate, acid dialysate, or stretching and irritation of the diaphragm (generally manifested as referred pain between the shoulder blades)
  Outflow failure due to a full colon, catheter obstruction, peritonitis, dislodged catheter, or absorption of initial small-volume exchanges
  Tunnel infections (involving the subcutaneous segment of the implanted catheter)

- Assess weight, blood pressure, vital signs, and temperature.

- Assess nutritional status. Check for signs of electrolyte imbalance or protein depletion.
- Assess for signs of fluid overload (e.g., increasing abdominal girth, respiratory distress, gallop rhythm on cardiac auscultation, pitting edema).
- Evaluate catheter placement. Pressure in the bladder area indicates that the catheter should be pulled out slightly. Epigastric pressure indicates that the catheter is entangled in the omentum. Rectal pressure is normal if the catheter is newly inserted, but the catheter may need to be withdrawn slightly if the pressure continues.

Environmental Assessment

- Determine whether the physical set-up at home is suitable for dialysis. Space will be required for supplies and equipment. Since the system drains by gravity, check that the bed or chair used during dialysis is positioned below the heater cabinet and above the weigh arm (if the client uses a cycler). Determine whether blocks will be needed to raise the client's bed, or whether a hospital bed will be required. Effluent can be discarded into the sewage system.
- Determine whether routine sanitary practices are followed in the home. Aseptic technique is mandatory to prevent local and systemic infections.

Planning Strategies

Potential Nursing Diagnoses

Fluid volume, alteration in: excess due to renal failure

Urinary elimination, alteration due to renal failure

Infection, potential for: due to indwelling peritoneal catheter

Knowledge deficit related to peritoneal dialysis and dietary management

Home maintenance management, impaired due to changes in elimination

Nutrition, alteration in: less than or more than body requirements

Bowel elimination, alteration in: constipation interrupting peritoneal dialysis

Expected Outcomes

Elimination of excess fluid using the peritoneum

Elimination of metabolic wastes using the peritoneum

Prevention of infection

Increased knowledge of home peritoneal dialysis and dietary management

Provision of adequate home care to promote optimal health

Maintenance of an adequate nutrition level

Promotion of normal bowel patterns

Health Promotion Goals

- The client and family will
  Perform peritoneal dialysis in the home setting safely
  Observe dietary modifications necessary for the person with chronic nephritis on a peritoneal dialysis program

Equipment*

Sterile gloves (optional)

Tape

Sterile 4 × 4s

Perforated sterile drape

Iodophor swab sticks

* Peritoneal catheter tray contains all necessary dressing equipment. For CAPD, add belt and pouch for attachment to abdomen. For CCPD, add automatic dialysate cycler.

Alcohol swab sticks (or peroxide)

Sterile cups or basins, 2 (if swab sticks are not prepackaged)

Sterile inlet cap

Dialysate tubing

Dialysate solution (at room temperature)

Outflow bag or bottle (as indicated by dialysis mode)

Interventions/Health Promotion

ACTION

Manual Dialysis

1. Warm the dialysate containers to room temperature. Remove the dialysis tubing from the protective package. Connect 2 flasks of dialysate to the tubing connectors and prime the tubing.

2. Wash hands thoroughly. Open sterile tray (if used) and use the wrapper as a sterile field. Pour solutions into the basins. If a sterile tray is not used, open the supplies using the individual wrappers as a sterile surface. Use a clean, dry nightstand or small table for opening supplies.

3. Remove the tape and soiled 4 × 4s, taking care not to touch the entry site of the catheter. Soak the catheter tip with 4 × 4s saturated in iodophor solution or thoroughly clean the tip with an iodophor swab.

4. Use a fresh iodophor swab or 4 × 4 to clean the insertion site. Clean around the catheter first, and move away from the catheter in increasing concentric circles. Discard the swab or 4 × 4 and repeat the cleaning procedure. Handle the catheter as little as possible, and always away from the entry site.

RATIONALE/AMPLIFICATION

If a warm-water bath is used, dry the containers before hanging to prevent water drops from contaminating the catheter. Warming dialysate will prevent abdominal discomfort from cold dialysate and will prevent lowering core body temperature. If additives are ordered to be added to the dialysate (e.g., heparin to prevent clotting, potassium chloride, antibiotics, or lidocaine for control of local discomfort), use sterile technique to add them to the dialysate before spiking the containers.

If sterile gloves are used, don them after removing the soiled dressings.

These techniques prevent contamination of the catheter entry site.

ACTION	*RATIONALE/AMPLIFICATION*
5. Disinfect the catheter with an iodophor swab or 4 × 4, moving from the insertion site toward the catheter tip. Discard the 4 × 4 and repeat. Insert the catheter tip through the perforation of the sterile drape.	The sterile drape will serve as a sterile field while the catheter is connected to the dialysis tubing.
6. Remove the catheter cap and secure the catheter to the primed dialysis tubing. Redress the catheter–client dialysis line connection with a dry, sterile 4 × 4 and tape.	Dry dressings allow the client to check for leaks. Wet dressings are also more conducive to bacterial growth.
7. Tear away and discard the sterile drape. Wipe the skin again with iodophor solution and apply a dry, sterile, occlusive dressing.	Use alcohol or peroxide to clean the skin if a sensitivity develops to iodophor. Coil the catheter beneath the dressing so that no part of the catheter is exposed.
8. Release the clamp and begin the infusion of dialysate.	Inflow is controlled by gravity.
9. On completion of inflow, clamp the tubing.	A period of approximately 10 to 20 minutes is allowed for inflow. Record vital signs every 15 minutes during the first dialysis and every hour thereafter if stable. The first exchange may be drained immediately to determine catheter patency.
10. Allow for the prescribed dwell time and then begin the outflow phase.	The dwell time is determined by the physician depending on the individual client needs.
11. Position the container below the level of the abdomen and allow the dialysate to return by gravity flow (Fig. 18-4).	If the return drainage slows down considerably, notify the physician unless the amount returned is greater than or equal to the amount instilled. Changing the client's position or raising the head of the bed or chair will help the return flow if the catheter is kinked or lodged against the peritoneum. Check for cloudy outflow, which can indicate infection. Blood-stained outflow may occur after the catheter has been inserted but should cease after a few exchanges. Brownish outflow can indicate bowel perforation. Amber outflow can indicate bladder perforation.

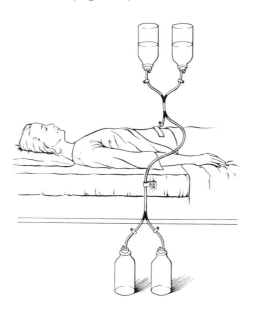

Figure 18.4
Manual peritoneal dialysis. After solution flows into patient, it remains *in situ* for length of time ordered by physician. Then clamps on lower bottles are opened and solution is drained.

ACTION	*RATIONALE/AMPLIFICATION*
12. On completion of the outflow, clamp the tubing. Record the amount infused and the volume returned on a flow sheet.	Notify the physician if the volume returned is 500 ml greater than the amount infused. Changes may be made in the infusion rate to prevent fluid imbalance.
13. If additional exchanges are not planned, prepare to disconnect the dialysis tubing. Remove the dressing and repeat the cleaning procedures for the catheter connection and the skin, using iodophor. Place a sterile drape under the catheter.	
14. Disconnect the dialysis line from the catheter and apply a sterile sealing cap to the end of the catheter. Discard the drape. Clean the skin with iodophor. Redress the site with a dry, sterile, occlusive dressing.	A transparent dressing can be used to dress the site. This allows inspection without having to remove the dressing. Site care for the dialysis catheter is similar for a right atrial catheter. (See Technique 24, Right Atrial Catheter, for illustrations.)

Continuous Ambulatory Peritoneal Dialysis

1. Check that the dialysate is at room temperature.	If warming is required because of client preference, use heating pads, place the tubing in a warm-water bath during inflow, or warm in a microwave oven. *Check the temperature carefully if using a microwave oven.*
2. Wash hands thoroughly. Remove the empty solution bag from the pouch that secures it to the body.	The dialysate remains in the peritoneal cavity for 4 to 6 hours. During this time, the bag used for inflow is rolled up and secured to the abdomen.
3. Position the client comfortably. Place the empty container below the level of the client's abdomen. Unclamp the tubing and begin the outflow phase. On completion of outflow clamp the tubing.	Allow approximately 15 to 20 minutes for outflow. Check vital signs at the end of 15 minutes.
4. Inspect the outflow for cloudiness or discoloration. Measure and record the amount returned.	Cloudiness or discoloration may indicate infection or perforation of abdominal organs. Compare the amount of outflow with the amount infused.
5. Remove the tubing from the outflow bag and spike a new dialysate bag. Hang the new solution bag and open the clamp to begin inflow.	Take care not to contaminate the port while connecting the tubing. Use a conveniently placed hook in the bedroom or bathroom to suspend the dialysate.

ACTION	**RATIONALE/AMPLIFICATION**
6. When the inflow is completed (10 to 20 minutes) clamp the tubing.	Leave a small amount of fluid in the bag. This will prevent air from entering the system and will facilitate drainage.
7. Fold the empty bag so that the entry port is folded to the inside. Secure the bag to the abdomen. Record the amount of dialysate infused.	
8. Change the inflow tubing every 24 hours. Change the catheter dressing at the same time, unless it becomes soiled earlier.	Replacing the tubing with fresh, sterile tubing is an infection-control precaution.

Continuous Cycled Peritoneal Dialysis

ACTION	**RATIONALE/AMPLIFICATION**
1. Spike the dialysate containers with the tubing spikes and prime the tubing. Clamp the tubing. Thread the tubing through the cycler.	Follow specific instructions provided in the manufacturer's handbook.
2. Connect the primed tubing to the catheter using the technique outlined under Manual Dialysis, above. Connect the remaining tubing to the weigh bag near the base of the machine.	
3. Set the time controls for inflow, dwell, and outflow times.	Clamps open automatically according to preset times to allow for the exchange.
4. Activate the cycler to begin the exchange.	An alarm system will be activated to alert the operator to inflow or outflow problems. Often a position change is all that is necessary to activate the alarm, such as if the client has rolled onto the catheter during sleep.
5. Allow the final exchange to dwell during the day. Remove the bag and tubing from the cycler and secure to the abdomen as for CAPD.	
6. Record the amount of dialysate used and returned and the number of exchanges.	
7. At the end of the day, thread the tubing through the cycler and allow for outflow. Secure the new solution bags and initiate the next exchange.	

Related Care

ACTION	**RATIONALE/AMPLIFICATION**
1. Administer antibiotics as ordered for peritoneal infection.	Antibiotics are usually administered daily during dialysis for 10 days. Oral antibiotics may also be ordered.

ACTION	*RATIONALE/AMPLIFICATION*
2. If the dressing remains dry and intact between exchanges, do not disturb. Redress the site if the dressing becomes soiled or wet.	

Education/ Communication

- Teach the client and family to

  Practice initiation and discontinuation of dialysis on a model of the catheter before performing the technique on their own catheter with supervision

  Use sterile technique to add heparin or other medications to the dialysis containers

  Set up the tubing and equipment for dialysis. Maintain and troubleshoot an automatic cycler if used. To prevent problems with the heater cabinet, always keep the dialysate stored at room temperature.

  Recognize impending problems that set off automatic alarms on the automatic cycler, such as kinking of the catheter during sleep, inadequate amount of drainage during the outflow time, or the catheter lodging against the peritoneum. Change position to alleviate these problems.

  Use strict aseptic technique during dialysis to prevent infection. Repeated peritoneal infections may result in the need for catheter replacement or loss of the peritoneum as an access route.

  Check each new container of dialysate for the correct concentration, leaks, or particles in the solution that could indicate contamination

  Use stool softeners or mild laxatives if necessary to prevent colonic distention that interferes with effective dialysis

Referrals and Consultations

- Refer the client to the physician if a peritoneal infection occurs or if the catheter requires repositioning.
- Refer the client and the family member who prepares the food to the dietitian for assistance in menu preparation and instruction on dietary restrictions.
- Refer the client for periodic follow-up by the physician.
- Ensure that the client knows to notify the home health nurse of any problems during dialysis or of any changes in urine output.

Evaluation of Health Promotion Activities

Quality Assurance/ Reassessment

- Culture the peritoneal fluid if infection is suspected and monthly.
- Check weight and blood pressure monthly.
- Check the catheter for patency monthly.

DOCUMENTATION

Charting for the Home Health Nurse
- Determine whether there is acceptance of peritoneal dialysis by the client and family.

Records Kept by the Client/Family

Vital signs, weight, and temperature before and after each dialysis treatment

Percent of the dialysate solution and the number of containers used

Amount of outflow

Number of exchanges required

Record of prescribed medications added to dialysate or taken orally

Record of any problems or signs of infection

Urine output

Health Teaching Checklist

Name of Care Provider _____

Relationship to Client _____ Telephone # _____

Taught by _____ Date _____

	EXPLAINED	DEMONSTRATED
Rationale and principles for dialysis	_____	
Dialysis procedure	_____	_____
Equipment maintenance	_____	_____
Signs and symptoms of complications	_____	
24-hour emergency number	_____	
Infection-control precautions	_____	_____
Dietary modifications	_____	
Importance of bowel training program	_____	
Medical follow-up	_____	
Insurance counseling	_____	

Product Availability

Dialysis supplies are available at medical-supply companies or home health agencies listed in the yellow pages of the telephone book. Dressings and tape are also available at drug stores.

The cycler is manufactured by Travenol Laboratories or Belmed, Inc. Check the medical-supply company for rental options.

Selected References

County CM, Collins AJ: Dialytic therapy in the management of chronic renal failure. Med Clin North Am 68(2):399–421, 1984

Denniston DJ, Burns KT: Home peritoneal dialysis. Am J Nurs 80(11):2022–2026, 1980

Nursing Photobook Series. Implementing Urologic Procedures, pp 134–143. Horsham, PA, Intermed Communications, 1981

19   Suprapubic Catheter

Background

A suprapubic catheter is inserted into the bladder through a permanent opening that has been surgically created to provide an alternate path for urine from the bladder. A retention catheter is inserted into the opening, which is usually located midway between the pubic bone and the umbilicus (Fig. 19-1). The skin from the abdomen is sutured to the bladder itself. Therefore, reassurance may be given that the catheter will not be inserted into the "wrong" place and harm done to the client.

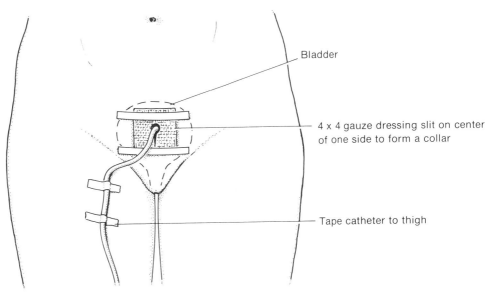

Figure 19.1
Illustration of placement of suprapubic catheter.

Assessment of Self-Care Potential

Client/Family Assessment

- Assess the willingness of the family members to assist in the procedure.
- Assess the fine motor movement of the family assistant to determine the ability to perform the catheterization procedure.
- Determine if the family will require outside assistance to care for the catheter successfully.
- Assess the feelings of the client and family toward the catheter.

Physical Assessment

- Assess the healing stage of the surgical site. Until healing has taken place, provide nursing assistance for catheter care. After healing has occurred, teach the family to care for the catheter.
- Assess for bleeding, drainage, or obstruction at the insertion site.
- Assess the condition of the skin surrounding the stoma for irritation, drainage, and/or bleeding.
- Assess the appearance of the urine as a baseline for future comparisons.
- Collect a urine specimen for laboratory analysis.

Environmental Assessment

- Assess the bed and main chairs/wheelchair used by the client to determine a method for hanging the urinary drainage bag. The bag must be below the level of the bladder at all times.
- Assess the bathroom area or other area with running water where equipment cleaning and drying may take place. The area should be clean and well lighted and have capability of hanging the unused bag to dry.

Planning Strategies

Potential Nursing Diagnoses

Infection, potential for

Urinary elimination pattern, altered

Skin integrity, potential breakdown

Sexual dysfunction, potential

Expected Outcomes

Prevention of urinary tract infection

Restoration of adequate urinary function by artificial means

Prevention of skin breakdown at catheter insertion site

Acceptance of client's altered body image and maintenance of desired level of sexual activity

Health Promotion Goals

- The client and family will
  Clean and redress the catheter insertion site daily and change the catheter monthly or as needed
  Irrigate the catheter daily
  Collect periodic urine samples for analysis
  Properly cleanse used equipment
  Perform effective odor control measures
  Maintain adequate fluid intake
  Verbalize feelings related to altered body image
  Adapt to necessary alterations of daily living
  Achieve independence of functioning related to urinary diversion
  Verbalize when to contact nurse or physician for assistance

Equipment

For daily cleaning
  Mild bacteriostatic soap
  Water for rinsing
  Nonabsorbent ointment (e.g., Diaperene)
  Scissors (clean)
  Sterile 4 × 4 dressing
  Hypoallergenic tape
  Paper bag (for discarded dressing)

For irrigation
  Sterile disposable irrigation tray with 30-ml or 50-ml irrigation syringe
  or
  Sterilized stainless-steel basin with sterile 30-ml or 50-ml irrigation syringe
  Irrigating solution (as recommended by physician)
  Catheter clamp

For catheter change
    Tray to include
        Sterile gloves
        Sterile drapes
        Specimen container
        Water-soluble lubricant
        Antiseptic solution
        Cotton balls
        Syringe with 12 ml of normal saline
    Foley catheter (silicon- or Teflon-lined)
    Collection bag and tubing for nighttime use
    Collection bag for leg attachment for ambulatory use (Fig. 19-2)

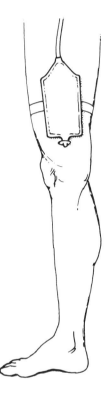

Figure 19.2
A leg-attached urine-collection device for use
when the client has a suprapubic catheter or an
indwelling catheter.

    Sterile 4 × 4 dressing
    Nonabsorbent ointment
    Bacteriostatic soap
    Protective pad or towel
    Paper bag (for discarded dressing and catheter)

EQUIPMENT MAINTENANCE   Water and distilled vinegar solution (1½ cups of vinegar to 2 quarts of water)
Commercial appliance cleaner

Interventions/Health Promotion

ACTION

RATIONALE/AMPLIFICATION

Irrigation

1. Wash hands carefully.

   Handwashing has been shown to prevent cross-contamination.

2. Assemble Equipment.

   This will prevent needless interruption of the procedure.

3. Withdraw required amount of irrigating solution into the sterile syringe.

4. Disconnect catheter from drainage tubing or leg-attached urinary collection device. Protect tubing opening with a sterile 4 × 4 pad or the cap provided.

   Covering the tubing prevents the entry of microorganisms into the collection device.

5. Connect syringe to the tubing and allow solution to flow in by gravity (Fig. 19-3).

   Irrigation is performed to ensure maintenance of patency of the catheter.

6. Clamp catheter if solution is to remain in the bladder for a period of time.

   The length of time that the irrigating solution is to remain in the bladder (if any) is usually specified by the physician.

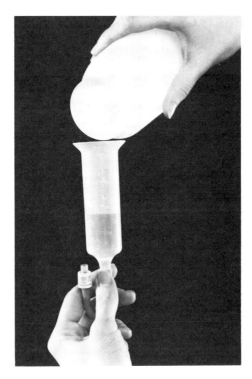

Figure 19.3
Irrigating the catheter, allowing fluid to flow into the bladder by gravity.

ACTION	*RATIONALE/AMPLIFICATION*
7. Reconnect the catheter to the tubing. At the end of the specified time, unclamp the catheter.	If a time is required for the solution to remain in the bladder, set an alarm to prevent forgetting to unclamp the catheter.
8. Allow the irrigating solution to drain by gravity.	If force is necessary to get a return of the solution, the nurse should be notified for assistance.
9. Repeat the irrigation daily or as ordered.	

Cleaning and Dressing the Insertion Site

1. Remove and discard soiled dressing into paper bag provided.	Proper disposal of soiled items prevents contamination.
2. Wash hands and assemble needed equipment.	Handwashing is an effective measure to prevent cross-contamination.
3. Clean the area around the catheter with a mild bacteriostatic soap and 4 × 4's or a sterilized cloth.	Mechanical scrubbing with an effective soap removes potentially infective organisms normally found on the skin.
4. Rinse with clean water.	Soap may be irritating to the skin if left in contact with the skin for a prolonged period of time.
5. Inspect the skin for irritation, purulent drainage, bleeding, or urinary leakage.	If any of these are present, advise the nurse and collect a urine specimen.
6. Apply nonabsorbent ointment around the stoma.	The nonabsorbent quality of the ointment keeps moisture away from the skin and helps to prevent tissue breakdown.
7. Reapply sterile 4 × 4, cut to center on one side to fit around the catheter like a collar.	This serves as a barrier to entry of microorganisms through the stoma and absorbs moisture.
8. Secure the 4 × 4 with hypoallergenic tape.	The tissue is already compromised due to moisture and frequent dressing changes. Allergic reaction to the tape may cause additional tissue breakdown and discomfort.
9. Repeat the procedure daily.	

Catheter Change

1. Place the client in a reclining or semireclining position on a protective pad or towel.	A pad or towel protects the bed linen or the surface of the reclining chair.
2. Make sure adequate lighting is present. Obtain a lamp if necessary.	Adequate lighting is necessary to illuminate the field of work to ensure proper placement of the catheter without contamination.
3. Provide for privacy.	Privacy promotes a feeling of respect for the client's dignity.
4. Maintain sterility throughout the procedure.	The bladder is very susceptible to infection, especially with an artificial opening so close to the surface.

ACTION	*RATIONALE/AMPLIFICATION*
5. Deflate the balloon by inserting a needle into the lumen at the end of the catheter. Remove the 10 ml of normal saline or sterile water. Remove the catheter and discard into the paper bag.	The inflated balloon holds the catheter in the bladder. When the balloon is deflated, the catheter slips out of the bladder easily.
6. Wash hands carefully. Place a nightstand or small table nearby for equipment.	Keeping the environment as clean as possible reduces the possibility of cross-contamination.
7. Open sterile Foley catheter tray without touching the inside of the wrapper.	The inside of the wrapper is sterile and will become the sterile field.
8. If the Foley catheter or other sterile equipment is packaged separately, open the packages, observing sterility, and drop the contents onto the sterile field.	All equipment must be kept sterile during the procedure.
9. Don sterile gloves. Open lubricant package and squeeze lubricant onto sterile field.	
10. Pour antiseptic or provided solution onto cotton balls.	
11. Cleanse stoma and surrounding area with cotton balls, using left hand (or nondominant hand). Do not allow this contaminated hand to touch the stoma or the catheter.	For left-handed persons, the opposite applies. This glove is now considered unsterile because it has touched the skin.
12. With the right hand (uncontaminated hand), grasp the catheter about 4 inches from the tip and dip the tip into the sterile lubricant.	Use of sterile lubricant reduces friction and facilitates insertion of the catheter.
13. Insert the catheter into the stoma until resistance is felt.	Observe for urine flow from the catheter.
14. Inflate the bulb of the catheter with normal saline (8 ml–10 ml).	The inflated bulb prevents the catheter from being removed from the bladder.
15. Collect a urine specimen (if desired).	Allow a few milliliters of urine to flow from the catheter into the sterile container.
16. Connect the catheter to the drainage apparatus. Check the collection bag to ensure that the drainage port is closed and there are no leaks.	A closed system is required to ensure that bacterial contamination is prevented.
17. Dress the stoma and catheter.	

ACTION	RATIONALE/AMPLIFICATION
Related Care	
1. Equip the client's bed with a hook on which to hang the urinary collection bag while the client is lying down.	Fashion a hook using a wire coat-hanger, or install a hook. Position the hanger so that the position of the receptacle is lower than the tubing and the bladder. Ensure that movement in bed is not restricted by tension on the catheter.
2. Wash bags and tubing not in use with cleansing solution or water and distilled vinegar solution.	These measures assist with odor control and in reducing the number of microorganisms in the system. The vinegar solution tends to make the rubber equipment brittle and discolors the plastic. These do not occur with Kay-Lux or other similar commercially available cleaning solutions.
3. Empty the drainage receptacle every 2 to 8 hours as needed.	Measure volume of urine using a graduated measure. Report to home health nurse an output of less than 720 ml for 24 hours.
4. Maintain fluid intake as recommended by the physician.	Adequate fluid intake reduces stone formation potential and promotes odor control.
5. Change to a different catheter composition if irritation of the stoma indicates a possible allergy to the catheter.	Silicon- or Teflon-lined catheters are expensive but last much longer than the simple rubber ones. Unless allergy dictates a change, select either the silicon or Teflon.

**Education/
Communication**

- Teach the client and family to
  Observe for changes in the character or odor of the urine (e.g., cloudiness, mucous threads, blood)
  Observe for patency of the system
  Position the collection device below the level of the tubing and the bladder
  Irrigate the catheter
  Redress the insertion site
  Change the catheter if a family member is capable and willing to do so
  Maintain the equipment correctly
  Make dietary alterations as needed, such as ensuring adequate fluid intake and drinking cranberry juice
  Measure intake and output and report urine volume reduction below 750 ml/ 24 hours
  Maintain sexual practices
  Continue previous lifestyle practices
  Verbalize feelings related to alterations in body image, sexual adjustments, and lifestyle alterations

Evaluation of Health Promotion Activities

Quality Assurance/ Reassessment

- Obtain urine specimen for urinalysis or culture if
  Changes occur in the character of the urine
  The client reports bladder pain or spasm
  Obstruction of the catheter occurs
- Periodically inspect the stoma and skin for irritation, drainage, and bleeding.
- Allow time and privacy to give the client and family the opportunity to verbalize feelings related to the suprapubic catheter and altered body image.

DOCUMENTATION

Charting for the Home Health Nurse
- Document progress of the client/family in assuming responsibility for the procedures.
- Note psychological responses related to the suprapubic catheter.
- Document results of urinalysis, condition of skin, and quantity of urine.

Records Kept by the Client/Family
General intake and output

Questions and concerns

Difficulties with any of the procedures

Health Teaching Checklist

Name of Care Provider _____

Relationship to Client _____ Telephone #_____

Taught by _____ Date _____

	EXPLAINED	DEMONSTRATED
Dressing of insertion site	_____	_____
Catheter irrigation	_____	_____
Changing of catheter	_____	_____
Dietary alterations	_____	
Monitoring intake and output	_____	
Maintaining equipment	_____	_____
Measures for odor control	_____	
Positioning of drainage receptacle	_____	_____

Product Availability

Catheterization equipment is available through any medical-supply agency. Commercially available cleaning solution is available from a hospital-supply agency. One example is Kay-Lux Appliance Cleaner, Kay's Health Care Center, 1-800-421-6455, South Gate, CA 90280.

Selected Reference

Brunner L, Suddarth D: Lippincott Manual of Nursing Practice, 4th ed, pp 470–472. Philadelphia, JB Lippincott, 1986

Food/Fluid

20   Breast-Feeding

Background

Breast-feeding is the nourishing of the infant from the mother's lactating breasts. It not only provides a natural form of nourishment for the infant, but also facilitates involution of the mother's uterus. Breast-feeding is considered a means of fostering the mother–child relationship. The precursor to breast milk production, *colostrum*, is a thin, yellowish fluid that fills the alveoli, ducts, and ampullae of the breasts. It is present immediately after birth and is replaced by milk several days later. Lactogenesis, or the formation of milk, is promoted by the infant's sucking and emptying the breasts of milk. With complete emptying of the breasts, the milk flows more freely and copiously in subsequent feedings. Fullness is produced in response to the infant's needs and is relieved by the infant's feeding.

Assessment of Self-Care Potential

Client/Family Assessment

- Assess the feelings of the family regarding breast-feeding. Note any signs of embarrassment about breast-feeding. Determine whether or not there is a tradition of breast-feeding in the family.
- Assess the emotional feelings of the client, since these may have a decided effect on lactation. Assess the motives for breast-feeding and reinforce the positive aspects of this feeding method.

Physical Assessment

- Assess the condition of the client's nipples to make sure that the infant is able to grasp the nipple and surrounding tissue in the mouth satisfactorily for successful sucking.
- Assess the client for engorgement of the breasts. Engorgement refers to excessive fullness of the breasts caused by buildup of milk, resulting in discomfort and possibly pain. The skin may appear shiny and the breasts may feel hard to the touch. Venous distention may be present, and the mother may relate that she feels throbbing pain in her breasts.
- Assess the adequacy of the breast-feeding mother to meet the infant's nutritional needs. Assess her knowledge of breast-feeding and her understanding of infection control and care of the breasts.

Environmental Assessment

- Assess whether a comfortable chair is available in which the mother may breast-feed the child. Determine if there is a small stool on which the mother may place her feet for comfort.
- Assess the sleeping arrangements in the home with the new baby. The cries of the infant may stimulate milk secretion. If the baby sleeps in the same room with the parents, intermittent crying during the night, which is common with newborns, may cause discomfort for the mother, who may experience a "let-down" of the milk each time the infant cries.

Planning Strategies

Potential Nursing Diagnoses

Knowledge deficit regarding breast-feeding technique

Anxiety

Alteration in nutrition, less than body requirements

Alteration in comfort, pain (acute) due to breast engorgement

Expected Outcomes

Understanding and proficiency in breast-feeding technique

Acquisition of self-confidence by the mother in her new role

Adequate nutrition of the infant as evidenced by growth and weight gains consistent with those expected of healthy infants

Prevention of breast infection and discomfort

Health Promotion Goals

- The client and family will
  Learn to meet the nutritional needs of the infant while maintaining a family schedule that is compatible with group needs
  Accept the infant as an integral part of their family
  Understand the needs of the nursing mother regarding nutrition, rest, and exercise
  Learn to recognize the signs of breast engorgement and gain an understanding of how to prevent or resolve it

Equipment

Soft cloth and warm water

Pillow

Comfortable chair and footstool

Nursing bra and nursing pads

Breast pump

Interventions/Health Promotion

ACTION	*RATIONALE/AMPLIFICATION*
1. For breast-feeding in the home environment, focus on the comfort and relaxation of the mother. If she is confident about breast-feeding, it will usually be a satisfactory experience.	Breast-feeding is related closely to the mother's emotions. If the mother believes she will fail, the chances are good that she will. However, with a little information and moral support, her self-confidence can be bolstered to the point that she will succeed in her breast-feeding efforts. The keys seem to be a positive attitude and a sincere desire to breast-feed her baby.
2. Show the mother how to assume a position of comfort for her and safety for the baby. The infant's body may be supported with a pillow. The infant's mouth should be at the level of the breast so that the entire nipple and areola can be taken into the mouth. The infant's trunk should be lower than the head. Assist the mother to position the infant with its abdomen against her abdomen (Fig. 20-1). The feet of the mother should be supported if she is sitting in a chair.	Proper support of the infant is important so that falls are prevented. The sucking action of the infant may be erratic and weak at first. The mother will need encouragement so that she does not become discouraged during these initial efforts. If her arms and feet are supported, she will be able to focus her attention on nursing the infant without worry about her own fatigue or discomfort. If the infant is in a position to reach the nipple easily, nursing may be done at the infant's own pace.

ACTION   **RATIONALE/AMPLIFICATION**

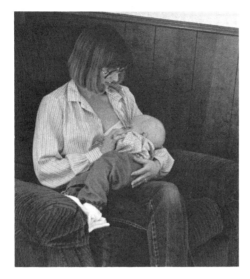

Figure 20.1

3. Caution the mother that initial breast-feeding efforts may cause some soreness of the nipples. The first breast-feeding periods should be about 3 to 5 minutes on each breast. This will increase gradually to 15 to 20 minutes. Initially, the infant should be allowed to nurse at both breasts during each feeding. Later the mother may choose to alternate breasts for each feeding. Explain and demonstrate, if necessary, how to break the infant's suction during feedings so that trauma to the nipple is avoided. Depress the areola near the infant's mouth until the suction is broken. The nipple may then be gently pulled from the infant's mouth.

The soreness from initial feedings will decrease as the nipples become toughened by subsequent nursing periods. If the infant is nursed at both breasts initially, soreness in one or both breasts may be prevented or reduced. The infant's mouth forms a vacuum seal over the nipple. Pulling the nipple out without breaking the seal may stretch the breast tissue and cause trauma to the nipple.

4. If the nipples become sore or if cracking and fissures of the nipple tissue occur, nursing may have to be discontinued for a short time until healing has taken place. The affected breast can usually be pumped with less discomfort than is involved in nursing. The infant may be allowed to nurse at the unaffected breast. However, care must be taken that the unaffected breast does not also become sore. Reassure the mother that the nipple will heal soon and normal nursing can be resumed.

Cracked and fissured nipples may become infected if not allowed to heal. The sucking action of the infant may irritate the sore nipple. Pumping the breast is considered less traumatic than nursing. The other breast must also be emptied to relieve engorgement since it fills simultaneously with the breast being pumped.

ACTION	*RATIONALE/AMPLIFICATION*
Related Care	
1. For flattened nipples or smooth nipples, advise the mother to compress the areola around the nipple gently with her thumb and forefinger or to massage the nipple lightly to make it stand up so the baby can grasp it. Brushing the finger or nipple against the infant's cheek is usually sufficient to stimulate the infant's rooting reflex, which causes the infant to turn toward the stimulus with mouth open.	To nurse successfully, the infant must be able to grasp not only the nipple but the surrounding breast tissue during nursing. The infant's rooting and grasping reflexes are usually sufficient to cause the nipple to project satisfactorily so that it may be secured in the infant's mouth for nursing.
2. Manual expression of milk from the breasts may be accomplished by grasping the breast tissue with the thumb on the upper portion of the breast and the forefinger on the lower portion. The thumb and forefinger are then used to compress the breast tissue gently but firmly. The thumb and forefinger are brought toward each other behind the areola, allowing the milk to flow out of the nipple. The hand does not touch the nipple or the milk during the process.	Manual expression of milk may be used to relieve tension on the engorged breast so the infant may grasp the nipple. The milk may also be expressed into a cup or bottle for later feeding. If the milk will be kept for longer than a few hours, it may be expressed into a plastic bag that can be sealed and frozen for later use. The hand does not touch the nipple or milk during manual expression, thus avoiding contamination. Manual and electrical breast pumps may be used. If the milk will be fed to the infant, it should be covered and stored in the refrigerator or freezer for later use. Breast pumps must be cleaned thoroughly after each use to prevent growth of microorganisms that might contaminate the milk.
3. If the breasts become engorged and the infant is unable to grasp the nipple, advise the mother to apply warm towels to the breast for 20 minutes before feeding time. Priming the breasts with a breast pump may also stimulate milk flow and allow the infant to grasp the nipple.	Warmth may relax the tension on the nipple enough for the infant to grasp it. If the areola is still too hard for the infant to grasp successfully, manually expressing a small amount of milk may relieve the congestion in the immediate nipple area and allow the infant to grasp the nipple and nurse successfully.

Education/ Communication

• Teach the client to
   Care for her breasts. Stress the importance of wearing a well-fitting support bra. These are available in all sizes and have a releasable cup that may be lowered for nursing. Nursing pads may be placed in the cup of the bra so that leaking milk will be absorbed without leaking onto clothing. These pads are available in disposable forms or may be made out of several layers of soft cloth sewn together. Emphasize the importance of changing the pads often, especially if leaking is profuse. The warm, moist environment is conducive to the proliferation of microorganisms. The nondisposable pads should be laundered between uses in hot, sudsy water and rinsed well.

Successfully nurse her infant. Stress the importance of careful handwashing before caring for the breasts or feeding the infant. The breast area should be wiped with a warm, damp washcloth prior to feeding the infant. Explain that the infant may suck intermittently with rest periods. Reassure the mother that the infant will nurse when hungry. The infant may suck lightly after the mother feels that the milk has stopped flowing. This seems to satisfy the infant's need to suck and should not be discouraged if the nipples are not sore. If possible, the infant will nurse most successfully if allowed to breast-feed when hungry.

Recognize the signs of the "let-down" reflex, which indicates that the client is ready to nurse her infant. Explain that her breasts will feel full and that she may feel a tingling sensation. Small amounts of milk may leak from the nipples. Explain how to express milk from the breasts manually (Fig. 20-2) as well as with a breast pump. Stress that milk should be stored in such a way that spoilage and contamination are prevented.

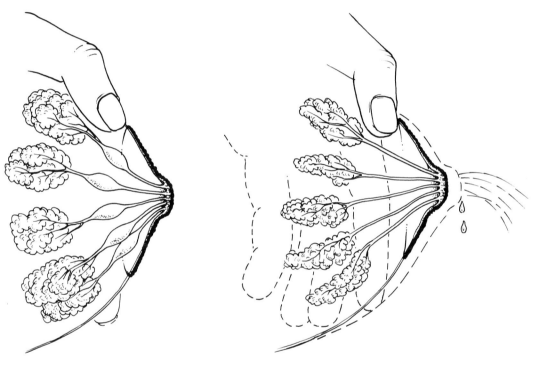

Figure 20.2

Take proper care of her health during the nursing period. Instruct the mother on maintaining an adequate diet during lactation. An additional 500 calories per day generally is considered to be a minimum requirement to meet the needs of lactogenesis and to maintain the mother's energy level. An additional 20 g of protein and 400 g of calcium are recommended. Phosphorus, iron, and water-soluble vitamins also should be increased during lactation. Fluid intake is important to the production of an adequate milk supply. A fluid intake of about 3000 ml is needed. Foods that should be avoided are those that cause digestive problems during the nonlactating state. There is controversy about the effect on the baby of the foods eaten by the mother. Encourage the mother to eat whatever she wishes but to be aware of the reaction of her nursing infant. If the food the mother eats seems to upset the infant, she may choose to avoid it until the lactation period is finished.

Understand the great variations among babies regarding their desire and ability to nurse. Some babies are slower than others in learning how to nurse; some begin nursing successfully immediately after birth and some must be coaxed and learn only after several weeks of persistence and patience. Since emotions are so closely tied to a successful nursing experience, continual reassurance may be needed to salvage the mother's self-image and her desire to nurse. Encourage her to resist the temptation to compare herself and her baby with friends and acquaintances and their babies.

Understand the importance of taking some time for herself. Emphasize to the new parents that an occasional bottle of expressed milk or formula will not hurt the baby and will allow them to have some time alone. Stress the importance of physical and psychological care of self, and encourage the new mother to spend some time away from the baby occasionally.

Referrals and Consultations

If the mother has difficulty in breast-feeding her child, she may be referred to support groups, such as the La Leche League, which can offer support and assistance.

Evaluation of Health Promotion Activities

Quality Assurance/ Reassessment

- Check the mother's breasts after she has nursed the infant to determine if they are being emptied. The breasts should be soft after nursing. Check for knots or hard lumps on the surface of the breast as well as in the axillae.
- Check the nipples for fissures or cracks. Observe for signs of bleeding. Watch the mother as she nurses to assess if the nursing action of the infant seems to cause discomfort.
- Observe the feeding to assess the breast-feeding technique. Watch to see if the infant has a firm grasp of the nipple, which allows compression of the surrounding tissue as well as the nipple. If the infant is sucking rapidly without swallowing, the infant may not be grasping the nipple adequately. Note whether the mother's breast tissue compresses the infant's nose, inhibiting breathing. This may be a factor in the infant who cannot nurse successfully.

DOCUMENTATION

Charting for the Home Health Nurse
- Note the appearance of the breasts and nipples at each visit to the nursing mother during the first several months after the infant's birth. If any problems are noted, document the recommendations as well as follow-up care. The chart should contain a progressive record of resolution of any problems identified.

Records Kept by the Client/Family
The mother may wish to keep a small chart regarding which breast to use in nursing the infant when she begins alternating breasts for each feeding. The tendency is often to place the infant on the dominant arm for nursing. Thus, a right-handed person may nurse the infant on the right side more frequently, especially if she cannot remember which breast was used at the last feeding. To prevent soreness and ensure that both breasts are emptied regularly, a small chart indicating which breast was used last may be hung in a convenient place, such as in the bathroom where the mother washes her hands before feeding the baby or near the infant's crib. This is usually not necessary once the breast-feeding regimen becomes established and the initial tenderness of the nipples subsides.

**Health Teaching
Checklist**

Name of Care Provider _____

Relationship to Client _____ Telephone # _____

Taught by _____ Date _____

	EXPLAINED	DEMONSTRATED
Positioning of baby for breast-feeding	_____	_____
Proper grasping of nipple by infant	_____	
Cleansing of breasts	_____	_____
Properly fitting support bra	_____	_____
Use of nursing pads	_____	_____
Importance of emptying breasts	_____	
Use of electrical breast pump	_____	_____
Use of manual breast pump	_____	_____

Product Availability

A well-fitting nursing bra may be purchased at maternity shops and many women's retail fashion shops. Nursing gowns that open in the front to facilitate nursing the infant are also available at these same stores. Nursing pads are available in most drug stores and pharmacies. Manual breast pumps may be purchased wherever infant supplies are sold, such as pharmacies or drug stores. Electrical breast pumps often may be rented from hospitals or hospital-supply houses.

21   Enteral Feeding Tube Insertion

Background

For people who require long-term nutritional support, enteral feeding is an option if there is sufficient healthy absorptive tissue in the gut. Enteral nutritional feeding programs are less expensive and have fewer complications than home parenteral nutrition (HPN), and they are easier for the client and family to manage.

The person will require intubation unless a surgical opening, such as a gastrostomy, has been made for feeding purposes. Enteral feeding tubes can be passed through the mouth or nose into the stomach or intestine, depending on the type of formula to be infused (see Technique 25, Tube Feeding). Nasogastric or nasoenteric feeding tubes are usually inserted for home enteral nutrition programs. Prior to the development of pliable, fine-bore, weighted feeding tubes, rubber or polyvinyl feeding tubes (16 French to 18 French) were the only option for enteral feeding. Although contraindicated for feeding purposes, these tubes are still commonly used. Large-bore feeding tubes are irritating to the gastrointestinal (GI) tract and cause pressure necrosis. They deteriorate when exposed to gastric juice, requiring frequent replacement. Furthermore, the large bore tends to cause incompetence of the gastroesophageal sphincter, thus increasing the chance of esophageal reflux and aspiration.

Several fine-bore, weighted feeding tubes are available (Fig. 21-1). Depending on the length of the tube inserted, they may be used for nasogastric feeding (90 cm, or 36 inches) or nasoenteric feeding (108 cm, or 43 inches). The bolus weight aids passage of the tube into the intestine and also helps anchor the tube after placement is confirmed. The size of the tube selected for enteral feeding should be the smallest through which the feeding will flow (7 French to 8 French for adults, infant feeding tubes for pediatrics). Smaller tubes (5 French or 6 French) and viscous formulas require a feeding pump to keep the tube open.

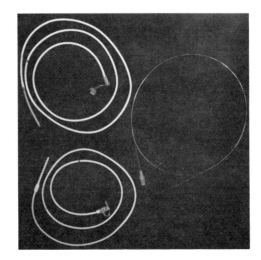

Figure 21.1

Intubation using fine-bore feeding tubes may be difficult because the tubes are very soft. Most are available with a stainless-steel stylet to stiffen the tube during insertion. Depending on the policy of the home health agency, the physician may be called on to reinsert a feeding tube if a stylet is used. Nurses experienced in the technique can successfully insert tubes with stylets. In some cases, tubes can be inserted without the stylet. Clients can insert their own nasogastric tubes before a feeding session and remove them at the end. Special instructions are necessary if the person is performing self-intubation using a stylet. This is not possible with nasoenteric tubes, which require a number of hours to reach the correct position in the intestine. The position is confirmed by x-ray film. A nasoenteric tube requiring reinsertion can be inserted by the home health nurse, and the position can be confirmed by an x-ray film at the physician's office or local emergency treatment center before feeding is started. Enteral feeding (gavage) can be given using an enteral feeding pump or by gravity using a feeding bag and administration set. Some practitioners still use bolus feeding, particularly for clients with head and neck problems. Bolus feedings are administered using the barrel of an irrigation syringe or a funnel attached to the feeding tube.

Assessment of Self-Care Potential

Client/Family Assessment

- Assess whether the client is capable of inserting the nasogastric (NG) tube before a feeding session.
- Determine whether the family is willing and able to assist the client in maintaining the tube and feeding program.
- Assess the client for problems accepting body-image changes that occur as a result of intubation. Observe for a decrease in socialization as a result of not being able to eat with family members.
- Determine if the family has been provided with insurance counseling. Check whether a third-party payor will reimburse the client for the cost of the feeding program.
- Assist the family to select feeding apparatus that they can easily handle. Check that the person can easily pour formula into the bag. Determine whether special tubing is required with the administration bag. Check that the feeding pump selected has a battery pack if the person will be ambulating during feeding. Determine whether the pump will be purchased or rented from a medical-equipment company. Check whether rental payments will be credited toward purchase.

Physical Assessment

- Assess GI system with emphasis on abdominal assessment.
- Determine if there is a history of food intolerance or allergies, or health problems with the GI tract.
- Determine that the tip of the tube is in the appropriate area in the GI tract (i.e., stomach or intestine).
- Assess the skin condition for pressure areas caused by taping the tube.
- Determine if the tube is ready for replacement (if it is left in continuously). When the tube is removed, check to see that it has not deteriorated from exposure to gastric secretions. Manufacturers recommend replacement of disposable fine-bore feeding tubes every 4 weeks. Red rubber feeding tubes will have a longer life.
- Determine the type of tube that will be best for the client. If the client is performing self-intubation, a red rubber tube may be the tube of choice. The dimensions of the tube will be larger, but it can be inserted without a stylet. If the tube is removed at the end of the feeding, consider red rubber tubes.

Environmental Assessment

- Determine a suitable area in the home for intubation and for cleaning the equipment. A bathroom is probably best if the client is performing self-intubation. Seating the client in a chair or in a high Fowler's position in bed is suitable if the nurse or a family member is intubating the person. The feeding can be administered while the client is seated in a comfortable chair or even while ambulating if the feeding pump has a battery pack. A semi-Fowler's position in bed is suitable if the feeding is administered at night.
- Check on a suitable place to give the feeding. The client may prefer to sit in the living room with the family or, if feeding at night, the client will be in bed.

Planning Strategies

Potential Nursing Diagnoses

Injury, potential for displacement of feeding tube into the lung

Comfort, alteration in: pain or discomfort during self-intubation

Skin integrity, impairment of: potential, due to taping of feeding tube

Oral mucous membranes, alteration in: dryness due to alternate feeding route

Self-concept, disturbance in: presence of feeding tube

Expected Outcomes

Prevention of complications of enteral intubation (e.g., displacement of tube, aspiration of stomach contents, or tissue necrosis caused by pressure of the tube)

Prevention of discomfort and trauma

Maintenance of skin integrity

Prevention of dryness of oral mucous membranes

Acceptance of body-image changes

Health Promotion Goals

- The client and family will
  Prevent complications of intubation
  Maintain the feeding tube
  Incorporate the feeding program into other activities of daily living
  Accept body-image changes that occur because the client has a feeding tube and is unable to eat with the family
- The client will
  Safely insert the NG tube prior to the feeding session (if appropriate)

Equipment

Feeding tube (with or without stylet)

Examination gloves (optional)

Benzoin

Hypoallergenic tape

Water-soluble lubricant (if tube not prelubricated)

Glass of water

Litmus paper (optional)

Disposable irrigation syringe

Stethoscope

Safety pin

Bathtowel to protect linen

If tube is to be inserted without stylet:

    Basin of ice chips

    Cotton swab (for fine-bore tubes only)

Interventions/Health Promotion

ACTION

1. Place the client in high Fowler's position or sitting in a chair. Protect the person's clothing or bed linen with the bathtowel. For gastric placement, determine the approximate length for insertion. Wash hands. Use clean examination gloves for intubation if the client has lesions of the mouth or lips.
   Measure the distance from the earlobe to the tip of the nose, and from there to the xiphoid process (NEX measurement).

   For enteric placement, add approximately 22.5 cm (9 inches) to the NEX measurement. Mark the appropriate point on the tube, or note the closest mark on the tube. If inserting a large-bore feeding tube, simply omit the steps involving the stylet.

2. If a stylet is being used with a prelubricated tube, activate the lubricant inside the tube by flushing it with water (Fig. 21-2). Insert the stylet, making sure it is locked in place behind the weighted tip.

RATIONALE/AMPLIFICATION

Herpetic whitlow, a painful viral infection of the pulp space of the finger, can be contracted from clients with oral herpes outbreaks.
Alternate method: Mark the 50-cm point on the tube. Insertion length is midway between the 50-cm point and the NEX measurement. Research has shown this to be more accurate. Marking the point on the tube enables the person inserting the tube to determine when the tube is in the correct place.

The technique for inserting a large-bore tube is similar to that for other tubes.

Prelubricated tubes are lubricated at the tip as well as within the lumen. Lubricant within the lumen makes withdrawal of the stylet easier and prevents accidental removal of the tube at the same time.

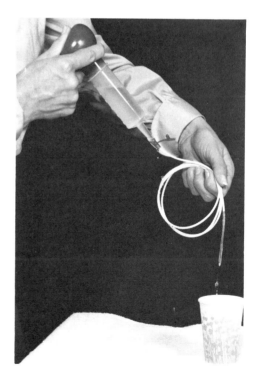

Figure 21.2

ACTION	RATIONALE/AMPLIFICATION
3. Activate the lubricant on the weighted tip by dipping it in water. If the tube is not prelubricated, apply water-soluble lubricant to the first few inches of the tube.	Use only water-soluble lubricant. Aspiration of mineral oil or other petroleum-based products can cause granulomatous pneumonia.
4. Check for the preferred nostril by having the client breathe through each nostril alternately. Insert the tube in the most patent nostril. Arrange a predetermined hand signal with the client to let you know if the client is having trouble speaking.	If a tube is accidentally passed through the vocal cords, the client will not be able to speak. This usually causes choking, but it may not be as apparent if using a fine-bore feeding tube.
5. Flex the client's neck. Pass the lubricated tip through the nostril and into the nasopharynx. Rotate the tube 180 degrees and encourage the client to swallow.	Giving small amounts of water through a straw may assist the passage of the tube. Stroking the throat may stimulate reflex swallowing in the unconscious person.
6. Pass the tube until the premeasured length is inserted. Do not force the tube against resistance. Pull back a few centimeters and try to pass it again. If this is not successful, remove the tube and report the problem to the physician.	
7. Ascertain the correct position of the tube in the stomach by injecting a small bolus of air into the tube while auscultating the left upper quadrant of the abdomen with a stethoscope.	The correct position is indicated by a "wooshing" sound as the air is injected. Some stylets are hollow and permit withdrawing stomach contents or inserting air without removing the stylet (flow-through stylet). If a flow-through stylet is not used, the stylet will have to be removed before checking placement. *Do not reinsert the stylet while the tube is in the client.* There is a risk of damaging tissue if the stylet exits through one of the terminal holes in the tube. If the stylet has been removed and the tube is not placed correctly, if more of the tube cannot be passed while the client swallows, it will have to be removed and reinserted.

ACTION

Place the end of the tube in a glass of water and watch for bubbles as the client inhales. Withdraw stomach contents from the tube using the irrigation syringe.

Check the contents with litmus paper to determine acidity.

8. Remove the stylet (if it is the flow-through variety).

   Prepare the skin with benzoin. Tape the tube to the nose avoiding pressure on the naris (Fig. 21-3). Attach the tube to the person's clothing with a safety pin and a tape tab.

RATIONALE/AMPLIFICATION

This is used to determine that the tube is not in the lung. Be careful not to allow the client to inhale water.

Acid turns blue litmus pink.

Use at least 2 methods to check for correct placement of tube.

Be sure that the tube is not removed simultaneously.

Pressure on the naris can lead to necrosis of the tissue. If enteric placement is desired, do not tape the tube to the nose because an additional length of the tube will need to be inserted.

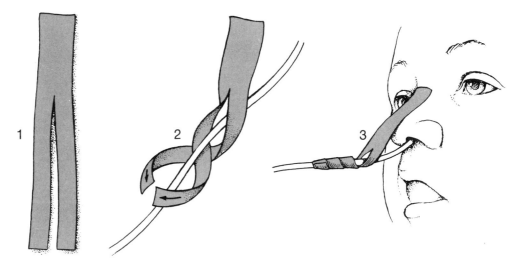

Figure 21.3

9. If enteric placement is desired, place the client on the right side in a semi-Fowler's position. Continue to insert the tube a little at a time, until the correct length has been inserted. Secure the tube to the nose. Obtain an x-ray film to confirm placement.

10. Connect the tube to the appropriate feeding apparatus.

    Irrigate the tube and cap it if feeding is not to be started.

This position encourages migration of the bolus weight into the duodenum. This usually occurs within 24 to 48 hours. An x-ray film can be obtained at a local emergency treatment center or physician's office.

Tube feeding can be commenced before the tube has migrated to the intestine if there is no contraindication to instilling formula into the stomach.

ACTION

RATIONALE/AMPLIFICATION

11. To insert a fine-bore tube without a stylet, place the tube on ice to stiffen.
    Place the uncovered end of a cotton-swab stick into the distal eye of the tube. Use the swab to stabilize the tube and aid in passing it into the nasopharynx (Fig. 21-4). Remove the swab. When the bolus falls behind the soft palate, the tube may be easily passed into the stomach.

Fine-bore tubes will stiffen somewhat, but this technique is not as effective as with large-bore tubes.

12. To insert a red rubber feeding tube, stiffen the tube on ice. Lubricate the tube with water-soluble lubricant. Insert the tube following the directions above, omitting the steps involving the stylet.

It is not necessary to use a cotton-tipped swab to stabilize the rubber tube. The tube has sufficient body after being placed on ice to pass easily into the pharynx.

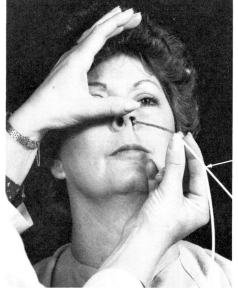

Figure 21.4
Insert end of a cotton-tipped swab into the terminal exit hole to stiffen the tube and pass the tube into the nasopharynx. Remove the swab and pass the tube into the stomach.

Related Care

Change the tube every 4 weeks or if signs of deterioration occur.

Changing disposable weighted feeding tubes every 4 weeks is recommended by the manufacturer.

Education/
Communication

- Teach the client and family to

    Cap feeding tubes that are placed in the intestine. These tubes are not re-moved between feedings.

    Check that the tube is in the correct position (see above) before instilling for-mula or medications. Obtain pediatric suspensions of medications, when possible, to make administration easier. Crush other medications and mix with ¼ cup of formula if they are compatible with dairy products. Give medications by pouring into the barrel of the irrigating syringe attached to the tube. Follow with at least ¼ cup of tapwater. Medications should not be added to formula in the bag. They would not be given at the correct time, and formula may be discarded or spilled.

    Remove the tube when instructed, by untaping the tube and removing it gently with one smooth motion. Protect clothing or bed linen with a bath-towel. Pinch the tube between the fingers while removing it to prevent leakage from the tube.

    Clean the tube by soaking in warm soapy water. Use an irrigating syringe to flush the tube. Rinse with tapwater and hang the tube to drain over the bathtub or shower door. When the tube is dry, place it in a plastic bag for future use. Discard tubes that have deteriorated.

    Rotate the tube daily and retape to prevent pressure areas on the nose. Use benzoin to protect the skin from the tape. Use hypoallergenic tape. Tape the tube without causing pressure to the nose.

    If using a weighted tube, select a tube that does not have a mercury bolus weight. Mercury requires special disposal procedures and should not be incinerated. Other tubes can be discarded in the household trash.

    Use tapwater to irrigate the tube before and after instilling medications or for-mula, or at least twice a day if feedings are on hold for any reason. Irri-gate with full-strength cranberry juice weekly if this intake is permitted. Cranberry juice cuts protein buildup in the lumen of the tube and helps keep the lumen open. Follow the juice with tapwater.

    Brush the teeth and use mouthwash regularly to help keep the mucous mem-branes of the mouth moist. Use a variety of mouthwashes and toothpaste to help prevent gustatory deprivation. If this is prohibited because of mouth surgery, provide mouth care with warm saline and cotton-tipped swabs or as instructed by the physician.

    Chew chewing gum (if permitted) to help keep the mouth moist and to satisfy gustatory needs. Buy sugar-free gum if the person is a diabetic. Expecto-rate oral secretions if swallowing is not possible.

    Prepare formula using clean utensils to prevent contamination. Refrigerate formula until ready for use.

- Teach the client to follow these additional instructions if inserting own feeding tube:

    Have the feeding tube and pump ready to go.

    Measure the length for insertion (NEX measurement) and mark the tube with a marking pen or strip of tape.

    If the tube is not self-lubricating, take 10 ml of water in a syringe with an equal amount of lubricant and insert the mixture into the tube to give body to the tube. If using a stylet, lubricate it and place it in the tube. Dip the bolus weight into the same mixture to lubricate it before insertion.

    If the person is unable to insert the tube without a stylet, remove the stylet when the tube is in the mid-esophagus, and continue advancing the tube into the stomach. (The use of stylets by clients at home is not recom-mended.)

Once the full length of the tube has been inserted, check the position by quickly inserting a small amount of air into the tube with an irrigating syringe. Confirm the tube position by feeling a gurgling sensation in the stomach or by listening over the stomach with a stethoscope. If preferred, confirm the position by taking 3 deep breaths while placing the tip of the tube in water and watching for bubbles. If bubbles appear, remove the tube, which may be in the respiratory tract.

Check that the tube is patent by flushing it with about ¼ cup of tapwater in the irrigating syringe.

Tape the tube securely to the nose and cheek. Use benzoin or other skin preparation to protect the skin.

Connect the feeding apparatus and complete the feeding. Flush the tube at the end of the feeding. Either cap the tube or remove it.

Age-Specific Modifications (Pediatric)

- For a nasogastric tube, measure the length of insertion from the tip of the nose to the ear, to a point midway between the xiphoid process and the umbilicus (Fig. 21-5).

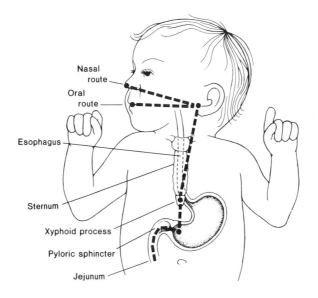

Figure 21.5

- Use a mummy or elbow restraint during intubation for infants and children.
- The tube is usually removed after each feeding. If the tube is to remain in place for an infant, use a mitten restraint and tape the tube securely.
- To place a tube in the intestine, turn the infant or child on the right side with the hips elevated for approximately 4 hours. After this time the child may be turned to the back, but not the left side. Continue to insert the tube a little at a time until the required length has been inserted. Tape the tube. Check the position of the tube with an x-ray film.
- Warm the formula to room temperature to prevent gastric spasms from cold formula. Control the flow of fluid into the stomach with a clamp on the feeding tube. Instill the formula very slowly to avoid overloading the stomach and precipitating vomiting.
- Position the child on the right side to facilitate the flow of fluid into the stomach. Elevate the child's head to lessen the possibility of aspiration. Leave the child recumbent following feeding to prevent "dumping syndrome."
- Check the infant for bradycardia due to a vagal reflex while the tube is inserted.

Referrals and Consultations

- Refer the client to the home health nurse if the tube is not patent and cannot be flushed with tapwater.
- Local clubs (ileitis, colitis, or ostomy clubs) may be of assistance to the client.
- The American Cancer Society has several self-help and group programs for terminal clients or clients with cancer.
- Contact a hospice program if the person has a terminal illness.

Evaluation of Health Promotion Activities

Quality Assurance/ Reassessment

- Periodically check client's technique if performing self-intubation.
- Check tube position during visits.
- Reassess family members' techniques for tube maintenance.

DOCUMENTATION

Charting for the Home Health Nurse
Ability of the client and family to assume self-care

Incorporation of the feeding program into activities of daily living

Abdominal assessment, bowel sounds

Condition of the skin

Assessment for dehydration, skin and mucous membrane condition

Body weight

Complications of the feeding program

Acceptance of self-concept changes

Records Kept by the Client/Family
Daily weight

GI problems (e.g., diarrhea)

Health Teaching Checklist

Name of Care Provider _____

Relationship to Client _____ Telephone #_____

Taught by _____ Date _____

	EXPLAINED	DEMONSTRATED
Tube insertion and maintenance	_____	_____
Self-management of the feeding program, including the feeding pump	_____	_____
Infection-control precautions	_____	_____
Checking daily weight	_____	_____
Complications to report	_____	

Product Availability

Feeding tubes, irrigating syringes, formula, and enteral feeding pumps (rental and purchase) are available at medical-supply companies (listed in the yellow pages).

(See Technique 22, Home Parenteral Nutrition, for feeding program vendors.)

Selected Reference

Barcia RM: Selection of enteral equipment. Nutritional Support Services 3(2):15–23, February, 1983

22   Home Parenteral Nutrition

Background

To improve the quality of life and to reduce the expense of an extended hospital stay, selected clients are being discharged on home parenteral nutrition (HPN) programs. Essential nutrients, electrolytes, vitamin B_{12}, vitamin K, folic acid, and trace elements are administered intravenously using a subclavian or right atrial catheter. Catheters such as the Hickman, Broviac, and Centracil have been developed for long-term use (see Technique 24, Right Atrial Catheter).

To ensure tissue building (anabolism), calories supplied by dextrose or intravenous lipids are infused with protein in the form of crystalline amino acids. Usually hypertonic dextrose is used as the calorie source, which means that the total parenteral nutrition (TPN) solution must be infused into a central vein to prevent phlebitis. The ideal calorie-to-nitrogen ratio is 150 to 200 calories to 1 gram of nitrogen (protein).

Lipids are infused two to three times a week to prevent essential fatty acid deficiency (EFAD). Intravenous lipids can be infused concurrently with the TPN solution if a double-lumen right atrial catheter is in use. Lipids can also be piggy-backed into the TPN line using a special Y-connector tubing, or they can be mixed with the TPN solution using a 3-in-1 system where a 24-hour supply of TPN is prepared. Intravenous lipids also supply calories. However, no more than 60% of calories should be supplied by fat.

Depending on the available vendors and the family resources, the client or family member can be provided with premixed TPN solution, which is stored in the refrigerator, or may be taught to mix the TPN solution at home. The least complex method that fits the client's needs is the best and offers the least risk of contamination of the solution. Premixed 3-in-1 solutions where a 24-hour supply is provided in one bag has potential for home use. A strict TPN protocol is mandatory to prevent complications, including infection and metabolic problems, which can occur if the rate of infusion is erratic. Use a low-pressure IV controller to monitor the rate of infusion.

Select candidates for home TPN carefully to implement a successful program. A supportive family environment is essential. The nutritional team must consider the need for long-term nutrition, whether the client's quality of life can be enhanced, and the person's prognosis. If the client's life expectancy is but a few months, a home TPN program is probably not feasible given the amount of education and training that is involved.

The teaching program should begin in the hospital. When the client is discharged to home care, evaluate additional learning needs. Teaching the client to infuse TPN at night allows freedom from the program during the day, and the client can resume some normal home activities or return to work. This time table should be implemented prior to discharge from the hospital, so that the client is stable before beginning HPN. Some people with chronic diseases may only require HPN during an exacerbation of the disease. If oral nutrients are contraindicated, the client will require HPN continually. However, if the person is permitted to eat, oral intake can supplement the HPN. Specific nutrients will be ordered by the physician in consultation with the nutritional team and home health nurse. Periodic laboratory parameters are used to evaluate the client's response to the HPN regimen.

Assessment of Self-Care Potential

Client/Family Assessment

- Assess the willingness and the ability of the client and family members to manage the home TPN program. A supportive family environment will enhance the chances for success of the program.

- Determine that the client or a family member has the physical and mental ability to manage the program. Assess the client for emotional stability and for compliance with the medical regimen. (Maintaining sterility of the system is mandatory.) Evaluate the client's strength, dexterity, hand/eye coordination, and so forth, to determine that physical limitations will not be a problem and to determine the appropriateness of equipment and supplies (e.g., the person with decreased grip strength due to arthritis may be better able to handle an IV bag rather than a bottle, which adds weight).

- Determine whether the client is eligible for Medicare or if another third-party payor will pay for HPN. Most third-party payors recognize the cost-effectiveness of HPN, but coverage is not automatic, and this should be determined prior to implementing the teaching program. Determine whether the client is aware of the fees prior to discharge to the HPN program, and whether insurance counseling has been provided.

- Determine what equipment will be purchased from the home health agency or other vendor, and what can be purchased by the client. If a HPN vendor is selected, assist the client to evaluate the services provided:
  Will an infusion pump be purchased by the client from a medical-supply company or rented from the HPN vendor?
  How is the formula mixed and how frequently will it be delivered to the home? What quality-control measures are in effect?
  Will a local hospital pharmacy mix the TPN, which can then be picked up by a family member?
  Will the vendor supply all tubings and dressings or will the client obtain these from the home health agency, hospital pharmacy, or medical-supply company?
  Is there a policy for returned supplies?
  What is the cost of supplies and formula? Assist the client to obtain requirements at the best price without compromising quality. The costs may range from $3500 to $5000 monthly.
  Will laboratory specimens be collected in the home or will the client have to travel to a laboratory? How quickly will laboratory results be obtained in the event that intervention is necessary?
  Does the vendor have a 24-hour on-call service or will the home health nurse be available? Assistance after hours is necessary because most clients infuse TPN at night to allow free time during the day.

- Obtain a consult with a dietitian periodically to assist in nutritional assessment, unless the client returns to an outpatient clinic on a regular basis where this is provided.

AGE-SPECIFIC MODIFICATIONS (PEDIATRIC)

- Determine whether the child will require home-bound instruction or whether return to school is possible. If TPN is infused at night, the right atrial catheter (RAC) can be capped and taped to the child's chest during the day.

- If the child returns to school, instruct the school nurse and homeroom teacher regarding emergency management of the right atrial catheter (see Technique 24, Right Atrial Catheter).

- Determine what activities the child will be engaging in. Discourage extremely rough activities to prevent dislodging the catheter. Moderate activity should be encouraged. Swimming is prohibited because of the chance of infection. If dust or dirt may be a problem, occlude the RAC dressing with an adhesive surgical drape (Steridrape).
- If the child is very active, heparinize the catheter more frequently to prevent clotting.
- Involve the child in the HPN program as much as possible.

Physical Assessment

- Assess the reason for which HPN is required. Persons who are unable to either consume or absorb nutrients may be candidates for HPN (e.g., chronic malabsorption problems, draining intestinal fistulas, short bowel syndrome, congenital atresia, burns, chemotherapy, following radiation therapy).

Chart 22-1. HOME TPN INFORMATION SHEET

Name:_____ History Number: _____

Sex: _____

Address: _____ Birthdate: _____

_____ Phone #: _____

Contact Physician: _____

Physician's Address: _____

Physician's Phone Number: (Office) _____ (Home) _____

Date TPN Started: _____ Date D/C or HTPN: _____

Date HTPN D/C: _____ Reason: _____

HTPN Supplier: _____

Pump: _____

Insurance—Primary: _____

Secondary: _____

Family Members and Relationship to Patient: _____

_____ _____

Home Assessment:

Diagnosis: _____

Clinical History of Illness: _____

_____

_____

_____

(Reprinted with permission from Nutritional Support Services, Volume 5, Number 3, March, 1985)

- Complete a physical assessment with emphasis on nutritional history and assessment:
  History: medical, social, diet, weight
  Anthropometrics: Height, frame size, weight, height-to-weight ratio, skin-fold measurements
  Biochemical data: serum albumin, transferrin, urinary nitrogen (see Charts 22-1 and 22-2)
- Determine to what extent the HPN can be supplemented by oral feedings, if any. For example, a person on chemotherapy, unless cancer of the GI tract has been diagnosed, will be able to eat to whatever extent food can be tolerated, and HPN will probably be used to supplement the oral diet. A person with chronic inflammatory bowel disease will only require supplemental HPN during an exacerbation of the disease.
- Assess the dressing change technique of the client or family member periodically. Observe the condition of the site and subcutaneous tract for redness, drainage, or swelling. Check catheter integrity.
- Monitor the client for thrombosis, sepsis, or catheter displacement. Assess heart sounds for murmurs due to tricuspid valve injury.
- Assess the client for complications related to TPN:
  Metabolic imbalances (hypoglycemia or hyperglycemia)
  GI disturbances (diarrhea or constipation)
  Electrolyte imbalance
  Recognize complications of TPN, and take appropriate action.

Chart 22-2. NUTRITIONAL ASSESSMENT FLOWSHEET

Name: _____

Date of birth: _____

Weight: _____ cm

Wrist Circumference: _____ cm

Usual Weight: _____ kg

Frame size: _____

Ideal Weight: _____ kg

BSA: _____ m²

Goal Weight: _____ kg

BEE: _____ Kcal/d

Somatic and Visceral Parameters									Estimated Requirements			Current Support						
									Calories			TPN				PO's		
Date	Wt	% Ideal	% Usual	MAC	TSP	AMA	A1b	TFN	BEE	Goal	Pro	CHO	Fat	Non-Pro Cal	Pro	Cal/Pro	Cal/Kg	Pro/kg

(Reprinted with permission from Nutritional Support Services, Volume 5, Number 3, March, 1985)

Environmental Assessment

- Assess the home for effective sanitary practices. Since HPN will require sterile procedures, cleanliness is essential. Is there a work area free from traffic, open windows, and dust where formulas can be prepared if the client is mixing the TPN solution? Limit housekeeping procedures such as vacuuming during dressing changes or while mixing HPN solutions.
- Determine whether refrigeration will be available for storage of premixed solutions. If a HPN vendor will be used, will refrigeration be supplied if necessary? Will there be an additional fee?

Planning Strategies

Potential Nursing Diagnoses

Nutrition, alteration in: less than body requirements

Fluid volume, alteration in: excess or deficit related to home IV infusion

Home maintenance management, impaired: related to alteration in nutrition

Infection (local or systemic), potential for: related to HPN program

Bowel elimination, potential alteration: constipation related to low residue; diarrhea related to high IV solute load (osmolality)

Self-concept, disturbance in: related to indwelling right atrial catheter and dietary modifications

Knowledge deficit: management of HPN program

Expected Outcomes

Achievement of an improved nutritional state relative to the nutritional problem

Maintenance of an adequate fluid volume

Increased client independence and self-sufficiency

Prevention of infection through appropriate care of the indwelling catheter and implementation of a safe feeding regimen

Regular bowel elimination pattern

Acceptance of body-image changes

Understanding of the management of the HPN program

Equipment

For infusing TPN
    IV tubing
    In-line IV filter
    Drip controller (with alarm that will sound when a preset volume is infused)
    Iodophor swab
    Rubber shod or padded clamp

For discontinuing infusion
    Iodophor swab
    Sterile injection cap
    Rubber shod or padded clamp

Interventions/Health Promotion

ACTION	*RATIONALE/AMPLIFICATION*
Infusing TPN	
1. Instruct the client to wash hands and assemble equipment.	The client will probably choose to infuse TPN at night during sleep.
2. If the client mixes the TPN solution	
• Choose a nonporous work surface such as a kitchen or bathroom bench.	The area should have minimum traffic and be free from drafts to prevent contamination.
• Wipe the area with alcohol and allow it to air dry.	This cleans the area and decreases the surface bacteria.
• Follow the manufacturer's directions in the package insert to mix the TPN.	
• Inspect bags, bottles, and other equipment for evidence of contaminants or cracks.	Contamination may be indicated by cloudy solutions or bacterial or fungal growth.
• Instruct the client not to use any suspicious fluids, but to return them to the vendor.	If solutions are contaminated, quality control should be investigated.
• Instruct the client on the correct use of tubings and syringes used in mixing the solutions. Discuss volume calculations, the order of mixing, and compatibility considerations.	Swirling the base solution after each addition minimizes incompatibility potential.
• Refrigerate the mixed solutions.	This minimizes instability and decreases the potential for bacterial proliferation.
3. Retrieve the TPN solution from the refrigerator 1 to 2 hours before infusing.	Cold solutions can cause hypothermia or venospasm. Premixed solutions supplied by HPN vendors should also be refrigerated until used.
4. Prepare the solution for infusion:	Most clients choose to infuse TPN at night to allow freedom during the day. The infusion takes about 10 to 12 hours. Caution the client to use sterile IV tubing for each infusion session to prevent contamination.
• Close the regulator clamp on the IV tubing and connect the in-line filter. Spike the IV bag or bottle.	
• Squeeze the drip chamber until it is half full.	
• Release the clamp and prime the tubing. Follow manufacturer's directions if there are any special instructions for priming the filter. Close the regulator clamp.	
• Thread the tubing through the drip controller.	Follow the manufacturer's instructions in priming tubing and threading the pump.

ACTION	RATIONALE/AMPLIFICATION

5. Infuse the TPN:
   - Clamp the catheter with a padded clamp. Remove the injection cap and wipe the end of the catheter with an iodophor swab.
   - Remove the protective covering from the IV tubing, and connect it to the catheter (Fig. 22-1).
   - Tape the connection (Fig. 22-2).

This prevents accidental disconnection during the night.

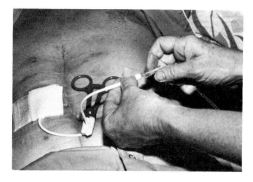

Figure 22.1
Note that the clamp is covered with tape to protect the catheter.

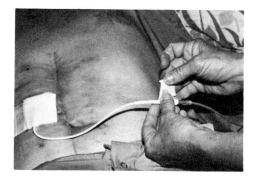

Figure 22.2
Taping the IV-RA catheter connection to prevent accidental disconnection.

   - Check the pump for the correct flow rate.

The flow rate will be ordered by the physician and will depend on the regimen that was established prior to discharge from the hospital. The first and last 2 hours of the infusion are usually run at a slower rate than the remainder of the infusion to prevent metabolic complications from sudden changes in the blood glucose level.

   - Remove the clamp from the catheter and open the regulator clamp on the tubing.
   - Start the pump and begin the infusion.

The pump alarms will alert the client to when it is time to change the container or when it is time to increase or decrease the rate.

6. Discontinue the infusion when it is completed:
   - Turn the pump off.
   - Clamp the catheter with a padded clamp. Close the regulator clamp on the IV tubing.
   - Disconnect the IV tubing from the catheter. Wipe the catheter tip with an iodophor swab.
   - Cap the catheter with a sterile injection cap.

Caution the client not to use the injection cap that was removed before the infusion. It may be contaminated.

ACTION	*RATIONALE/AMPLIFICATION*
• Heparinize the catheter (see Technique 24, Right Atrial Catheter).	
• Redress the catheter and tape it to the body.	A female client may coil the catheter and tuck it in her bra rather than tape it to her chest.

Related Care

1. Draw blood at least monthly to monitor the progress of the HPN program.	The following laboratory determinations will be required: blood glucose, electrolytes, blood urea nitrogen, creatinine, transferrin, albumin, total protein, cholesterol levels, prothrombin and partial thromboplastin times, hemoglobin and hematocrit, complete blood count, and liver function.
2. Change the IV tubing every 24 hours if the HPN is continuous.	This decreases the chance of infection.
3. Redress the catheter every 48 hours.	
4. Monitor blood glucose using self glucose monitoring and/or urinalysis for sugar and acetone (see Technique 39, Blood Glucose Monitoring, and Technique 41, Urine Glucose Testing).	If unstable, notify the physician. The client may require insulin or a rate change. This can also signal infection.

Education/ Communication

• Teach the client and family to

Call the home health nurse on call to answer any questions or help with problems. As the client becomes more competent, these calls will be reduced to a minimum.

Be sure to have blood drawn for monthly studies to monitor progress of the HPN regimen

Change the dressing every 48 hours or if wet or soiled (see Technique 24, Right Atrial Catheter).

Change the injection cap every 3 days if TPN is piggy-backed using the injection cap. Use a new tubing and filter every 24 hours.

Deal with RAC complications (see Technique 24, Right Atrial Catheter).

Monitor and treat complications of TPN, such as hyperglycemia or hypoglycemia

Hyperglycemia: signs and symptoms include nausea, weakness, thirst, headache, urine sugar greater than 0.5% and elevated blood sugar. Insulin may need to be added to the infusion, or the rate of infusion may have to be decreased. Prevent hyperglycemia by maintaining prescribed drip rate and never trying to catch up if the rate slows. Use aseptic techniques to prevent infection. Test for glucose tolerance before discharge from the hospital. Monitor blood sugar levels monthly.

Hypoglycemia: signs and symptoms include sweating, pale skin, palpitations, nausea, headache, shaky feeling, blurred vision, and feeling hungry. Drink a glass of juice or water with 2 teaspoons of sugar or honey immediately. Tell the family member to place a piece of hard candy or a teaspoon of honey under the tongue if the client is too drowsy to drink liquids. Prevent hypoglycemia by not stopping TPN too abruptly. Insulin in the infusion may require adjustment. Monitor blood glucose levels monthly. Keep hard candy or honey in the house in case of hypoglycemia.

Check the catheter periodically to ensure that blood is not backing up in the catheter. This will occur if the injection cap is not secured. Clamp the catheter and remove the injection cap. Replace it with a sterile injection cap and reheparinize the catheter.

Monitor for infection by checking the catheter site for signs of infection during dressing changes and taking a daily temperature to check for elevation. Signs and symptoms of infection include redness, swelling or drainage at insertion site, temperature above 100 °F (37.7°C), chills, sweating, lethargy, urine glucose levels greater than .5%, and unstable blood sugars. Report these signs immediately to the home health nurse. Prevent infection by adhering to HPN protocols.

Obtain and record a daily weight for the first 2 weeks on the HPN program (to check for fluid overload) and 3 times a week thereafter. Weigh daily at the same time, using the same scales, and wearing a similar amount of clothing.

Record oral intake (if applicable)

Infuse TPN at night and cap the catheter during the day to allow the client freedom from the HPN program. This goal must be achieved gradually to avoid sudden glucose shifts. The schedule is best achieved while the client is in the hospital with constant supervision. Adjustments can then be made during the HPN program.

- Teach the client and family that

  The pump alarms will alert them if the pump or infusion requires attention or if the bag or bottle is empty

  HPN can be infused during the day if they are anxious about not being awakened at night

  Feeling uncomfortable because meals cannot be shared with others is a normal reaction to the body-image changes that occur with HPN programs

Referrals and Consultations

- Tell the client to report any problems with the catheter or HPN program to the home health nurse as soon as possible.

- Refer the client with cancer to the American Cancer Society for assistance such as providing dressing equipment for catheter dressing changes.

- Refer the child in school to the homeroom teacher or school nurse if problems with the catheter develop while the child is at school.

- Refer the home-bound child to the home-bound education program in the local school district.

- Suggest the client obtain the *Lifeline Letter*, c/o Oley Foundation, 214 Hun Memorial, Department N85, Albany Medical Center, Albany, NY 12208, for information on support groups.

Evaluation of Health Promotion Activities

Quality Assurance/ Reassessment

- Periodically observe the caregiver's catheter care and infusion technique to ensure adherence to infection-control and safety standards. Inspect the site for signs of infection. Monitor daily temperatures.

- Monitor weight gain or maintenance.

- Culture the catheter insertion site if drainage is present.

- Refer an infected catheter to the physician to evaluate it for possible removal.

- Periodically evaluate the patient's antithrombin III level to assess thrombosis potential. (Low levels enhance clot formation. Wafarin sodium, 1 mg daily, effectively restores normal antithrombin III levels without significantly prolonging the prothrombin time.)

- Evaluate storage techniques for premixed TPN solutions.
- Evaluate service if a HPN vendor is employed to provide TPN solutions or equipment.

DOCUMENTATION

Charting for the Home Health Nurse

Progress of the client/family in assuming responsibility for the procedures

Physical parameters including weight, vital signs, nutritional assessment, blood glucose monitoring, urinalysis results, and laboratory work. Use a flowsheet to document progress (Chart 22-3).

Changes in the formula or rate of administration (Chart 22-4)

Psychological responses of the family and client regarding lifestyle and body-image changes

Chart 22-3.   LABORATORY DATA FLOWSHEET

Name: _____

LAB	NORMS	Date	Date
Na	135–145 mEq/L		
K	3.2–4.8 mEq/L		
Cl	98–108 mEq/L		
CO_2	21–30 mEq/L		
BUN	7–21 mg/dl		
Creatinine	0.7–1.4 mg/dl		
Glucose	75–110 mg/dl		
Albumin	3.5–5.0 g/dl		
Transf	200–400 g/L		
PreAlb	10–40 mg/dl		
Ca	8.7–10.2 mg/dl		
Phos.	2.3–4.3 mg/dl		
Mg.	1.6–2.2 mEq/L		
Bili.	0.2–1.2 mg/dl		
Alk. Phos.	30–110 U/L		
SGPT	5–35 U/L		
SGOT	5–35 U/L		
Iron	45–160 ug/dl		
Cu	80–120 ug/dl		
Zinc	45–160 ug/dl		
B-12	300–1000 pg/ml		
Folate	3–15 ng/ml		
PT	9.8–13.8 secs.		
Hgb	(M) 14–18 (F) 12–16 g		
Hct	(M) 40–54 (F) 37–47%		
WBC	5000–10,000/mm^3		
TLC	1500/mm^3		

(Reprinted with permission from Nutritional Support Services, Volume 5, Number 3, March, 1985)

Chart 22-4.   HTPN FORMULA SHEET

	Date	Date
Infusion—time —rate		
Taper—time —rate		
Liters/day		
Home vs. Pharm Mix		
Fat		
Dextrose		
Protein		
Na		
K		
Cl		
Ca		
Mg		
Phos		
Zn		
Cu		
Mn		
Cr		
Se		
Vitamins		
Insulin		

*Components added by patient

(Reprinted with permission from Nutritional Support Services, Volume 5, Number 3, March 1985)

Adaptation of the client to independence from the hospital and dependence on the home health-care provider

Condition of the insertion site and patency of the catheter

Coverage of expenses by third-party payor or private pay

Records Kept by the Client/Family

Daily weight until stable, then 3 times a week

Temperature measurements

The amount and rate of TPN infused

Complications or problems

Record of the client's oral intake if applicable

Health Teaching Checklist

Name of Care Provider _____

Relationship to Client _____ Telephone #_____

Taught by _____ Date _____

	EXPLAINED	DEMONSTRATED
RAC catheter care	_____	_____
Rationale for HPN	_____	
Mixing the formula (if applicable)	_____	_____
Storage of the formula	_____	_____
Managing the IV pump	_____	_____
Managing the TPN regimen	_____	_____
Metabolic and catheter-related complications, and treatment	_____	
Record keeping	_____	
Changes in lifestyle	_____	

Product Availability

HPN VENDORS

National
Travacare
Abbott
American Continue Care
Home Health Care of America
Home Nutritional Support

Local
Community Corporation
Hospital-based programs

Regional
Community Alimentation
HOMED
Home Medical Support Services
New England Critical Care

Selected References

Baptista RJ: Home TPN: Patient identification, formula generation, teaching methods and home vendor selection. Nutritional Support Services 4(2):71–75, February, 1984

Decker K: Home parenteral nutrition: Evaluating community services. Nutritional Support Services 4(4):15–16, April, 1984

Grant JP, Davey JA, Grabowski V, Payne N, Sparks W: A home total parenteral nutrition monitoring system. Nutritional Support Services 5(3):16–18, March, 1985

Wilhelm L: Helping your patient settle in with TPN. Nursing '85 15(4):60–64, April, 1985

23   Infant Nutrition

Background

The sucking and swallowing reflexes are present at birth. Feeding time meets the infant's need for closeness and tactile stimulation. After the second month of life, the infant begins to equate mother with food. Feeding schedules vary: the newborn usually eats about 5 times a day and should soon sleep through the night. After age 3 months, the infant will be able to swallow with less tongue protrusion. At this age, the infant will recognize the bottle as a source of food and will not readily accept a cup. Feeding the infant should fit into the everyday schedule of the family. The infant may be fed by breast or bottle, or by a combination of both. A major goal of home care is to provide the family with the confidence to meet the nutritional needs of the infant with a minimum of disruption to normal routine.

Assessment of Self-Care Potential

Client/Family Assessment

- Assess the feelings of the family regarding the newborn. Determine if the baby was planned and anticipated or if the birth was unplanned and perhaps viewed as an inconvenience.
- Assess the feelings of the family toward feeding of infants. Some families have a tradition of breast-feeding their children. Those in the family who do not follow this practice may be looked upon with disfavor. There are also families in which breast-feeding is considered inappropriate and inconvenient to schedules and socialization. The mother who decides to breast-feed in this family may be regarded as unusual and inconsiderate of the rest of the family.
- Assess the schedule and priorities of the family. If the new mother will return to work very soon after birth, infant feeding may be affected.
- Assess the knowledge level of the new family regarding methods of feeding, how often to feed, and how to handle feeding problems.
- Assess the financial resources of the family. Determine if the family is able to purchase prepared formula and disposable bottles. Assess their knowledge of the various types of formulas and the relative expense of each.

Physical Assessment

- Assess the infant's abilty to take food orally. If the infant was born in a hospital, this will have been established. However, the introduction of new foods takes place in the home. Assess sucking and swallowing abilities. If the infant has physical disabilities that inhibit sucking and swallowing, assess the degree of disability and the needs of the family in regard to the infant's condition.
- Assess the adequacy of the breast-feeding mother to meet the infant's nutritional needs. Assess her knowledge of breast-feeding and her understanding of infection control and care of the breasts.

Environmental Assessment

- Assess the kitchen area where formula will be prepared. Assess the type of formula selected for feeding and the storage facilities. Determine if the home has a refrigerator in which to keep the formula cold. Determine if they have a dishwasher or water hot enough to clean and disinfect the bottles used.
- Assess the feeding area for the infant. Determine whether the infant will be fed in a communal group with the family. Assess the level of understanding of the family regarding the socialization needs of the infant and the relationship of the feeding process to early socialization.

Planning Strategies

Potential Nursing Diagnoses

Alteration in nutrition, potential for more or less than body requirements

Alteration in bowel elimination, diarrhea or constipation due to introduction of new foods

Expected Outcomes

Adequate nutrition as evidenced by weight gains consistent with expected patterns

Prevention of gastrointestinal problems

Introduction to and acceptance of a wide variety of foods

Health Promotion Goals

- The client and family will
  Meet the nutritional needs of the infant while meeting the socialization and affection needs as well
  Include the infant as an interacting member of the family group with individual needs and potential for contribution
  Assist the infant to develop an acceptance of a variety of foods to promote a well-balanced diet
  Learn how to feed the infant safely and to evaluate the infant's tolerance of new foods

Equipment

Formula or food (See Technique 20, Breast-Feeding, for consideration of breast-feeding the infant.)

High chair and bib (for finger foods)

Child's feeding utensils (for solid foods)

Interventions/Health Promotion

ACTION	RATIONALE/AMPLIFICATION
1. Advise the mother to wash her hands before feeding the baby. Provide a comfortable chair, preferably one with arms (Fig. 23-1). Check to be sure that the baby is clean and dry before feeding.	Microorganisms found on the hands of adults may be injurious to the infant, whose immune system is immature. Handwashing will remove most of these microorganisms. Providing a position of comfort for the mother with the arms supported makes the feeding session more enjoyable and relaxing for mother and baby.

ACTION   **RATIONALE/AMPLIFICATION**

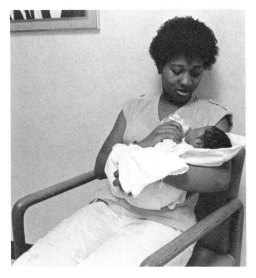

Figure 23.1

2. Show the mother how to hold the infant snugly in the crook of her arm. The bottle is held with the other hand. The arm supporting the infant's head may be rested against the arm of the chair. The infant's head should always be kept on a higher plane than the rest of its body (Fig. 23-2).

Holding the infant during feeding promotes a feeling of trust and security in the infant. If the infant's head is held higher than the rest of the body, there is less chance of the infant choking because gravity will facilitate swallowing.

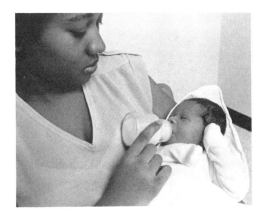

Figure 23.2

3. Gently insert the nipple along the infant's tongue. The opening in the nipple should be large enough for the feeding to flow smoothly, but it should not be so large that excessive formula fills the infant's mouth. The bottle should be held at an angle so that the nipple is always filled with formula.

The infant's sucking efforts should result in adequate feeding. If the opening in the nipple is too small, aggressive but unproductive sucking will soon tire the infant. If the opening is too large, the infant may become choked. If the nipple becomes filled with air, the infant will suck and swallow the air, resulting in gastric discomfort.

ACTION	*RATIONALE/AMPLIFICATION*
4. Feed the infant slowly. Allow an opportunity for the removal of swallowed air during the feeding by removing the bottle and "burping" the baby. Place the infant against either shoulder and gently pat the middle and upper back. The infant may also be placed in a sitting position with the head supported or in the prone position with the head supported to facilitate breathing (Figs. 23-3, 23-4, and 23-5). Gentle patting or stroking of the infant's back is sufficient to assist the infant in removal of swallowed air. This procedure may be done at the beginning of the feeding, after 1 oz of formula has been fed, and after the feeding has been completed.	Air trapped in the gastrointestinal tract can cause cramping and discomfort. Slight pressure on the infant's stomach and gentle patting or stroking of the back will aid in the removal of this swallowed air. Too much pressure or too vigorous stimulation may cause regurgitation. Since the infant's neck muscles are immature, the head of the infant must be supported.

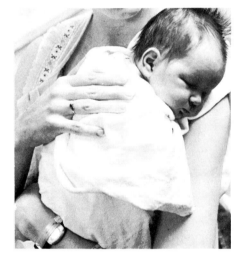

Figure 23.3

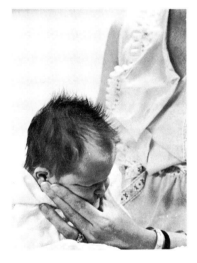

Figure 23.4

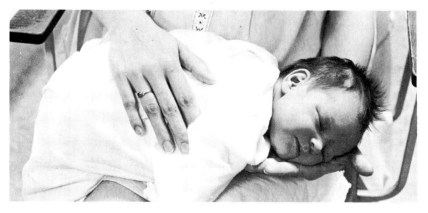

Figure 23.5

ACTION

5. Advise the mother to avoid over-feeding the infant. The formula should be at room temperature or slightly warmer. Ready-to-feed formulas at room temperature do not require warming. Refrigerated formulas should be warmed by heating the bottle of formula in a pan of water. The formula should feel warm to the touch when dropped onto the inner aspect of the mother's arm. After feeding, allow the infant to rest quietly.

6. As the infant grows older, new foods will be introduced. Advise the mother to introduce new foods by offering the new food first in a small amount, such as 1 or 2 spoonfuls. At subsequent meals the new food can be given in greater quantities. New foods should be started one at a time.

7. The sitting infant may be fed in a high chair at the family table. Place the infant in the chair and secure the restraining strap immediately. Allow the infant to touch the food and to engage in self-feeding as much as possible.

RATIONALE/AMPLIFICATION

Overfeeding causes abdominal discomfort and regurgitation. Cold formula may cause abdominal cramping. Allowing the infant to rest after feeding minimizes the danger of overtiring and allows the infant's energy to be channeled to digestion.

The introduction of new foods not only broadens the child's diet, but also offers an opportunity for the child to experience new tastes and textures. It also provides an opportunity to test for allergies. If the child does have an allergy, the reaction may be less severe if only a small quantity of the food is given. If more than one new food is offered at the same meal, it is impossible to differentiate which of the new foods may be causing the allergic reaction.

The greatest risk in the use of high chairs is the possibility of the infant falling. If the tray of the high chair is removed to place the infant in the chair, restraint of the infant is necessary while retrieving and reattaching the tray. The active infant can slip from the grasp of a distracted adult very suddenly. Constant attention to the possibility of falls is the best prevention. The desire to touch and explore food is a natural part of an infant's development.

Related Care

Formula Preparation

1. Before preparing formula, careful handwashing is essential. Clean the area where the formula will be prepared thoroughly with a clean damp cloth.

2. Follow the directions on the formula package when preparing. Although many packages still contain the directions for sterilizing the water before diluting powdered or concentrated formula, sterilizing is

Microorganisms may contaminate the feedings through direct contact with unclean objects.

Sterilization of tap water may decrease the normal fluoride content and should be avoided unless there is a chance that the tap water may be contaminated.

ACTION	*RATIONALE/AMPLIFICATION*
not recommended unless the sanitation conditions in the home may compromise the safety of the newborn. In these cases, sterile water should be used. Sterilized water may be purchased or tap water may be sterilized by boiling it in a clean pan for 5 minutes. Under normal circumstances, the formula may be diluted with unsterilized tap water. The pediatric nurse practitioner or pediatrician will usually prescribe the type of formula to be used.	
3. Formula should be at room temperature for feeding. The ready-to-feed bottle does not require refrigeration and may be fed to the infant as soon as it is opened. Reconstituted formula may be prepared with water at room temperature and may be fed at once. Refrigerated feedings should be warmed to room temperature by placing them in boiling water for a few minutes.	The infant usually prefers feedings that are of a consistent nature. As the infant grows older, formula directly from the refrigerator may be acceptable. Refrigerated formula should be heated to room temperature rather than removing it from the refrigerator and allowing it to warm to room temperature slowly, since microorganisms can grow during the time it takes for the milk to warm up.
4. Milk solids can coat the sides of the bottle during heating of the formula. If the bottles are not cleaned immediately after use, this film will adhere to the sides of the bottle and may result in contaminated formula. To prevent this, rinse the bottle, cap, and nipple immediately after use and place them to soak in warm, soapy water until they can be washed.	Contamination with heat-resistant organisms may cause digestive problems for the infant because these microorganisms are transmitted through the contaminated formula.
5. Bottles, nipples, caps, and collars should be washed with warm, soapy water and rinsed well in hot water. A brush may be used to remove milk solids. This should be done in a clean basin. The bottles may also be washed separately from other dishes in the dishwasher. Water should be forced through the hole in the nipple to ensure that the opening is cleaned.	Water and soap are usually sufficient to remove most microorganisms. The water in the dishwasher should be hot enough to ensure that the bottles are cleaned efficiently, or the bottles should be cleaned with a brush before being placed in the dishwasher.

ACTION

RATIONALE/AMPLIFICATION

6. Proper storage or disposal of unused portions of formula is very important. Cover unused portions of cans of formula and store them in the refrigerator for no longer than 24 hours. Open containers of powder may be covered and stored in a cool, dry place indefinitely. Unused portions of feedings should be discarded. If several bottles of formula are prepared at one time, those not used immediately may be stored in the refrigerator until needed.

Refrigeration will retard the growth of microorganisms. Open containers of liquids should not be kept longer than 24 hours because of the danger of spoilage and contamination. After a bottle of formula has been warmed to room temperature and the formula fed to the infant over a period of 30 minutes to 1 hour, the chances of contamination are great. These unused feedings should not be kept for later. It is safer to use a new bottle of formula for each feeding.

Age-Specific Modifications

Low-birth-weight infants require special skill and patience during feeding. These infants tire easily, and they generally must be fed smaller amounts at more frequent intervals. Encourage the family to adjust to the infant's needs and abilities. Techniques for stimulating the infant to eat include gently pressing the nipple against the roof of the infant's mouth, gently lifting the infant's chin during feeding, and changing the infant's position frequently. Reassure the family that the infant's low birth weight is no indication that the infant will always be small.

Low-birth-weight infants expend a great deal of energy on metabolism as their immature organs attempt to adjust to extrauterine life. The additional energy required to suck on the bottle or breast will soon deplete the infant's energy resources. Patience and understanding are essential in adequately nourishing these special infants.

**Education/
Communication**

• Teach the client and family to
Successfully feed the infant. Explain the procedure for "burping" the infant. Be sure that the family understands that very gently patting and stroking the infant's back is sufficient to assist the infant in removing the trapped air. Caution them against vigorously hitting the infant's back because this may cause structural damage to the infant's back and ribs and may cause regurgitation.
Observe the infant's tolerance to feedings. Explain how to determine if the formula is being ingested too quickly or too slowly. Show them how to change the rate by changing the size of the hole in the nipple.
Understand the importance of holding the infant during every feeding. The primary developmental task of the infant is the development of trust. The tactile stimulation and the closeness of the parent who is feeding the infant promote feelings of trust and enhance the parent–infant relationship. Discourage the practice of propping the bottle.

Safely and effectively prepare infant feedings. Encourage frequent handwashing, especially before preparing the feeding and before feeding the infant. Be sure the family understands the differences among the various commercial formulas. It is essential that the dilution instructions accompanying the formula be followed correctly. If too much diluent is added to the concentrated formula, the infant will not be receiving the required amount of nutrients. Underdilution may cause an increase in renal solute, with ensuing dehydration.

Understand the special needs of the low-birth-weight infant. Explain that a flexible schedule is essential with frequent feedings. Encourage the family to be patient and flexible. Above all, assist the mother who has guilt feelings about having produced an infant who has problems to see the positive side of the situation. Emphasize that being small at birth is in no way indicative of the future size of the child or adult.

Identify when to introduce new foods to the growing infant. Encourage the family to follow the schedule recommended by their pediatric care provider. Emphasize the need to provide a well-balanced diet. The tendency is to give the baby those foods that are tasty and desired; however, these are usually fruits and foods to which sugar has been added. Although these foods may have a place in the child's diet, it is important for the child to gain an acceptance of vegetables, meats, and cereals.

Referrals and Consultations

In order to conserve strength and build up the autoimmune system, the low-birth-weight infant may stay in the hospital for several weeks after the mother comes home. After discharge from the health-care center, follow-up by a neonatal nurse practitioner may be of help to the new mother faced with a special child with special feeding problems.

Follow-up visits to a pediatric nurse practitioner or a pediatrician will help ensure that the infant is gaining weight and growing at the expected rate. These visits also allow the infant to be monitored for normal development and immunizations.

Evaluation of Health Promotion Activities

Quality Assurance/ Reassessment

One of the best indicators of adequate nutrition is weight gain. The newborn will usually lose several ounces immediately after birth; however, for the next few years, the infant will steadily grow and gain weight. Periods of weight loss are usually associated with illness. If the infant loses weight for no apparent reason, a pediatric nurse practitioner or pediatrician should be consulted.

- Evaluate the understanding of the family regarding preparation and storage of formula by checking the refrigerator when visiting the home. Formula bottles should be covered. Ready-to-feed formula does not require refrigeration unless it has been opened. Concentrated formula should be mixed according to the package directions. Observe the mother mixing the formula to ascertain her understanding of the proper procedure.

- Observe care of used bottles. After a feeding, the bottle should be emptied and soaked in hot water. Observe the cleaning of the bottles to determine whether they are cleaned in a dishwasher on the hot cycle or manually with hot, sudsy water and a bottle brush capable of reaching to the bottom of the bottle.

- Observe the family during meals. Determine the role of the infant or small child in the social structure of mealtimes. Observe the manner in which the child is encourged to experiment with new foods and to be involved in the meal.

DOCUMENTATION

Charting for the Home Health Nurse
- Record the weight and height of the child at each visit. Such a record will provide an opportunity to determine if the child is following expected patterns.

Records Kept by the Client/Family
If dietary problems are anticipated or experienced, the family may be asked to keep a record of the dates when new foods are introduced to the infant and the amounts of the new foods given. This record can be kept in a small spiral notebook and can be used by the home health nurse or pediatric care provider to assess the child's nutritional schedule.

Health Teaching Checklist

Name of Care Provider _____

Relationship to Client _____ Telephone #_____

Taught by _____ Date _____

	EXPLAINED	DEMONSTRATED
Type of feeding		
Bottle	_____	
Breast	_____	
Technique for preparing the feeding	_____	_____
Technique for feeding	_____	_____
Technique for "burping" the baby	_____	_____
Importance of holding the infant for feeding	_____	
Possible feeding problems		
Regurgitation	_____	
Cramping	_____	
Choking	_____	
Cyanosis	_____	

Product Availability

Formulas may be purchased in most grocery stores in powder, concentrate, and ready-to-feed forms. If the infant requires a special type of formula, it can usually be ordered through a pharmacy or hospital.

24

Right Atrial Catheter

Background

Clients requiring long-term venous access for medication administration, cancer chemotherapy, or total parenteral nutrition (TPN) may be dismissed from the hospital with indwelling right atrial catheters (RAC) specifically developed for long-term home care use. Hickman, Broviac, and Centracil catheters are the most commonly used. The Hickman and Broviac catheters are similar in design, except that the lumen of the Broviac catheter is smaller than that of the Hickman. A double-lumen Hickman catheter is also available, providing one route for continuous infusion and a second lumen for intermittent use.

The Hickman and Broviac catheters are placed surgically in the operating room. The catheter is advanced through a long subcutaneous tunnel into the superior vena cava or right atrium. The catheter design is similar to the Tenckhoff catheter used for home peritoneal dialysis and features a Dacron mesh cuff that assists in stabilizing the catheter in the subcutaneous tissue (Fig. 24-1). Eventually, fibrous tissue will infiltrate the cuff. The location of the exit site away from the venipuncture site decreases the risk of infection of the vascular system. The Centracil catheter does not have a cuff.

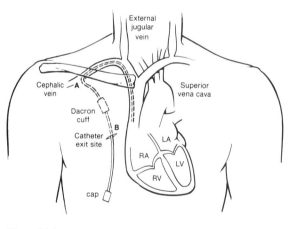

Figure 24.1
Right atrial catheter.

Catheters not used for continuous infusion are heparinized periodically to prevent clotting. Strict sterile technique is mandatory when changing the dressing or the injection cap to prevent infection and septicemia.

Assessment of Self-Care Potential

Client/Family Assessment

- Assess the willingness and the ability of family members to assist the client in caring for the catheter. Sterile technique is more difficult to maintain if the client has to perform the dressing changes. Determine whether using sterile gloves or a "no touch" technique will be more suitable for dressing changes.
- Determine how much assistance from the home health nurse will be needed for the family to care for the catheter successfully.

- Determine whether the client's altered body image has been accepted by the client and family. Feelings about the catheter will depend on the reason for the insertion of the catheter. For example, if the client is suffering from cancer many other issues will intervene, such as the fear of dying.
- Estimate whether the client or family can meet the expenses of the equipment involved in caring for the catheter site. Trying to cut costs inappropriately, such as saving sterile 4 × 4s from an opened dressing tray, may lead to breaks in sterile technique. Is third-party payment available?
- Determine which equipment will be provided by the home health agency and what can be purchased from a local pharmacy by the family.

Physical Assessment

- Assess the insertion site and subcutaneous tract for redness, swelling, or purulent drainage. Check for signs of thrombosis.
- Assess for catheter integrity, including displacement. Assess heart sounds for cardiac murmurs due to tricuspid valve injury.
- Monitor vital signs for signs of infection (e.g., increased pulse rate, elevated temperature).
- If client is receiving chemotherapy, assess for complications of the drugs.
- If the client is on TPN, assess for local, systemic, and metabolic side-effects (see Technique 22, Home Parenteral Nutrition). Monitor daily weight.

Environmental Assessment

- Assess the home environment for cleanliness. If standard sanitary practices are not followed in the home, the client may be at less risk if the dressings are performed on an outpatient basis or by the home health nurse personally.
- Determine a suitable area for dressing changes. Avoid areas where aerosols may be used or areas by open windows where dust can be a problem. All vacuuming and cleaning procedures should be completed 2 hours before giving catheter care to allow dust to settle. If a reading lamp is to be used to provide extra light, damp dust the lamp periodically.
- Determine that suitable handwashing facilities are available adjacent to where catheter care will be given. Provide paper towels if a supply of freshly laundered towels cannot be provided.

Planning Strategies

Potential Nursing Diagnoses

Infection (local or systemic), potential for: related to indwelling central venous catheter

Home maintenance management, impaired

Knowledge deficit related to indwelling RAC

Self-concept, disturbance in body image, related to indwelling RAC

Expected Outcomes

Prevention of local or systemic infection

Maintenance of a patent right atrial catheter free from infection

Understanding of protocols for caring for the right atrial catheter in the home setting

Acceptance of body-image changes

Health Promotion Goals

- The client and family will
  Redress the catheter site, using strict sterile technique, every other day, when soiled or wet, and if the dressing comes loose
  Implement appropriate protocols in caring for the right atrial catheter

Equipment

For dressing change and site care
    Paper bag for disposal of dressing
    RAC disposable dressing tray, or individually wrapped alcohol prep sponges,
        iodophor prep swab sticks, precut 2 × 2s, iodophor ointment (unit dose),
        sterile pickups, sterile plastic clamp, scissors (cleaned with alcohol)
    Tape or transparent dressing
    Optional: Steridrape (transparent adhesive surgical drape) or foam postoper-
        ative dressing (Op-Site)

For emergency kit (in a resealable plastic bag)
    Plastic clamps
    Syringe of premixed heparin solution, or heparin solution, 5-ml syringe in
        sterile package, Needles (20 gauge × 1 inch, 25 gauge x ⅝ inch) in sterile
        packages
    Alcohol and iodophor prep pads (2 each)
    Roll of 1 inch tape
    Sterile injection cap

For heparinizing the catheter
    Tubex syringe and unit-dose heparin flushes, or heparin solution, 5-ml
        syringe, 25-gauge and 20-gauge needles
    Alcohol and iodophor wipes
    (A standard strength for a heparin flush has not been determined. If a pre-
        mixed flush is not used, use 1 unit of heparin to 1 ml of saline. Premix
        this in a vial and label for client use.)

For catheter removal
    Clamp
    Suture set (if applicable)
    Sterile 4 × 4s
    Sterile specimen container
    Sterile culture tube (if applicable)
    Dressing supplies

For clearing a clotted catheter
    Clamp (Centracil uses a 10-cm extension tube with built-in plastic slide
        clamp.)
    Sterile saline for injection
    Heparin solution (or unit-dose heparin flush)
    5-ml syringes (2)
    Sterile replacement injection cap
    Iodophor and alcohol wipes
    Sterile gloves
    Sterile towel

For changing the injection cap
    Clamp
    Sterile replacement injection cap
    Alcohol and iodophor wipes

For catheter repair
    Clamp
    Iodophor wipes
    Alcohol wipes
    Hickman repair kit containing catheter tubing, splicing sleeve, tube of adhe-
        sive, syringe, blunt needle (Repair kits are steam autoclaved. Autoclave
        kits ahead of time so they will be available in an emergency.)
    Sterile injection cap
    Sterile surgical gloves (2) (if used)
    Sterile towel
    Sterile suture set, or sterile scalpel or scissors
    Sterile 4 × 4s
    Mask (optional)

Interventions/Health Promotion

ACTION	RATIONALE/AMPLIFICATION
1. Assist the client to a comfortable, semireclining position. Place an open paper bag close by.	Select a well-lighted area in the home to permit adequate inspection of the catheter. The paper bag will be used for discarding the old dressing and used swab sticks.
Wash hands thoroughly.	Use a freshly laundered hand towel or paper towel to dry your hands.
2. Place the dressing tray on a clean, dry surface. Unwrap the tray without touching the inner, sterile contents, or open individual packages leaving the contents on the inner, sterile surface.	The inside of the wrapper will be used as a sterile field. Be careful not to touch the inside of the wrapper with anything, including the dressing that is removed.
3. Remove the old dressing and discard it in the paper bag. Check the site for signs of infection (redness or drainage).	Take care not to place tension on the catheter during removal of the dressing. This could dislodge the catheter. Do not touch the catheter insertion site while removing the dressing (Fig. 24-2). This would contaminate the site.

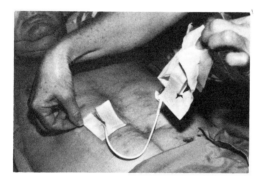

Figure 24.2
Removing the soiled dressing from the Hickman catheter using a "no-touch" technique.

ACTION	RATIONALE/AMPLIFICATION
4. Wash and dry hands. Put on the sterile gloves.	The sterile gloves will be the first item in the sterile package. An alternative method is to use a "no-touch" technique in place of sterile gloves. The insertion site is dressed using sterile pickups. The distal end of the catheter can be touched with the ungloved hand, but *not* the insertion site.
5. Remove an alcohol swab stick from its package. Clean the site using a circular pattern starting at the catheter insertion site and finishing about 4 cm away from the catheter insertion site. Check the swab stick for color or debris.	This prevents a soiled swab stick from coming in contact with the insertion site. Alcohol is used to defat and disinfect the skin. Hydrogen peroxide can be substituted for alcohol to clean around the catheter.

ACTION	RATIONALE/AMPLIFICATION
Discard the swab in the paper bag without touching the bag with the gloved hands. Repeat the cleaning process until there is no color on the swab stick. Allow the alcohol to dry.	
6. Repeat the cleaning technique using iodophor swab sticks. Use 2 swab sticks to clean the site (Fig. 24-3). Clean the first 8 cm of the catheter using the remaining swab stick. Allow the iodophor solution to dry.	Iodophor is used to disinfect the skin surrounding the insertion site. Clean away from the insertion site. Do not blot the iodophor solution from the skin. It is effective while in contact with the skin.

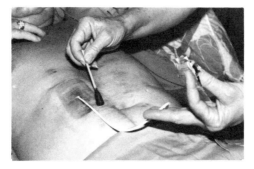

Figure 24.3
Cleaning around the Hickman catheter using a "bull's eye" pattern with the insertion site at the center.

ACTION	RATIONALE/AMPLIFICATION
7. Apply a small amount of iodophor ointment directly over the insertion site. Dress the insertion site using precut 2 × 2s, using the sterile pickups or the gloved hand. Coil the excess catheter on the 2 × 2s to prevent accidental removal (Fig. 24-4).	Iodophor ointment retards the growth of bacteria and fungus.

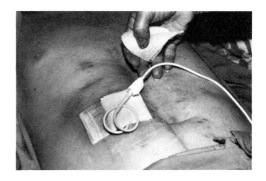

Figure 24.4
Coiling the Hickman catheter to prevent accidental removal if tension is applied to the catheter.

ACTION	RATIONALE/AMPLIFICATION
8. Cover the insertion site and the surrounding area with the clear plastic dressing (Fig. 24-5).	Alternative: cover the site with 4 × 4s and tape. If a draining wound or tracheostomy is present, cover the dressing with a Steridrape to waterproof the site. Give tracheostomy care before dressing the catheter to minimize the chance of coughing and contamination of the site. Do not change any other dressings at the same time as the RAC. This must be a separate technique to minimize the chance of infection.

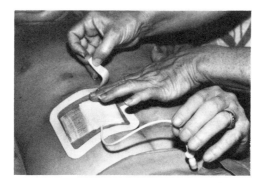

Figure 24.5
Dressing the Hickman catheter using a transparent dressing.

ACTION	RATIONALE/AMPLIFICATION
Tape the catheter securely to the chest or, if foam postoperative dressing is used, clip the corners of the dressing and double back about 2 cm of the foam dressing to form a pocket. Coil the catheter and place it in the pocket (Fig. 24-6).	This prevents tension on the catheter and accidental removal. Avoid putting any type of adhesive-backed tape or dressing directly on the nipple. Taping the catheter to the chest rather than coiling it under the dressing facilitates home management and presents less chance of disturbing the catheter during catheter care procedures.

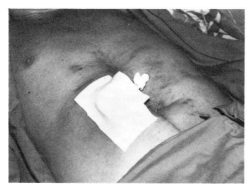

Figure 24.6
Excess catheter is coiled and retained in a tape "pocket" built into the dressing.

ACTION	RATIONALE/AMPLIFICATION
9. Remove the gloves and place them on the used dressing tray. Rewrap the tray and discard it in the paper bag. Close the paper bag securely and discard it in the trash.	Do not retain any unused items on the tray for later dressing changes. Always use wrapped, sterile supplies to prevent infection.

ACTION	*RATIONALE/AMPLIFICATION*

Related Care

Wrap the catheter with a piece of tape 1 cm wide, about 4 cm from the injection cap. When clamping the catheter, place the clamps over the tape.

This protects the catheter from damage caused by clamping it.

Heparinizing the Catheter

Heparinize the catheter daily:
- Clean the top of the heparin solution bottle, first with an alcohol wipe and then with iodophor.

This keeps the catheter patent.
This disinfects the rubber stopper.

- Assemble a sterile syringe and 20-gauge needle. Remove the cover from the needle and withdraw 2 cc of air into the syringe.
- Insert the needle into the center of the heparin vial and insert the 2 cc of air into the vial. Turn the bottle and syringe upside down and allow 2 ml of the heparin solution to flow into the syringe.

Alternative: if unit-dose heparin flushes are used, allow one flush to reach room temperature. Insert the preloaded barrel into the Tubex syringe, and remove the needle cap. Expel any air before injecting the catheter with the heparin flush.

- Remove the needle and syringe from the bottle and replace the needle cover. Remove the 20-gauge needle from the syringe and discard. Replace it with the smaller 25-gauge needle.
- Remove the needle cover and expel any air from the syringe. Replace the needle cover and let the heparin come to room temperature.

This takes approximately 20 minutes. Do not place the syringe in direct sunlight to warm. This can destroy the heparin.
Allow the iodophor to dry.

- Clean the injection cap of the catheter with an alcohol wipe, followed by iodophor.
- Insert the needle into the injection cap as far as it will go.

To avoid damage to the injection cap, use only the 25-gauge needle in the injection cap.

- Slowly inject the heparin solution into the catheter.
- Clamp the catheter gently on the taped section.
- Remove the needle and syringe and unclamp the catheter.

Avoid the plastic connector on the end of the catheter.
Removing the needle and syringe without clamping the catheter can cause blood to back up into the catheter and cause it to clot.

- Secure the catheter to the chest with tape.

Be sure the catheter is not kinked to prevent clotting.

Catheter Removal

Remove the catheter when ordered by the physician:

- Clamp the catheter and withdraw it using steady, even pressure.

If a Centracil catheter is used, clip the sutures securing the catheter before withdrawing the catheter.

ACTION

- Using sterile scissors or a scalpel, clip the tip of the catheter and allow it to drop into a sterile container.
- Deliver the specimen to a laboratory for culture. Obtain a sensitivity report if the culture is positive.
- Control the minimal amount of bleeding caused by the removal of the cuff with local pressure and a sterile 4 × 4.
- After removal, clean the site and apply iodophor ointment and a sterile dressing.
- Inspect the catheter to determine that the complete length was removed.

Clearing a Clotted Catheter

Attempt to clear a clotted catheter:
- Don sterile gloves. Drape the catheter with a sterile towel.
- Clean the distal end of the catheter and injection cap with alcohol and iodophor.
- Remove the injection cap, taking care to maintain the sterility of the catheter tip.
- Connect a syringe directly to the catheter and attempt to withdraw the clot. *Do not flush the catheter.*
- Maintain suction on the catheter until blood is observed in the syringe. Clamp the catheter over a piece of tape.
- Cap the catheter with a sterile replacement injection cap.
- Remove the clamp and heparinize the catheter.

Changing the Injection Cap

Change the injection cap weekly before heparinizing the catheter:
- Gently clamp the catheter where the piece of tape has been placed on the catheter.
- Grasp the end of the catheter between the index finger and thumb. Clean the connection with the alcohol wipes for 1 minute, followed by iodophor. Allow the iodophor to air dry.
- Open the package containing the replacement cap and leave it in the bottom half of the package.

RATIONALE/AMPLIFICATION

Obtain a separate culture of any drainage if present.

The Centracil catheter does not have a cuff. Pressure at the site will still be required.

This disinfects the catheter.

Flushing the catheter can release the clot into the circulation, causing an embolus.
If blood flows freely into the syringe, the clot has been removed. Clamping the catheter over a piece of tape protects the catheter.

For a Centracil catheter clamp the catheter using the plastic slide clamp on the extension tubing.
This disinfects the catheter. Use friction.

ACTION	*RATIONALE/AMPLIFICATION*
• Unscrew the old injection cap and discard it. Pick up the new cap, touching only the outside rubber part. Remove the protective cap from the insertion end of the new cap and discard it. Screw the new injection cap on the catheter, being careful not to touch the tip of the catheter or the injection cap.	If the new injection cap is accidentally contaminated, discard it and use a fresh package.
• Heparinize the catheter.	

Catheter Repair

If a sterilized repair kit is not immediately available

• Place a piece of tape on the catheter close to the chest wall and clamp the catheter.	
• Insert a 14-gauge intravenous angiocath into the damaged catheter and remove the stylet. Tape the angiocath securely and flush it with heparin solution.	The catheter can be used while the repair kit is obtained or the flush syringe left in place.

Catheters damaged more than 4 cm from the chest wall can be repaired as follows:

• Flush the catheter with heparin solution. Clamp the catheter close to the chest wall over a piece of tape.	The tape protects the catheter from damage from the clamps.
• Create a sterile field using the sterile towel. Open sterile 4 × 4s, alcohol and iodophor wipes, sterile scissors or scalpel, and new injection cap onto the sterile field.	
• Wear a mask and sterile surgical gloves.	
• Clean the catheter with alcohol wipes followed by iodophor.	
• Change to another pair of sterile gloves and remove the powder from the gloves with a sterile alcohol wipe.	Glove powder weakens the adhesive used for catheter repair.
• Load the syringe barrel with 1 ml of adhesive and insert the plunger into the barrel. Attach the blunted needle to the syringe. Set aside for later use.	
• Using the scalpel or scissors, cut the catheter just proximal to the damaged section (Fig. 24-7). Trim the replacement tubing to the required length.	When the catheter is repaired, the catheter should extend no more than 15 cm to 20 cm from the chest wall.

ACTION	RATIONALE/AMPLIFICATION
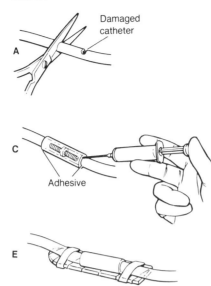	

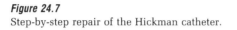

Figure 24.7
Step-by-step repair of the Hickman catheter.

• Connect the damaged catheter and the replacement tubing with the connector.	Insert the connector all the way to the center ridge to make sure the repair will be secure.
• Apply adhesive liberally over the area of the center ridge. Slide the loose splicing sleeve on the replacement segment over the connector.	The center ridge should be in the center of the splicing sleeve.
• Inject adhesive under the sleeve from both ends.	
• Roll the sleeve in your fingers to spread the adhesive. Wipe the excess with a 4 × 4.	
• Replace the sterile injection cap.	
• Splint the joint with a protected tongue blade and tape for 48 hours.	This protects the joint until the adhesive achieves maximum strength. *Do not use the catheter for infusion for 2 hours after the repair.*
• Before using the catheter, remove any air remaining in the replacement segment with a syringe until blood fills the entire segment. Flush the catheter with heparin solution.	

**Education/
Communication**

• Teach the client and family to

Perform all RAC catheter care that is within their capabilities

Carry an emergency kit at all times when away from home

Check temperature and pulse daily to monitor for infection

Observe the site daily for signs of infection if using a transparent dressing

Inspect the site during the dressing change if using tape for the dressing

Wash hands thoroughly and dry with a freshly laundered towel before performing any catheter care procedure

Heparinize the catheter daily unless a continuous infusion is in progress.

Keep the heparin solution or unit-dose heparin flushes in the refrigerator.

Bring to room temperature before use.

Change the injection cap weekly to prevent infection or leakage from the catheter

Prevent accidental cutting of the catheter. Do not use scissors around catheter.

Hold pressure on the site with sterile 4 × 4s if the catheter is accidentally removed

Always use smooth-edged clamps when clamping the catheter to prevent damage

Clamp the catheter if it is damaged or develops a leak or if the injection cap is accidentally disconnected. Tape the catheter above the leak, and clamp it at the taped site.

Take tub baths and avoid getting the dressing wet. Wetting the dressing can cause an infection.

Temporarily discontinue strenuous activities requiring use of the arms to prevent accidental catheter removal (e.g., golf, racquet ball, tennis). Substitute less strenuous activities such as brisk walking.

Notify the home health nurse immediately if the catheter is damaged or accidentally removed, or if signs of infection are noted. A damaged catheter must be repaired as soon as possible to prevent clotting.

- Reassure the client and family that
  The only real emergency is blood leaking from the catheter. This is no longer an emergency situation once the catheter is clamped.
  Catheter care can be accomplished with minimal lifestyle changes
  Negative feelings about the catheter are normal. Allow time and privacy for the client to verbalize feelings about altered body image and lifestyle changes.

Referrals and Consultations

- Tell the client to report any problems with the catheter to the home health nurse as soon as possible. The nurse will determine whether a medical consultation or culture of the catheter is necessary. If the nurse or physician is unavailable in an emergency, refer the client to a local emergency room. Make emergency telephone numbers available.

- Refer the client on cancer chemotherapy to the American Cancer Society for assistance in providing equipment for dressing changes.

- Refer the pediatric client to the homeroom teacher or school nurse if problems with the catheter develop while at school. Teach appropriate school personnel how to deal with an emergency situation, and tell them how to contact the home health nurse for assistance.

- Refer the pediatric client who is too ill to remain in school to the homebound education program.

Evaluation of Health Promotion Activities

Quality Assurance/ Reassessment

- Periodically observe the caregiver's catheter care technique to ensure adherence to infection-control and safety standards. Inspect the site for signs of infection.

- Culture the catheter insertion site if drainage is present.

- Refer an infected catheter to the physician to determine possible removal.

DOCUMENTATION

Charting for the Home Health Nurse

Progress of the client/family in assuming responsibility for the procedures

Psychological responses of the family and client regarding lifestyle or body-image changes

Condition of the insertion site and patency of the catheter

Ability to purchase the required equipment

Health Teaching Checklist

Name of Care Provider _____

Relationship to Client _____ Telephone #_____

Taught by _____ Date _____

	EXPLAINED	DEMONSTRATED
Rationale for RAC placement	_____	
Dressing technique	_____	_____
Infection control techniques	_____	_____
Skin care	_____	_____
Changing the injection cap	_____	_____
Heparinizing the catheter	_____	_____
Complications to report	_____	
Emergency care	_____	
Preparation when away from home	_____	
Giving TPN using the RAC (if appropriate)	_____	
Cancer chemotherapy schedule, side-effects, and treatment	_____	
Modifications in ADL (if any)	_____	
Emergency measures for homeroom teacher/school nurse (pediatric)	_____	
(if appropriate)	_____	

Product Availability

Leur Lock Extension Set
(For use with Centracil)
Quest Medical, Inc.
Carrollton, TX 75006

Hickman Catheter Repair Kit
Evermed
PO Box 296
Medina, WA 98039

Selected References

Anderson MA, Aker SN, Hickman RO: The double-lumen Hickman catheter. Am J Nurs 82(2):272–275, 1982

Vogel TC, Mckimming SA: Teaching parents to give indwelling C.V. catheter care. Nursing '83 13(1):55–56, 1983

25   Tube Feeding

Background

Because of escalating health-care costs and changes in third-party payment for hospitalization (e.g., DRGs), many people are candidates for home nutritional support programs. Some degree of malnutrition occurs in conjunction with many health problems, including anorexia, malabsorptive or hypermetabolic conditions, radiation therapy, or cancer chemotherapy. Protein–calorie malnutrition leads to problems with cell-mediated immunity, an increased chance of infection, and delayed wound healing.

Tube Feeding Routes

For persons requiring nutritional support, tube feeding is a more physiologic, safer, simpler, and comparatively more economical alternative to home parenteral nutrition (HPN). If the absorptive surface of the gut is intact, enteral feeding is an option. The feeding route can be established by surgical placement of a feeding tube or by inserting a tube through the nose into the stomach (nasogastric tube) or intestine (nasoduodenal or nasojejunal tube). The development of fine-bore, pliable, weighted feeding tubes has facilitated long-term enteral feeding. To place a tube into the intestine, a tube with a bolus weight is required. Intestinal motility carries the tube through the pylorus and into the intestine. Methods of surgical tube placement include gastrostomy, jejunostomy, and esophagostomy. Depending on the specific surgical procedure, some gastrostomy tubes can be removed between feedings.

Enteral Feeding Formulas

There are several categories of commercially available formulas: blenderized, milk-based, lactose-free, complete formulas with predigested nutrients, special formulas for persons with liver or renal disorders, and modular feedings such as protein that can be used to individualize feedings. The small intestine is more sensitive than the stomach to both the volume and osmolality of the formula. Enteric (intestinal) feedings consist of predigested nutrients, are usually low in osmolality, and must be delivered at a continuous rate when infused directly into the intestine. Isotonic formulas are more easily tolerated and do not have to be diluted as much as hypertonic formulas. Obtain specific formula information from the individual supplier.

Administration of Enteral Feedings

Formula may be delivered by either gravity drip or an enteral feeding pump that is either volumetric or peristaltic in design (Fig. 25-1). Choose a pump that has a suitable alarm system if the client will infuse formula at night. A pump equipped for battery operation enables the client to ambulate during feeding. Continuous drip administration with a feeding pump provides optimal utilization of formula and avoids the complications associated with bolus feeding methods (e.g., gastrointestinal upsets and aspiration of formula). In certain circumstances, bolus delivery of formula might be the delivery method of choice if the person can tolerate it and if it fits in with the lifestyle. Some practitioners, particularly for persons with head and neck problems, still deliver bolus feedings using large-bore tubing and a funnel or barrel of an irrigating syringe. An alternative is to use a feeding bag and tubing and drip the formula over 20 to 40 minutes at 4-hour to 6-hour intervals throughout the day. This is recommended to prevent any side-effects from having a high-nutrient feeding reach the stomach so quickly.

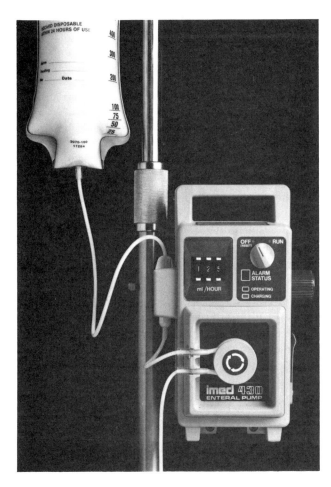

Figure 25.1
Enteral feeding pump with feeding bag and tubing. (Courtesy
of IMED Corporation)

The adult client is usually started on half-strength feedings at 50 ml/hour and advanced to full-strength feedings the next day if tolerated. The feedings are increased by 10 ml/hour/day, until 120 ml/hour/day is reached. Daily contact with the dietitian or home health nurse is mandatory during this regulation period. Once the client is regulated, the number of hours can be decreased while the volume is increased, thus allowing the person some freedom from the feeding regimen. This is known as *cyclic feeding*. For example, the client may be tube fed for 12 hours and off for 12 hours. If the client learns self-intubation, this allows returning to work or school.

Terminology

Gastrostomy: Surgical opening into the stomach for feeding purposes

Esophagostomy: Surgical opening into the esophagus with placement of a tube into the stomach for enteral feeding

Jejunostomy: Surgical opening into the jejunum with placement of a tube for enteral feeding

Continuous feeding: Formula is delivered at a constant rate using an administration bag and tubing connected to the feeding tube. The rate can be controlled by gravity or an enteral feeding pump.

Intermittent feeding: Formula is infused at 4- to 6-hour intervals throughout the day using an administration bag and tubing or large-bore tubing and a funnel.

Cyclic feeding: The client is advanced from continuous feeding to an increased rate over fewer hours (e.g., 12 hours on, 12 hours off). This allows some freedom from the feeding regimen.

Assessment of Self-Care Potential

Client/Family Assessment

- Assess the willingness and the ability of the family and client to assume self-care activities related to the feeding program. Determine whether the client will be able to learn self-intubation. Self-intubation is most appropriate when feedings are delivered into the stomach. Placing the tube into the intestine requires special techniques and x-ray confirmation.

- Assess the client's lifestyle to help determine the feeding regimen that will be most appropriate. People who work or go to school may prefer to feed themselves at night.

- Determine whether the client is entitled to third-party reimbursement for a home feeding program. Check that insurance counseling has been provided. If the client is not covered by private insurance or Medicare, determine whether community programs will provide aid.

- Assist the client to determine a vendor to supply the feeding pump, supplies, and formula. Check whether the vendor supplies a refrigerator, whether there is a 24-hour emergency service, and whether there are satisfactory quality-control checks.

Physical Assessment

- Complete a periodic nutritional assessment. Determine the client's response to the nutritional program and attainment of nutritional goals. Check for normal bowel sounds. Check residual feeding periodically to ensure proper absorption of feeding.

- Determine the route of the feeding (i.e., nasogastric, nasoenteric, or surgically placed feeding tube). Determine the type of formula that is required (e.g., blenderized or commercially prepared, elemental or other special formula).

- Determine whether the client has a history of lactose intolerance or renal or liver disorders requiring special formulas. Check whether the client has any risk factors associated with poor nutritional status (e.g., NPO for 10 or more days, anorexia, alcohol abuse, or severe burns). Check whether the client is a diabetic.

- Assess the client's condition to determine whether oral nutrition is permitted. If so, the client will be able to eat as tolerated, in addition to the nutritional supplements. Determine a calorie count including both formula and additional food and fluids.

- Check the client's weight during visits.

- Assess the following clinical parameters by monthly monitoring: blood glucose, electrolytes, blood urea nitrogen, creatinine, transferrin, albumin, total protein, cholesterol levels, prothrombin and partial thromboplastin times, complete blood count, and liver function. Check the urine for sugar and acetone every 4 to 6 hours for the first 48 hours of the feeding program. If the results are negative, this may then be discontinued in nondiabetic clients.

Environmental Assessment

- Check the home for facilities to prepare formula. Cleanliness is mandatory to prevent contamination of the formula. A blender can be used to prepare the formula at home using specified food products. If facilities are not available for preparation and refrigeration, the client can use commercially prepared formulas that are ready to feed. Ready-to-feed formula is more expensive than blenderized feedings prepared at home.
- Ensure that suitable bathroom scales are available for daily weights.

Planning Strategies

Potential Nursing Diagnoses

Nutrition, alteration in: less than body requirements due to health problem requiring tube feeding

Infection, potential for: from bacterial contamination of feeding formula

Skin integrity, impairment of: potential due to securing feeding tube with tape or irritation by gastric or intestinal fluids

Oral mucous membranes, alteration in: dryness due to inability to ingest food and fluids normally

Self-concept, disturbance in: body image, due to change in eating patterns

Social isolation, due to changed eating patterns and inability to participate with family and friends at mealtimes

Expected Outcomes

Achievement of nutritional objectives (weight gain or maintenance)

Prevention of infection

Prevention of skin trauma

Maintenance of integrity of oral mucosa

Acceptance of body-image changes

Substitution of appropriate social activities for mealtime interaction

Improvement in wound healing (if appropriate)

Health Promotion Goals

- The client and family will
  Deliver gastric or enteric feeding formulas safely and according to the nutritional plan
  Accept body-image changes associated with the tube and feeding program
  For pediatric clients, safely feed an infant with sucking, swallowing, or regurgitation problems

Equipment

For continuous, cyclic, or intermittent feeding:
  Formula-administration bag and tubing
  Enteral feeding pump
  Ice, if bag has an ice compartment

For bolus feeding:
  Funnel or barrel of irrigation syringe
  Wide-bore administration tubing
  5-in-1 barrel connector (to connect tubing to feeding tube)

For gastrostomy or jejunostomy tube feeding:
  Either continuous or bolus feeding set-up
  A & D ointment or ostomy product (to protect skin)
  Stomahesive (if skin is excoriated)

For tube placement check:
  Irrigation syringe
  Litmus paper
  Stethoscope
  Glass of water

Interventions/Health Promotion

ACTION	*RATIONALE/AMPLIFICATION*
1. After the feeding tube is inserted, make the client comfortable in a semi-Fowler's position. Wash hands and assemble equipment on a nightstand or TV tray.	The head must be elevated at least 30 degrees during feeding to prevent regurgitation of formula.
2. For continuous or intermittent feeding, assemble the administration tubing and feeding bag. Clamp the tubing. Fill the feeding bag with the required amount of formula and hang the bag over the client's head. Prime the tubing and thread the tubing through the feeding pump, following the manufacturer's directions.	Use a picture hook on the wall or fashion a hook from a coathanger and hang it over a door to suspend the feeding bag. Priming the tubing removes air and prevents infusing air into the stomach.
3. Check the position of the tube: • Listen over the abdomen with the stethoscope while rapidly inserting a small amount of air into the tube.	Gurgling will be heard (and felt by the client) if the tube is in the stomach. Checking placement is not as important with surgically placed tubes (e.g., gastrostomy) because the tubes are sutured in place. Check the position in the stomach if the gastrostomy is the type where the tube is removed between feedings.
• Aspirate stomach contents and check with litmus paper.	If the tube is in the stomach, contents will be acid. If the tube contents are alkaline, the tube may be in the intestine or the esophagus. (Blue litmus paper turns pink in acid solutions.) Aspirating stomach contents is difficult with small-bore feeding tubes.
• Place the end of the feeding tube in a glass of water and watch for bubbling during respiration.	Be careful not to allow inhalation of the water should the tube be in the lungs.
4. Connect the tubing to the feeding tube. Set the pump rate and commence the infusion. Set alarm parameters (if appropriate). Refill the bag when the pump alarm goes off to alert the client that the bag is empty.	Do not add formula to formula already in the bag. This could promote bacterial growth. Irrigating the tube prevents blockage caused by formula.
5. When the infusion is completed, turn the pump off. Disconnect the feeding tube. If the tube is to remain in place, irrigate it with about 25 ml of lukewarm tapwater. If the tube is to be removed and reinserted for the next feeding, untape the tube, clamp it between the fingers, and remove it gently and steadily.	Clamping the tube between the fingers prevents spilling formula from the tube as it is removed. Surgically placed tubes are not usually removed between feedings.

ACTION	*RATIONALE/AMPLIFICATION*
6. For bolus feeding, instead of using an administration set, connect the barrel of an irrigation set to the feeding tube. Fill the barrel with formula while clamping the feeding tube between the fingers. Release the tube and allow the fluid to flow into the stomach.	Clamping the tube prevents instilling air into the stomach.
Elevate the barrel above the client's head so that the fluid flows slowly. Refill the barrel before it is completely empty. When the feeding is complete, irrigate the tube with tapwater and reclamp or remove.	This prevents complications from rapid administration of concentrated nutrients into the stomach.
7. When feeding the client with a surgically placed feeding tube (e.g., gastrostomy), recap the tube following the feeding. Clean the skin around the tube with warm, soapy water and rinse with warm tapwater. Apply skin-protecting ointment. Redress if necessary.	
If the skin is excoriated, cut Stomahesive to an appropriate size and apply to the skin.	Stomahesive or similar products allow the skin to heal by protecting it from stomach or intestinal secretions.

Related Care

1. Check residual feeding periodically: • Aspirate the residual formula from the tube. Reinstill the formula unless there is more than 100 ml. If more than 100 ml, consult the physician to consider reasons for delayed emptying.	
2. Irrigate the tube with about 25 ml of lukewarm tapwater in an irrigating syringe: Every 4 hours if not on a continuous drip	Irrigation prevents blockage of the tube by formula.
Every 6 hours when on a continuous drip Anytime the feeding is interrupted or the feeding container is changed Before and after each feeding	Periodic irrigation while the person is on a continuous drip assists in preventing buildup of formula inside the tube. Periodic irrigation with cranberry juice (if permitted) is also effective.
3. Soak the feeding tube (if removed between feedings) and administration set in warm, soapy water. Rinse with tapwater. Hang equipment over the shower door or bathtub to dry. Store in a plastic bag until ready for use. Feeding equipment such as the barrel of the	Correct cleaning of the equipment is important to prevent bacterial growth in the formula. If the client is receiving continuous feeding, replace and clean the administration set daily.

ACTION	RATIONALE/AMPLIFICATION
syringe and formula containers can be cleaned the same way or washed in a dishwasher.	
4. If the pump is used on battery power, recharge it between feedings.	
5. Remove and replace the feeding tube every 4 weeks or if deterioration of the tube is noted.	Inspect the tube for signs of deterioration and discard if necessary.

Age-Specific Modifications (Pediatric)

1. Give formula at room temperature.	Taking the chill from the formula prevents colic.
2. If bolus feeding is used, give small amounts of formula frequently.	The amount will depend on the age of the infant or child. For infants, the feeding regimen will be similar to a regular feeding schedule.
3. Use an enteral pump specifically designed for infants if continuous feeding is used.	Continuous feeding of infants requires a pump that can deliver small quantities of fluid accurately.
4. Restrain the infant's hands or place in mittens if the tube is to be left in place.	
5. Restrain the infant using a papoose board or elbow restraints during intubation.	
6. Position the child on the right side after feeding to hasten emptying of the stomach.	This prevents aspiration of feeding.
7. Take care not to introduce air into the stomach during the feeding procedure.	Air in the stomach will cause colic.
8. Provide a pacifier to meet the infant's sucking needs. Touch and cuddle the infant as the condition allows to meet mothering needs.	

**Education/
Communication**

• Teach the client and family to
Maintain the feeding tube and nutritional program
Use infection-control precautions to prevent bacterial contamination of the formula. Use correct handwashing techniques. Prepare the formula using clean utensils. Store the formula in the refrigerator until 30 minutes before use, when it can be removed from the refrigerator and allowed to warm to room temperature. This is only necessary if the client is sensitive to cold solutions. Use ice to keep formula cool if administration bag has an ice compartment. Change the bag and tubing as directed.

• Teach the client to
Expect a decreased frequency to bowel movements due to decreased residue in the feeding. Treat constipation with stool softeners as ordered by the physician. An exercise program will help also.

Ambulate and exercise as able. This improves the person's general health and promotes anabolism (tissue building). Ambulation will not dislodge the feeding tube.

Insert own feeding tube (as appropriate)

Referrals and Consultations

- Refer the client to a dietitian for assistance in assessing nutritional status and in determining goals of nutritional therapy.
- The client or family should report constipation or diarrhea to the home health nurse.
- Emergency problems with the feeding pump should be referred to the vendor.

Evaluation of Health Promotion Activities

Quality Assurance/ Reassessment

- Determine how well the client has integrated the feeding program with the lifestyle.
- Assess the family's and client's response to body-image changes attributed to tube feeding and the loss of socialization opportunities at family mealtimes.
- Evaluate for complications of enteral feedings (nasogastric or nasoenteric): pneumonia due to aspiration of formula, diarrhea due to feeding-related or nonfeeding-related causes, constipation due to low-residue feedings, fluid and electrolyte disturbances due to high protein-to-water ratio or high glucose content of the feeding, gastric distention due to paralytic ileus, or hyperglycemia or hypoglycemia due to erratic administration rates.
- Evaluate possible causes of diarrhea: formula delivered too rapidly or formula too concentrated; decreased natural flora secondary to antibiotic therapy or secondary to medications.
- Assess bowel program if constipation is a problem.
- Periodically check the client's urine for sugar and acetone.

DOCUMENTATION

Charting for the Home Health Nurse

Calorie count including the nutritional supplement and food or fluid ingested

Weight chart

Vital signs

Physical assessment with emphasis on nutritional assessment

Complications of the feeding program (e.g., gastrointestinal disturbances, metabolic problems such as hypoglycemia or hyperglycemia)

Laboratory work profile; urinalysis

Records Kept by the Client/Family

Amount and type of food/fluids ingested in addition to the nutritional supplement

Daily weight taken at the same time each day while wearing similar clothing

Health Teaching Checklist

Name of Care Provider _____

Relationship to Client _____ Telephone #_____

Taught by _____ Date _____

	EXPLAINED	DEMONSTRATED
Feeding techniques	_____	_____
Maintenance of equipment	_____	_____
Preparation and storage of formula	_____	_____
Infection control precautions	_____	_____
Self-intubation	_____	_____
Daily weights	_____	
Periodic laboratory work	_____	
Possible complications of tube feeding	_____	
Recording oral intake	_____	_____
Importance of exercise	_____	
Integration of the feeding program into the activities of daily living (ADL)	_____	
24-hour telephone number for pump service or problems	_____	
24-hour telephone number for home health nurse	_____	

Product Availability

Feeding equipment and pumps are available at medical-supply companies listed in the yellow pages of the telephone book. (See Technique 22, Home Parenteral Nutrition, for vendors.)

Selected References

Cataldo CB, Smith L: Tube feedings: Clinical applications. Columbus, OH, Ross Laboratories, 1980

Griggs BA, Hostetler C: Tube feeding reconsidered. NITA 4(6):409–413, Nov/Dec, 1981

Persons C: Why risk TPN when tube feeding will do? RN 44(1):35–41, January, 1981

Persons CB: Enteral nutrition: State of the art. In Zschoche D (ed): Mosby's Comprehensive Review of Critical Care. St Louis, CV Mosby, 1986

Hygiene

26 Artificial Eye, Removal and Insertion

Background

An eye prosthesis is used after enucleation to preserve the integrity of the eye socket and to enhance appearance. Enucleation involves surgical removal of the eyeball itself following trauma or disease. Since the eye socket is then a closed cavity, it provides a warm, dark environment that is conducive to proliferation of microorganisms.

Assessment of Self-Care Potential

Client/Family Assessment

- Assess the length of time the prosthesis has been worn by the client.
- Assess the familiarity of the primary care provider with the removal, cleansing, and insertion process.

Physical Assessment

- Assess the integrity of the eye socket. Determine the cause of the enucleation and note any resulting physical problems that might interfere with the client's ability to adapt to wearing the prosthesis.
- Assess the condition of the eye prosthesis. Note any chips or cracks.
- Assess the condition for which the client is being seen in the home care setting. If it is unrelated to the eye prosthesis, assess the impact of this condition on eye care.
- Assess the condition and appearance of the other eye.

Environmental Assessment

- Assess the cleansing area to determine if a flat work surface is available that will provide for the safety of the prosthesis in case it is dropped.
- Assess the presence of clean water in the home for cleansing the prosthesis.
- Assess the lighting in the client's room to determine if it is adequate for proper observation of the eye socket and for facilitation of the insertion and removal process.

Planning Strategies

Potential Nursing Diagnoses

Potential for impairment of skin integrity

Potential for injury

Knowledge deficit of family members regarding caring for the prosthesis

Self-care deficit regarding ability to care for prosthesis

Expected Outcomes

Prevention of infection and trauma to the eye socket

Preservation of the integrity and quality of vision in the other eye

Reinforcement of proper care and maintenance of prosthesis

Promotion of feelings of security and competence in those persons responsible for caring for the prosthesis

Health Promotion Goals

- The client and family will
  Clean the prosthesis and eye cavity daily
  Remove and insert the artificial eye in such a way that trauma to the skin is prevented and the prosthesis is not damaged
  Feel comfortable in handling the prosthesis
  Use proper technique in inserting and removing the prosthesis
  Preserve the integrity of the other eye

Equipment

Prosthesis container

Warm water (110° F)

Soft gauze or cotton ball

Suction cup to remove eye (optional)

Interventions/Health Promotion

ACTION	*RATIONALE/AMPLIFICATION*
1. Assist the client to a sitting or side-lying position. Allow the client to participate in or direct the procedure as much as possible. Remind the care provider that handwashing should precede and follow eye care.	It is important to reduce the chances of eye infection, which can be spread by contaminated hands and equipment.
2. Pull the lower eyelid down over the cheekbone with the thumb and exert slight pressure on the lower portion of the eyelid to release the suction. The eye should pop out. (An alternate method is to use a small suction cup applied directly to the prosthesis. Use a slight rocking motion to break the suction.)	Suction holds the prosthesis in the eye socket. Care must be taken not to drop or damage the eye as it is removed from the eye socket.
3. To clean the prosthesis, wash gently in warm water and dry with gauze pads. Hold the eye over a basin or cloth while it is being cleaned to prevent breakage in case it is dropped.	All crusts and secretions should be removed from the eye. The eye must not be dropped because breakage or chipping could occur, resulting in discomfort or trauma when the eye is reinserted.
4. Clean the eye socket by spreading the lids apart and washing out the inside with moist cotton balls or gauze pads. Wipe from the inner aspect of the eye toward the outer portion. Be sure to clean inside folds and crevices. Remove all crusts and secretions. Dry the socket with dry pads in the same manner.	The folds of the eye may harbor microorganisms. If the tear ducts remain intact, crusts may form. It is important to wipe away from the duct openings, which are in the inner portion of the eye socket.

ACTION	*RATIONALE/AMPLIFICATION*
5. Insert the eye by separating the lids with the thumb and forefinger (Fig. 26-1). Holding the prosthesis between the thumb and forefinger of the other hand, gently insert it into the socket in natural alignment (Fig. 26-2).	The eye has been made to fit into the socket. It should slide naturally into position. When released, the lids should close over the prosthesis in a comfortable and natural manner.

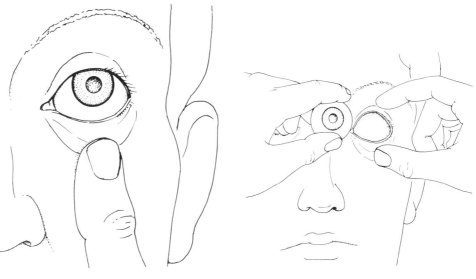

Figure 26.1 *Figure 26.2*

Education/ Communication

- Teach the client and family to

  Properly perform care of the prosthesis and socket

  Provide privacy while the prosthesis is out of the eye. Any type of prosthesis is a highly personal matter. If the client requires assistance to perform tasks that normally are done alone, embarrassment may be a consequence. Stress the importance of privacy during the period when the prosthesis is out of the eye.

  Adhere to a schedule for cleaning the eye to ensure that it is done regularly and correctly

  Observe the condition of the socket to detect signs of trauma and infection. Be sure that the client and family know the signs of infection and trauma, which may indicate the need for further treatment or a change in technique.

  Observe the condition of the prosthesis to detect nicks, cracks, or chips

  Be comfortable with handling the eye in a safe and efficient manner

Referrals and Consultations

Problems with the eye socket may necessitate referral to an ophthalmologist. If the condition of the prosthesis is poor, a new one may be needed. Eye prostheses are very expensive and should be obtained only from a reputable prosthetic expert.

Evaluation of Health Promotion Activities

**Quality Assurance/
Reassessment**

- Observe the technique of the primary care provider to ensure that the procedure is being done correctly and safely.
- Ask the client if the eye care that is being administered is satisfactory. Most clients have taken care of their own prostheses for many years and are in a position to offer excellent feedback as to the technique and skill of the care provider.

DOCUMENTATION

Charting for the Home Health Nurse
Documentation should include periodic assessment of the eye prosthesis and the eye socket. Any problems should be noted, with their disposition.

Records Kept by the Client/Family
Encourage the family to write down any comments or problems that they may have during the removal, cleaning, and insertion process.

**Health Teaching
Checklist**

Name of Care Provider _____

Relationship to Client _____ Telephone #_____

Taught by _____ Date _____

	EXPLAINED	DEMONSTRATED
Removal of prosthesis	_____	_____
Reinsertion of prosthesis	_____	_____
Cleansing of eye prosthesis Method	_____	_____
Safety factors	_____	_____
Cleansing of the eye socket Method	_____	_____
Infection-control factors	_____	_____

Product Availability

Cleansing products, such as gauze pads or cotton balls, may be obtained from any drug store. The storage container may be any type with a tight-fitting lid that can be cleaned thoroughly, such as a commercial whipped cream or butter tub container. It should be clearly marked so that it will not be inadvertently thrown away.

27 Baths, Cleansing

Background

Bathing is used to cleanse the body of dirt and debris that accumulate due to direct contact and elimination of waste through the skin. The cutaneous glands continually secrete substances onto the skin. Sebaceous glands are found on all skin surfaces except the palms of the hands and soles of the feet. They produce an oily secretion called *sebum,* which forms an oily layer over the skin and helps keep it soft and waterproof. The major sweat glands of the axillae, areola of the breast, and anogenital area secrete a milky, sticky secretion that is decomposed by the action of bacteria normally found on the skin. This decomposition causes the distinctive odor of sweat. Accumulation of natural body secretions may cause body odor and may provide a satisfactory medium for colonization of bacteria.

There are three types of baths for the client who is confined totally or partially to bed: the complete bed bath during which the client is completely bathed in the bed; the abbreviated bed bath during which only the parts of the client's body that, if neglected, might cause illness, odor, or discomfort are washed (such as the face, axillae, genitalia, anal region, back, and hands); the partial bath, which may take place at the sink, tub, or shower, when the client bathes to the extent needed or desired with assistance as required.

Assessment of Self-Care Potential

Client/Family Assessment

- Assess the degree of cleanliness of the family members to identify the priority placed on bathing.
- Assess the family hierarchy and power system to determine who makes the decisions and who provides the care during illness.

Physical Assessment

- During the bath is an excellent time to do the physical assessment of the client to determine nursing diagnoses and progress of current therapy.
- Assess the physical condition of the client to determine what type of bath will be safest and most successful in achieving the purposes of cleanliness and refreshment. If the client will get up to go to the bathroom for bathing, assess the need for assistance to and during the bath.
- Assess the condition of the skin during bathing. Assess the adequacy of the body's temperature-regulating mechanism as evidenced by sweating. Assess dryness of skin and any special needs to determine the desired frequency of bathing and agents used.
- Assess the client's range of motion and any limitations.

Environmental Assessment

- Assess the presence of hot and cold running water. Assess sanitation in and around the home.
- Determine the presence and location of bathing facilities if the client can get up to the tub or shower. Assess the physical layout of the home to determine if assistance apparatus (such as wheelchair, walker, crutches, etc.) will fit into the bathing area.

Planning Strategies

Potential Nursing Diagnoses

Self-care deficit, bathing/hygiene

Disturbance in self-concept

Potential for injury

Potential for impairment of skin integrity

Expected Outcomes

Cleansing of the client's body

Stimulation of systemic and local circulation

Maintenance of muscle tone

Improvement of self-esteem and self-image

Health Promotion Goals

- The client and family will
  Understand how to safely and efficiently cleanse the client or assist the client in self-cleansing
  Assist the client in preserving skin integrity and full range of motion
  Maintain the client's autonomy and self-concept
  Learn how to promote comfort and relaxation during bathing
  Understand how to assess and encourage range of motion
  Encourage the client's independence

Equipment

Bathtowel, washcloth, and soap

Lotion and powder, if desired

Bath basin and small table or stand

Toilet articles

Wheelchair, walker, cane, or crutches for assisted ambulation to the bathroom

Interventions/Health Promotion

ACTION	*RATIONALE/AMPLIFICATION*
Bed Bath	
1. Before the bath, explain the procedure to the client. Involve the care provider in making decisions about the best way to accomplish the bath. Determine where to fill the bath basin and where it can be safely set during the bath. A small table or stand near the bed will enable the basin to be moved to the desired location during the bath. Be sure to warm the room before beginning the bath. Wash hands before assisting with the bath.	The client and family will be most familiar with their surroundings in regard to the best way to bathe the client. Participation in decision-making also enhances self-esteem and promotes compliance with procedures.

ACTION

2. Protect the bed linens by placing a large towel or soft blanket under the client before bathing. A large piece of plastic may be placed under the towel to protect the mattress if it is not waterproof. Remove the top covers and place a light bath blanket over the client. Raise the bed to its highest level if the client is to be bathed by the caregiver.

3. Fill the basin with warm water (115°F). Change the water as often as necessary to maintain the desired temperature.

4. Fold the washcloth around the hand by laying the open hand, palm side up, on the cloth and folding each side over and the top down (Figs. 27-1 to 27-4). Tuck the top under the palm side to secure it (Fig. 27-5).

RATIONALE/AMPLIFICATION

Plastic is an irritant when in direct contact with the body. It should be separated from the client by some type of material. Several smaller towels may be used if a large towel is not available. The client must be protected from chilling during the bath. Raising the bed to its highest level prevents the need to stoop, which can cause back strain.

Warm water tends to relax muscles and increase circulation by dilating the blood vessels. Excessive heat may cause burns.

The dangling ends of the washcloth are annoying. Folding the cloth keeps it warmer longer.

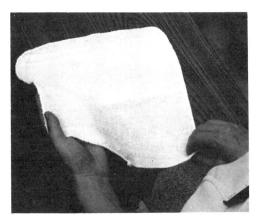

Figure 27.1

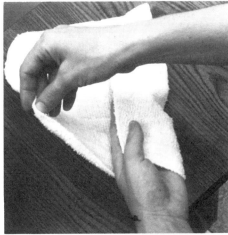

Figure 27.2

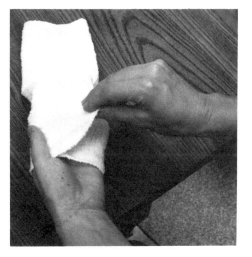

Figure 27.3

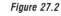

Figure 27.4

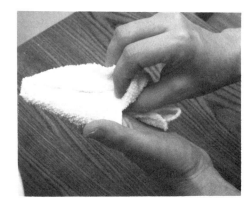

Figure 27.5

ACTION	*RATIONALE/AMPLIFICATION*
5. Use soap to promote cleanliness unless the client objects or has excessively dry skin. Rinse the skin thoroughly so that all soap is removed.	Soap decreases surface tension and allows more efficient cleaning. Soap may cause irritation, however; it should be kept away from delicate tissues, such as the eye, and should not be left in contact with the skin for prolonged periods. Lotion may be used in place of soap.
6. Use firm, gentle strokes to clean the client's skin. Cleanse contaminated areas last. The suggested sequence for the bath is face, arms, hands, axillae, chest, abdomen, legs, feet, back, perineum, and anal region. Each area should be dried as soon as it is cleaned. If the client is able to clean the genital area, then assist as necessary. If not, clean the female perineum gently between the labial folds and the surrounding area. Wash with soap and rinse thoroughly. Dry the area completely. In the uncircumcised male, the foreskin must be retracted and the glans rinsed and dried gently (see Related Care, below). Change the bath water as often as necessary to ensure that the client is cleaned without transferring microorganisms from dirty areas to clean areas.	Firm, gentle strokes stimulate muscles and aid circulation. Following the suggested sequence will reduce the chance of spreading microorganisms from the contaminated areas to the clean areas. Immediate drying reduces the chance of chilling.
7. Immerse accessible body parts, such as the hands and feet, in the basin of bath water (Fig. 27-6).	Immersion aids in dissolving contaminants, removing debris, softening nails, and refreshing the client.

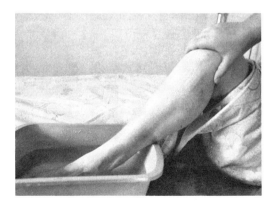

Figure 27.6

ACTION

8. Do not allow skin to rub against other skin areas. After cleaning the thighs, apply powder or cornstarch and a pillowcase or soft cloth to keep the thighs from rubbing together. If the client is obese and has a fold of abdominal flesh that protrudes over the pubic area, clean and dry the area thoroughly. Apply powder and a soft cloth to the area so the two skin surfaces do not rub against each other.

RATIONALE/AMPLIFICATION

By keeping the skin clean and dry and preventing skin areas from touching, it should be possible to prevent chapping and skin irritation.

Abbreviated Bath

The abbreviated bath follows the same principles as the bed bath. The sequence for bathing is face, hands, axillae, back, genitalia, and anal region.

The abbreviated bath serves to clean and refresh the more acutely ill client who cannot tolerate the bed bath procedure or the client who does not need an entire bath.

Partial Bath

1. Determine the easiest route and method of getting the client to the bathing area. A straight-backed kitchen chair may be most beneficial for the client who must sit down during the bath. A water-resistant stool or chair may be placed into the shower so the client may sit down. Warm the room before transporting the client to it.

Many homes are not built so assistance devices will readily fit through doors and around corners. If this appears to be a problem, rehearse the transport procedure with the equipment before the client actually attempts to travel to the bathing area. If the wheelchair will not go through the doors or around the corner, an alternative method must be devised. When the client is actually transported to the bathing area, it should be ensured that there are no environmental obstacles.

2. Someone should remain with the client who is unsteady or weak. If the client remains alone in the bathing area, some means of calling for help must be devised, such as a bell or a whistle.

The safety of the client during transport and bathing must be of paramount importance.

Related Care

1. During or after the bath is usually a desirable time to change dressings and perform other care related to cleanliness and a basic sense of well-being, such as shaving, hair wash, and mouth care.

Leaving the client within a clean environment encourages self-esteem and self-concept. If several procedures can be done at one time, the client can conserve energy as well.

2. Move all body parts through their full range of motion during the bath unless contraindicated.

Active and passive exercises prevent contractures and improve circulation.

ACTION

RATIONALE/AMPLIFICATION

3. In the uncircumcised male, the foreskin over the glans must be retracted for adequate cleansing. The foreskin should be retracted as far as possible. Allow water to run gently over the glans to remove the cheesy debris that builds up in this area. Gentle washing with a soft cloth may be necessary to fully clean the glans. Allow the client to perform this care or show the care provider how it is done.

Retraction of the foreskin stretches the opening to ensure that urination is not compromised. Accumulation of debris under the foreskin may lead to infection.

4. Hand care is essential for the debilitated client. Trim the fingernails when necessary, using manicure scissors. Smooth the edges of the nails with a file or emery board. If the client is immobile or rigid, the fingers tend to push into the palms of the hands as contractures form. Clean between the fingers and dry thoroughly. Do passive exercises and place a small rolled towel in the hand to help preserve normal positioning and decrease rigidity.

If the fingernails are not trimmed, they may causes scratches or become ingrown. If the fingers become tightly drawn up in a rigid contracture, they will become painful and difficult to keep clean. Exercise and patience are needed to prevent paralysis and infection.

Age-Specific Modifications

Bathing an Infant

1. Place all equipment within reach at the bedside. Fill the tub or basin half full of warm water (115°F). Remove the infant's clothing. Close diaper pins and place them out of reach. Perform the bath in the usual location used by the mother unless contraindicated. If the usual bathing area is not safe, use this opportunity to teach safety precautions to the care providers.

Having all equipment within reach eliminates delays during the bath. Since babies tend to place everything in their mouths, closing and storing the diaper pins safely reduces the chance of accidents. If the bath is as near normal as possible, the infant may be less frightened by the presence of different persons.

2. Place the infant in the tub, supported and secured at all times by the care provider's hand. Using a clean cloth, wash the infant's eyes and face first. Wash the skin over and around the eyes from the inner to the outer aspect with a different portion of the clean cloth for each stroke.

The skin over and around the eyes is washed to remove surface debris that might enter and contaminate the eye. The eye itself is not washed because it is too delicate and sensitive. To cleanse the eye, sterile irrigation is the method of choice. Using a clean portion of the cloth prevents cross-contamination.

ACTION	*RATIONALE/AMPLIFICATION*
3. Wash the areas of the infant that are dirty. Proceed from head to toe as needed.	The hands, knees, and feet of the crawling infant are usually dirty. The genital area is usually washed during every bath to remove potential irritants. The rectal area is always bathed last to prevent contamination of the rest of the body with flora that is normal to the rectum.
4. Grasp the infant with a towel for removal from the tub. Wrap the infant in a towel and dry well. Dress the infant.	Handling the wet infant with a towel reduces the chances of accidents.

Bathing a Child

1. Place the bath articles on a table top out of reach of the small child. Involve the parents or care provider in the bath as much as possible. The older child should be encouraged to participate as much as possible.	Safety is enhanced if the child cannot reach small articles, such as diaper pins. All equipment needed for the bath should be gathered in advance so that it is not necessary to interrupt the bath. The small child is *never left alone in the bath basin.* The older child should be attended as much as necessary, but should be encouraged and praised for self-help efforts.
2. Fill the bath basin two-thirds full of warm water (115°F). Change the water as often as needed to keep it the proper temperature.	The warm temperature will relax muscles and stimulate circulation without burning the child.
3. Place the child into the bath basin or set the child on a padded surface near the basin, keeping a secure hold constantly. Allow the child to play in the water, if desired. Bathe the child from top to bottom, cleansing the rectal area last.	Young children are usually very active. When the child's skin is wet, securing against falls becomes an even greater challenge. Use a towel to secure the child during the bath.

Education/ Communication

- Teach the client and family to

  Adequately perform a bath in bed or in the bathing area to cleanse the client without tiring or endangering anyone. Explain the need to conserve the debilitated person's strength while maintaining cleanliness and a sense of well-being. Explain the proper body mechanics involved in lifting or assisting the client to and from the bathing area.

  Assess the need for bathing of the client. The bedfast client should have a full bed bath every day. If drying of the skin is a problem, recommend that the client be bathed with soap and water on one day, and on alternate days skin lotion and water may be used. Lotion may be applied with a washcloth in the same manner as soap.

  Understand the safety precautions involved in bathing. Of primary importance is the prevention of falls. Water on a surface increases the chance of slipping and falling. Adhesive strips are available for the bottom of the bathtub or shower to help in preventing falls. Handrails may be applied to showers and tubs to aid the client in getting in and out. Chairs and stools placed in showers may prevent the client from becoming fatigued.

Understand and apply the principles of cross-contamination relating to bathing clean areas before contaminated areas. This is an excellent opportunity to explain why cleaning after elimination should be from front to back so that rectal flora will not be introduced into the genital area.

Perform range-of-motion exercise and promote adequate circulation to all parts of the client's body

Understand the unique needs of infants in relation to cleanliness. Explain that there is a trend away from daily ritualistic bathing of healthy infants. Daily bathing removes many of the natural oils that lubricate and protect the infant's delicate skin. Application of baby oils may cause dermatologic problems because of the presence of perfumes and other additives. The current trend is to wash only those areas of the infant that are soiled. If the infant soils a diaper, wash the genital and buttocks area. If the infant gets food on both face and arms, wash those particular areas. Stress to the family the desirability of bathing only those areas that are soiled.

Test the bath water for proper temperature by feeling the water on the inner aspect of the wrist. Advise the parents of small children that they should never add hot water to their child's bath with the infant in the tub. If the water gets too cool, the infant should be removed, the warmer water added, the water temperature checked, and the infant returned. Prevention of burning from hot water is also necessary for older clients. Explain to the care providers of persons with visual or sensory impairment the importance of checking the temperature of the water before the client enters the tub. If the water becomes too cold, the care provider must be the one to warm the water in a safe manner. Use of nozzle extension units or hand-held shower heads may help eliminate the chance of burning the client by accidentally turning on the hot water.

Evaluation of Health Promotion Activities

**Quality Assurance/
Reassessment**

- Assess the adequacy of the bathing technique by the physical appearance of the client. Such parameters as odor, visible dirt, itching, and dermatologic reactions may indicate that the bathing procedure is inadequate.

- Determination of the frequency of bathing should be left largely up to the client's needs and wishes and the abilities and desires of the family. If the family members bathe only once a week when they are well, they may not understand why they must bathe daily when ill. Base recommendations regarding frequency of bathing on the physical and emotional needs of the client rather than on tradition.

DOCUMENTATION

Records Kept by the Client/Family

If the client is being bathed on a schedule, it may be advisable for the family to keep a list of the days on which the client is bathed. A small note pad with the day listed and any problems may enable the care provider(s) to remember questions that arise during the bath.

Health Teaching Checklist

Name of Care Provider _____

Relationship to Client _____ Telephone #_____

Taught by _____ Date _____

	EXPLAINED	DEMONSTRATED
Safety precautions—falls	_____	
Safety precautions—water temperature	_____	
Transportation of client to tub/shower	_____	_____
Techniques for bathing	_____	_____
Observation of skin	_____	_____
Range-of-motion exercises	_____	_____
Proper body mechanics	_____	_____
Constant attendance during infant bath	_____	
Bath sequence to avoid contamination	_____	_____

Product Availability

Adhesive strips for the bottom of bathtubs or showers are available at most department and drug stores. Hand-held shower heads are also available at these same places as well as at appliance stores.

Baths, Therapeutic

Background

Therapeutic bathing involves immersing the body or body part(s) in water of varying temperatures or in water with emollients added. Types of therapeutic baths include the sitz bath and the emollient bath. The sitz bath involves immersion of the body from mid thigh to iliac crest in warm water (115°F). Emollient baths involve immersion of the body in tepid water (95°F to 110°F) that contains an added emollient agent, such as 3 cups of oatmeal, 1 lb of cornstarch, 8 oz of sodium bicarbonate, or specific prescribed medications. An emollient is a soothing or softening agent that is applied locally for palliative purposes.

Assessment of Self-Care Potential

Client/Family Assessment

- Assess the level of understanding of the client and family regarding the need for and mechanics of the therapeutic bath.
- Assess the financial situation of the family to determine their ability to purchase necessary supplies for the bath.
- Assess the level of cooperation that may reasonably be expected from the care provider. Determine what priority the therapeutic bath will likely be given in the everyday scheme of activities.

Physical Assessment

- Assess the condition for which the therapeutic bath has been ordered. If the bath is for a topical condition, determine the extent of the condition to serve as a baseline for assessing the effectiveness of the therapy.
- Assess the client's ability to get into the tub or onto the basin for the bath. Determine agility and physical mobility in relation to getting to the bathing area.

Environmental Assessment

- Assess the bathing facilities in the home. Assess the route to the bathing area and potential impediments to the client's progress, such as throw rugs or sharp corners. Assess the condition and cleanliness of the tub. If the client has an open wound, the tub may have to be cleaned and disinfected before bathing.
- Assess the presence of hot and cold running water in the home.

Planning Strategies

Potential Nursing Diagnoses

Actual or potential impairment of skin integrity

Alteration in comfort: pain due to dermatologic condition

Disturbance in self-concept regarding body image

Expected Outcomes

Stimulation of tissue formation by increased circulation

Promotion of suppuration

Increased peripheral dilation

Relief of pain

Relaxation of muscles

Promotion of positive self-image

Health Promotion Goals

- The client and family will
  Understand the safety precautions involved in therapeutic bathing
  Learn how to prepare the bath and successfully bathe the client
  Relieve the condition for which the treatment is designed

Equipment

Bathtub or portable sitz tub

Water of indicated temperature

Bath thermometer

Medication, if prescribed

Rubber or plastic ring for sitz bath, if indicated

Washcloths and towels

Interventions/Health Promotion

ACTION	*RATIONALE/AMPLIFICATION*
Sitz Bath	
1. Clean the bathtub with a cleanser and disinfectant, such as bleach or ammonia. Rinse thoroughly.	If the client has an open wound or sores, it is essential that cross-contamination be avoided by cleaning the tub.
2. Fill the bathtub to a level of about 3 to 4 inches (Fig. 28-1) with warm water (115°F).	The water should be warm enough to promote peripheral vasodilation and comfort, but not so warm as to burn the client.

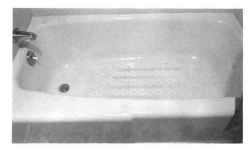

Figure 28.1

3. Assist the client to sit on a rubber or plastic inflated ring if rectal or perineal sutures are present (Fig. 28-2).	Direct pressure on the operative area may cause pain or pressure.

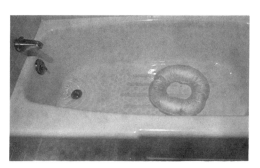

Figure 28.2

ACTION	RATIONALE/AMPLIFICATION
4. Elevate the client's feet and legs, if possible, so that only the rectal–genital area is in the water. Place a plastic basin or rust-proof metal stool in the tub and pad it with a towel. Assist the client to elevate both feet and rest them on this cushioned area.	Local vasodilation of the lower extremities will draw blood away from the perineal area.
5. Maintain consistent water temperature by adding warm water throughout the procedure. Take care not to burn the client during addition of warm water. *Do not add hot water.*	Fluctuations in water temperature can cause cardiovascular stress. Addition of hot water could cause burning.
6. Allow the client to remain in the tub for 10 to 20 minutes or as prescribed or desired.	Maximal benefit is obtained in the first 10 to 20 minutes. Prolonging the bath may tire the client.
7. Place a blanket or towel around the client's shoulders while in the tub to prevent chilling.	Chilling causes vasoconstriction, which may counteract the desired effects of the procedure.
8. Check on the client frequently during the bath. Counting the pulse midway through the bath may give an indication of the client's cardiovascular condition.	Changes in temperature of the environment may cause cardiovascular reactions. An irregular pulse may indicate stress and should be an indicator to stop the bath.

Emollient Bath

ACTION	RATIONALE/AMPLIFICATION
1. Fill the tub one half to two thirds full of tepid water (95°F to 110°F). Add the emollient material and mix it into the water.	Warm water will promote vasodilation, which may increase itching. Tepid water will allow soaking without increasing itching.
2. Assist the client into the tub. As much body surface as possible should be submerged. Apply the emollient solution to the areas that are not submerged with light, gentle strokes of a soft washcloth.	Assistance may help prevent falls. The aim of the bath is to apply as much of the emollient to the skin surface as is possible. The medium for achieving this purpose is the water. The greater the surface area reached by the water, the more effective the therapeutic bath.
3. Allow the client to soak in the emollient bath for 20 to 30 minutes so that the skin is coated but chilling is prevented.	Clients with skin conditions may be more prone to chilling than other persons.
4. Pat the skin dry with a soft towel. Do not rub the skin.	Brisk rubbing will increase the discomfort of itching.

ACTION	*RATIONALE/AMPLIFICATION*
Related Care	
Soiled dressings should be removed prior to the bath and discarded in a paper or plastic sack. If the inner dressing adheres to the wound, it may be soaked off in the tub.	As the healing process progresses, the sticky surface of the wound hardens and adheres to any material next to it. When the material is forcefully removed, it disturbs clot formation and may cause bleeding and pain. Soaking the dressing free is less traumatic and less painful.

Education/ Communication

- Teach the client and family to

  Safely and effectively prepare and carry out the sitz or emollient bath. Stress safety precautions such as assisting the client into and out of the tub. Adhesive strips on the bottom of the tub may help prevent falls.

  Understand the desired effects of the bath. Emphasize that the reason for the bath is not to clean the client but to relieve pain and/or itching. Explain that warm water causes an increase in the amount of blood coming to an area, and this effect of the sitz bath promotes healing of wounds. Also, emphasize that this influx of blood is not desirable in clients with dermatologic conditions because it increases itching; therefore, tepid water is preferred for emollient baths. Stress the importance of avoiding temperature extremes, and discourage brisk rubbing of affected areas.

  Accept the disfigurement that often accompanies dermatologic conditions. Help the client and the family accept the skin condition by avoiding the tendency to stare or show signs of revulsion. Demonstrate accepting behavior by looking at the client rather than the lesion or affected area. Use a matter-of-fact attitude and answer questions without hesitation. Allow the client to verbalize feelings about the disfigurement.

  Prevent contamination of the susceptible areas. Caution the client to keep hands and fingers away from wounds. Stress the importance of avoiding scratching in dermatologic conditions. Show the family how to clean the bathtub before and after the client takes a bath. If the client has had rectal surgery, a sitz bath may be recommended after every bowel movement for cleaning and pain relief.

Referrals and Consultations

Severe itching from dermatologic conditions may cause emotional distress. If this becomes severe, psychological counseling may be needed.

Evaluation of Health Promotion Activities

Quality Assurance/ Reassessment

- Reassess the condition of the wound at frequent intervals to ensure that healing is proceeding as expected. Be especially observant of any signs of infection, such as redness, pus, failure of parts of the incision to close properly, and a foul odor.

- Note the progress of the skin condition. Determine if it is spreading or receding. Note any signs of infection from scratching. The client's fingernails should be short to prevent accidental scratching.

DOCUMENTATION

Charting for the Home Health Nurse

A progress chart of the skin condition may help indicate whether current management is effective. Any ancillary problems, such as infection or emotional distress, should be noted.

Progress notes regarding healing of an incision or wound should also be kept. It is especially important to note the presence or absence of signs and symptoms that indicate proper or improper healing.

Records Kept by the Client/Family

The family may be asked to keep track of how many sitz or emollient baths the client takes each day or week as an indicator of the effectiveness of the treatment. They should be instructed to take this information when they visit the primary care provider for follow-up visits.

Health Teaching Checklist

Name of Care Provider _____

Relationship to Client _____ Telephone #_____

Taught by _____ Date _____

	EXPLAINED	DEMONSTRATED
Sitz bath		
Safety precautions	_____	_____
Water temperature	_____	
Depth of water	_____	_____
Propping of client's feet	_____	_____
Length of bath	_____	
Emollient bath		
Safety precautions	_____	_____
Product to be used and amount	_____	_____
Water temperature	_____	
Application of emollient mixture to parts of the body not submerged	_____	_____
Proper drying procedure	_____	_____

Product Availability

Oatmeal, cornstarch, and sodium bicarbonate are available in any grocery store. Portable sitz baths are available at hospital-supply houses.

29   Contact Lenses, Insertion and Removal

Background

Contact lenses are preformed visual aids that fit directly onto the eye itself. Lenses may be either hard, soft, or semisoft. They may be corneal or scleral lenses. They may be used to correct vision or to protect sensitive eye surfaces. Lenses may be removed daily or may be worn for extended periods, depending on the type of lens.

Assessment of Self-Care Potential

Client/Family Assessment

- Assess the length of time the client has worn contact lenses. Determine if there have been any problems with the lenses.
- Assess the familiarity of the family members with the type of lenses the client wears and their understanding of the cleaning procedure and safety precautions.
- Assess the understanding of the family regarding the safety precautions involved in inserting and removing contact lenses.

Physical Assessment

- Assess the condition of the client's eyes. Do both a gross and ophthalmoscopic examination to detect irregularities of or trauma to the eye surface as well as the inner eye.
- Assess the lenses themselves for nicks, cracks, and fit. Determine the method used to tell the right from the left lens.
- Assess the physical condition of the client that is necessitating nursing intervention. Determine if the condition warrants restriction of contact lens use during the healing process.
- Assess the ocular condition for which the lenses were originally prescribed when determining if the client can go for a period of time without the lenses.

Environmental Assessment

- Assess the area where contact lenses are cleansed. Determine the presence of handwashing facilities. Observe the cleansing equipment in order to assess the client's adherence to protection against infection and contamination.
- Assess the positioning of the client's bed or chair if the lenses are to be removed by someone else. Proper lighting is essential in order to ensure proper placement of the suction device or to position the lenses properly.
- Assess the floor and bed linens before removing the lenses. If the floor is carpeted, a newspaper may be placed over the carpet during insertion and removal if there is a chance that the lens may be dropped (such as might occur when a family member is attempting insertion or removal for the first time).

Planning Strategies

Potential Nursing Diagnoses

Potential for injury to eye tissue

Alteration in comfort due to improper placement of lenses

Knowledge deficit regarding insertion and removal technique

Expected Outcomes	Prevention of infection or trauma to the eyes
	Proper insertion and removal of the contact lenses
	Prevention of loss or damage to the lenses
	Education of family regarding proper technique

Health Promotion Goals

- The client and family will
  Learn proper insertion technique with emphasis on the importance of placing the correct lens in the correct eye
  Learn proper removal technique so that the eye surface is not traumatized
  Understand the importance of adequate cleansing of the lenses to prevent infection of the eye
  Store the lenses properly to prevent loss, damage, or confusion

Equipment

Contact lenses

Cleanser for lenses

Suction cup for removing contact lenses

Case or container for storing lenses with separate compartments labeled right and left for the lenses

Interventions/Health Promotion

ACTION

RATIONALE/AMPLIFICATION

Cleansing the Contact Lenses

1. Advise the client and family to engage in thorough handwashing before cleansing, inserting, or removing the contact lenses. Use the method of lens cleaning that the client is used to if it is considered effective and safe.

   Debris on the hands may easily be transferred to the lenses. These small particles feel very uncomfortable when compressed between the lens and the eye surface.

2. Cleanse the lens before insertion into the eyes. Place a stopper in the bottom of the sink (Fig. 29-1). Open the lens container while holding it in the sink well below the rim. Remove one lens with the tip of the finger. The damp lens will adhere to the finger. Identify whether it is the left or right lens. Wet the lens with slowly running water and a small amount of lens cleaner (Fig. 29-2). Rub the lens between the thumb and forefinger. Rinse with tap water. Insert this lens before cleansing the other.

   Soaking the lens will loosen the dirt and debris that accumulate from normal wearing. This must be removed from the lens before it is inserted into the eye. If the sink is plugged, accidental loss of the lens down the drain may be prevented. Holding the lens container below the rim of the sink will prevent accidental spilling or slipping of the container during opening. Lenses are usually marked so that the left may be discerned from the right. This may be done by a small dot in the corner of one lens. Ask the client how the lenses are marked. Each lens is made to correct the vision in the corresponding eye; they are not interchangeable.

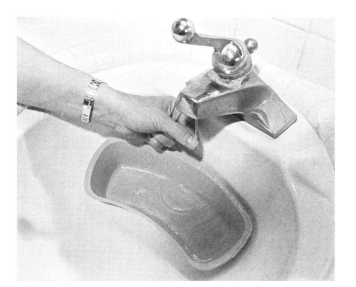

Figure 29.1

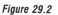

Figure 29.2

ACTION

3. Some types of soft lenses require special soaking solution and special equipment. Usually the soaking solution of choice in these machines is sterile normal saline. Some types of lenses are left in the eyes for extended periods.

Lens Insertion

1. *Soft lens insertion:* hold the lens with the edges between the thumb and forefinger. Apply a drop of wetting solution. Flex the lens slightly with finger pressure (Fig. 29-3). Position the client with head tilted backward.
   Separate the upper and lower eyelids with the thumb and index finger of the hand not holding the lens. Gently place the lens on the cornea directly over the pupil, covering the iris, the colored portion of the eye. Ask the client to blink a few times; then visually assess the placement of the lens.

RATIONALE/AMPLIFICATION

The minerals in normal tap water may harm some of the equipment used in lens cleaning. Advise the family to consult the manufacturer's recommendations regarding care of lenses and equipment.

Lenses are moistened before insertion to facilitate placement and decrease discomfort once the lens is in place.

Holding the eyelids apart will help decrease the urge to blink, which will interfere with the insertion process.

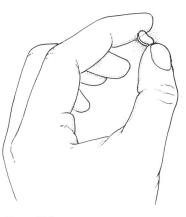

Figure 29.3

ACTION

RATIONALE/AMPLIFICATION

2. *Hard lens insertion:* balance the hard lens on the index finger (Fig. 29-4). Spread a drop of wetting solution onto both sides with a gentle massaging motion between the finger and thumb. Position the lens on the index finger and proceed as with soft lens insertion (Fig. 29-5).

The hard lens looks like a clear disk on the eye and is easily visible with the eye.

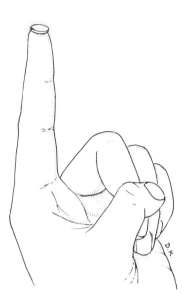

Figure 29.4

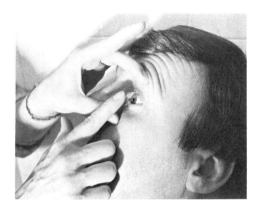

Figure 29.5

3. *Positioning of the hard lens after insertion:* place both forefingers at the eye orbit top and bottom. Gently push through the eyelids to guide the lens into proper position.

The lens floats on a thin watery surface on top of the eye. It will move easily if pushed gently. Once the lens is in proper position, it will stay in place.

Lens Removal

1. Use manual removal for corneal lenses only. Place the tip of the forefinger of one hand horizontally on the lower lid below its margin. Place the top of the forefinger of the other hand on the upper lid above its margin and observe to determine if the lens is visible. Manipulate the two lids against each other in a scissoring motion while the client closes, opens, and rolls the eye. The lens should slide out between the lids.

Pressure on the edges of the lens can cause it to pop out. Care may be taken not to lose the lens by placing a towel or colored sheet over the top of the client under the chin to catch the lens and make visualization easier.

ACTION

RATIONALE/AMPLIFICATION

2. Remove the hard contact lens with a suction cup if the client cannot participate in the removal process (Fig. 29-6). Be sure that the surface of the suction cup is free of dirt and grease. With the forefinger, pull the lower lid of the eye downward. Apply the suction cup to the lens and rock the lens gently to release the vacuum. Remove the lens from the eye in a outward and downward movement. If the vacuum cannot be released from the bottom part of the lens, raise the client's upper eyelid and attempt to release the vacuum at the upper edge of the lens. Remove the lens by pulling gently upward and outward. Apply a drop of wetting solution to the eye to facilitate removal of the lens.

Dirt and grease on the suction cup may adhere to the lens and cause discomfort when the lens is reinserted. The lower lid should not be pulled so far downward that the upper lid is drawn taut against the top of the lens. This will impede the removal process. All edges of the suction cup must be in contact with the lens to create the suction needed to remove the lens. Wetting the lens may ease the vacuum and facilitate removal of the lens.

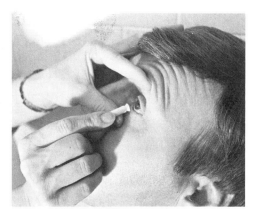

Figure 29.6

Education/ Communication

• Teach the client and family to
  Care for the lenses in a safe manner
  Insert and remove the lenses in a manner that promotes comfort and safety
  Adhere to precautions that will help prevent infection, such as proper cleansing technique
  Recognize when vision problems indicate the need to have the lenses reassessed and perhaps have the prescription changed

Referrals and Consultations

Symptoms such as eye discomfort, headaches, and changes in vision may indicate the need to see the prescribing ophthalmologist or optometrist.

Evaluation of Health Promotion Activities

Quality Assurance/ Reassessment

• Observe the family remove, cleanse, and reinsert the contact lenses to assess the adequacy of technique.

• Ask the client if the contact lens technique is satisfactory.

• Observe the eyes for any signs of trauma or problems relating to the contact lenses.

• Observe the contact lenses to determine if they are clean and intact. Observe the lenses in the client's eyes to determine placement and assess proper insertion into the correct eyes.

DOCUMENTATION

Charting for the Home Health Nurse
Regular notations regarding the state of the eyes and any problems relating to the contact lenses should be made on the client's record.

Records Kept by the Client/Family
If the lenses are cleaned on a regular schedule other than daily, notation on a calendar may help the client and family remember when the lenses were cleaned last and when they are due for cleaning again.

Health Teaching Checklist

Name of Care Provider _____

Relationship to Client _____ Telephone #_____

Taught by _____ Date _____

	EXPLAINED	DEMONSTRATED
Insertion procedure	_____	_____
Removal procedure	_____	_____
Cleansing procedure	_____	_____
Identification of which eye the lens fits	_____	_____
Proper storage	_____	_____
Safety precautions	_____	_____

Product Availability

Storage containers may be purchased at most drug stores and optical companies. Lens cleaner and moisturizer are available in most grocery and drug stores. Special electrical lens cleaners may have to be ordered through an optical company. Suction cups generally come with lens-carrying cases or may be purchased at most drug stores.

30   Douche

Background

Douche involves irrigation or flushing of the vaginal canal. It may be done to cleanse and disinfect the vagina and adjacent parts or to apply medication to relieve local discomfort. It is also used to reduce offensive odors emanating from the vaginal area. *Trichomonas* is a genus of protozoa that normally inhabits the vagina in small numbers without causing any problems. If the normal environment of the vagina is altered, which happens with certain drugs or infections, the protozoa may proliferate, with resulting symptoms including an irritating discharge with a foul odor and itching and burning of the vaginal area. Douche may be used to treat this and other vaginal conditions. In the past, douche was used indiscriminately by many women as a general hygiene measure to promote a feeling of freshness. This practice is no longer recommended because frequent douching may upset the delicate microbial balance in the vaginal canal. Douche has not been proven to be an effective method of contraception.

Assessment of Self-Care Potential

Client/Family Assessment

- Assess the financial resources of the family to determine if reusable douche equipment should be purchased or if they can afford to purchase commercial disposable douches.
- Assess the client's familiarity with douches. Ask the client if she has douched before, how often, and why.

Physical Assessment

- Assess the condition for which the douche is being done. If it is for application of medication or as a therapeutic aid, be sure that the proper prescription is understood. If it is for odor control and prevention of infection, reassess periodically to determine effectiveness.
- Assess the physical condition of the client. Determine if she can go to the bathroom and administer or assist with administration of the douche. Assess her range of motion to determine if she can assume a comfortable position in the bed to perform the douche.

Environmental Assessment

- Assess the home for an adequate area to perform the douche in privacy. If the client can go to the bathroom, this is the ideal place to perform the douche. If not, develop a system to notify family members when treatments are being done that might prove embarrassing to the client so that privacy can be ensured.
- Assess the bedroom to determine where the douche container may be set or hung so that it is 12 inches above the level of the client's vagina.

Planning Strategies

Potential Nursing Diagnoses

Alteration in comfort due to pain and itching

Self-care deficit regarding feminine hygiene

Expected Outcomes

Prevention or successful treatment of vaginal infection

Elimination of odors

Relief of pain and discomfort

Education of the client and family regarding the procedure

Health Promotion Goals

• The client and family will

Learn how to administer the douche in a safe and efficient manner. They will understand the desired frequency as well as the expected results. They will follow proper procedure and adhere to safety precautions.

Provide for the client's comfort by eliminating odors and relieving discomfort and itching

Determine the most effective location for performing vaginal irrigation. They will work together to determine the best position for the client to assume to gain maximum effects of the douche.

Understand that the indiscriminate use of douching may cause more problems than it solves. They will use douching only as prescribed or as needed to provide a pleasant environment for the client.

Equipment

Commercial douche kit or reusable douche container, tubing, and nozzle

Gloves, if desired or if a contagious condition is present

Several towels to pad the bed, and an additional small towel

Bath blanket or sheet for draping

Basin of warm water, soap, and a washcloth

Cotton balls and antibacterial solution

Water-soluble lubricant

Irrigating solution (such as tap water, normal saline, sodium bicarbonate solution consisting of 1 to 2 Tbsp sodium bicarbonate to 1000 ml water, or vinegar solution consisting of 8 ml vinegar to 1000 ml water. Special medicated solutions may be prescribed.)

Bedpan or commode

Stand on which to hang solution

Interventions/Health Promotion

ACTION	*RATIONALE/AMPLIFICATION*
1. If the client is able, she may go to the bathroom and douche while sitting on the commode or standing in the tub. Assist as necessary with gathering equipment and helping the client to the bathroom.	The ambulatory client will probably prefer to perform the douche in the bathroom where procedure and clean-up can be done efficiently and quickly.

ACTION

RATIONALE/AMPLIFICATION

Be sure that the bathroom is warm before the client begins the procedure. Stand by to assist if the client needs help. After the douche, the client should cleanse and dry her vulva before returning to bed.

2. If the douche must be done in bed, pad the bed so that the linen will not be soiled. Be sure that the client is warm and free of drafts. Wash hands before beginning the procedure.

When the irrigation fluid returns from the vagina, it is possible that it will leak onto the bed. Linen protectors will prevent soaking the bed linen and the mattress.

3. Fill the douche container with the desired or prescribed solution, which should be warm to the inner aspect of the wrist, approximately 105°F. Place the douche container on a towel on the bedside table. Attach the tubing and nozzle and place them on the clean towel. Also, bring to the bedside a basin of warm water, soap, and a cloth.

Solutions that are too hot may harm the mucous lining of the vagina and upset the normal vaginal flora. If the tray is set up before beginning, the client will not have to sit on the bedpan for extended periods. The vaginal area is not sterile. However, since infection of the vagina is common, every effort should be made not to introduce pathogenic organisms into this area. For this reason, all equipment should be clean.

4. With the client in the dorsal position on a bedpan, drape her with a bath blanket or bath sheet.

Even in the privacy of the client's own home, sensitivity to her modesty and need for privacy should be shown.

5. Cleanse the perineal area with soap and warm water before beginning the douche.

Cleansing promotes a feeling of cleanliness and reduces the number of microorganisms on the skin.

6. Place a towel over the client's pubic area. Pour the antimicrobial solution over the washcloth and cotton balls. Using the towel to pull the skin slightly taut and to separate the labia, cleanse the genitalia with the cloth, using a downward stroke. Repeat 3 or 4 times using a different portion of the cloth for each stroke.

The towel will be used to provide a feeling of modesty and to get traction against the skin as the labia are cleaned. A different cotton ball must be used for each stroke because the rectal area is considered contaminated. Any item that enters this area must not be reintroduced into the clean area.

ACTION	RATIONALE/AMPLIFICATION
7. Identify the vagina. Lubricate the douche nozzle with a water-soluble jelly. Insert the douche nozzle into the vagina (Fig. 30-1). Hold or hang the irrigation container about 12 inches above the level of the vagina. Cleanse the vaginal folds by gently moving the douche tip forward and backward along the vaginal tract. The douche container may be hung from the back of a chair or from a clothes rack. It may be suspended from a curtain rod by means of a bent hanger.	The lubricant will reduce the friction as the nozzle enters the vagina. Friction may cause trauma to delicate and inflamed tissue. The pressure with which the solution enters the vagina is determined by the level of the container from which it flows. The higher the container, the more pressure exerted by the fluid as it enters the vagina. Excess pressure is undesirable. The fluid should not be held over 12 inches above the vagina. The walls of the vagina are muscular folds that allow expansion during intercourse and childbirth. To cleanse the folds, the nozzle must be rotated and moved along the wall. The slight pressure exerted by the solution entering through the nozzle is sufficient to cleanse between the folds.

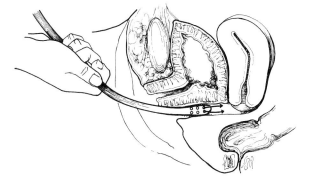

Figure 30.1

ACTION	RATIONALE/AMPLIFICATION
8. After all of the solution has been instilled, elevate the head of the bed or place some pillows behind the client's back so she is in a semi-sitting position and the solution can flow into the bedpan. After the solution has stopped flowing from the vagina, assist the client off the bedpan and dry her genital area thoroughly. Clean the equipment and store it in an area that is free of contamination. The equipment may be placed in a plastic trash bag for storage.	If the client's shoulders are elevated to an area above her hips, the solution will flow back by gravity. All of the solution should be returned to prevent it being expelled later, resulting in soiling of bed linen and gown. The genital area must be dried thoroughly to prevent chapping or irritation. Since this is a clean procedure, the equipment must be cleaned well before being stored. If debris is left on the nozzle, microorganisms may colonize and cause infection when introduced into the vagina during the next procedure.

ACTION	RATIONALE/AMPLIFICATION

Prepackaged Douche

1. Prepare the client as described previously.

2. Read the directions on the package to determine if gentle shaking is indicated. Remove the outer safety wrapping.

   Always read the directions on the douche package to ensure that maximum benefit is obtained from the product. Follow manufacturer's directions.

3. Insert the nozzle of the container into the vagina in a forward and slightly downward direction. Squeeze the douche container to evacuate the contents into the vagina. Allow the solution to return as with a reusable douche.

Related Care

A perineal wash may be used in lieu of the douche periodically, depending on the reason for the douche. Commercial products, such as Peri-Wash, are poured over the perineal area.

Peri-Wash is a soothing solution that promotes healing of chapped tissue and cleansing.

Education/ Communication

- Teach the client and family to
  Administer the douche in an efficient manner without unnecessary exposure of the client
  Adhere to safety precautions regarding douche administration. Emphasize the importance of using only warm solution, never hot. Explain the principles or pressure on a liquid when recommending that the solution be instilled with the bag at a level 12 inches above the client.
  Understand the basic female anatomy and physiology. Explain that the vagina is a muscle that exists in folds. Proper cleansing involves washing between these folds which is possible by rotating the nozzle and placing a small amount of pressure on the solution as it enters the vagina. At this time it is important to mention the importance of cleansing from front to back. Explain that the rectal area is considered contaminated due to the presence of bacteria and microorganisms that normally inhabit this area without problems. However, when these organisms are transmitted to susceptible areas, such as the vagina and urethra, they may cause infection. Translate this information into advice regarding cleansing after toileting. This is especially important for those who provide care to infants. Cleansing during diaper change should occur from front to back.
  Properly care for the douche equipment. Stress the importance of preventing cross-contamination. Show the family how to clean the nozzle, tubing, and container with hot sudsy water. The equipment must then be rinsed carefully and allowed to dry completely before storing in such a manner that contamination is prevented.

Referrals and Consultations

If the client develops a vaginal infection, which is characterized by redness, foul odor, itching, and drainage, referral to a gynecologist or nurse practitioner may be indicated.

Evaluation of Health Promotion Activities

Quality Assurance/ Reassessment

Effectiveness of a cleansing douche can be assessed by elimination of any odors and by the comfort of the client.

Effectiveness of a medicated douche may be assessed by observation of the progress of the condition for which the douche was given. If the condition disappears, the need for further douching should be assessed carefully.

DOCUMENTATION

Charting for the Home Health Nurse
The condition for which the douche was prescribed should be noted on the client's health record. A continuing reassessment of the condition should be done.

Records Kept by the Client/Family
The records kept in the home should reflect the frequency of douches, the type of solution, the amount of solution instilled, and any problems.

Health Teaching Checklist

Name of Care Provider _____

Relationship to Client _____ Telephone #_____

Taught by _____ Date _____

	EXPLAINED	DEMONSTRATED
Location of douching procedure	_____	_____
Type of equipment		
Commercial, disposable douches	_____	_____
Reusable equipment	_____	_____
Positioning for douche	_____	
Preparation of solution	_____	_____
Preparation of equipment	_____	_____
Client preparation		
Draping	_____	_____
Cleaning labia	_____	_____
Importance of downward strokes	_____	
Administration of solution		
Height of container (12 inches)	_____	_____
Lubrication of nozzle	_____	_____
Rotation of nozzle	_____	_____
Elevation of upper torso to evacuate solution	_____	_____
Clean-up of client	_____	_____
Cleaning and storage of equipment	_____	_____

Product Availability

Commercial douches may be purchased at most drug stores and pharmacies. Reusable douche equipment may be purchased at many pharmacies and at hospital-supply houses. Peri-Wash is made by the Sween Corporation and may be purchased at drug stores and pharmacies.

31　Eye Care

Background

The eye, the organ of vision, is extremely sensitive and susceptible to trauma and infection. The eyelids are the protective, movable sheaths of tissue located in front of the eyeball. The lacrimal glands secrete tears, which serve as a natural lubricant for the eyes and wash away debris. Eye care may involve application of medicated drops or ointments, application of a patch or compresses, or irrigation to remove foreign particles, treat infection, or prepare the eye for surgical intervention.

Assessment of Self-Care Potential

Client/Family Assessment

- Assess the level of understanding of the client and family regarding the client's eye condition. Determine if the condition is contagious and whether precautions must be taken against transmitting the disease to others.
- Assess the ability and willingness of family members to administer eye care.
- Assess the familiarity of the client with the room in which most of the time will be spent. Assess ability to move from room to room, especially to the bathroom.

Physical Assessment

- Assess the physical condition for which the client is receiving eye treatments. Determine if special precautions are necessary.
- Assess the ability of the client to cooperate with eye procedures that may require tilting of the head or a side-lying position.
- Assess the presence of photosensitivity in the client, which may accompany some eye conditions.

Environmental Assessment

- Assess the lighting in the client's room to determine if additional light is needed to perform eye care.
- Assess the arrangement of the client's room to determine the best location for the equipment that will offer the least likely opportunity for contamination and the easiest access.
- Assess the room in which the client will spend the majority of time. Determine if it is neat and uncluttered to prevent accidents as the visually impaired client moves around the room.

Planning Strategies

Potential Nursing Diagnoses

Potential for injury

Potential for impairment of skin integrity

Knowledge deficit regarding administration of eye care

Expected Outcomes

Treatment of the eye condition without injury to the eye

Localization of the condition to one eye or to one person

Satisfactory resolution of the eye problem

Education of family regarding proper eye care

Health Promotion Goals

- The client and family will
  Cleanse the eyes daily to prevent crust formation
  Learn how to irrigate the eye safely and effectively
  Adhere to a schedule of irrigation that is most conducive to healing
  Instill eye drops and ointments in a safe and efficient manner
  Apply a patch in the proper manner to provide comfort and to protect the
    eye
  Know what symptoms to report to the physician

Equipment

Eye patch, pads, and ½-inch tape

Eye medications

Eye irrigation device (eyedropper, soft rubber bulb syringe, or commercially pre-pared irrigation device)

Irrigation solution

Cotton ball or gauze pad

Interventions/Health Promotion

ACTION

1. Wash hands carefully before ad-ministering any type of eye care.

2. Cleanse the eyes by gently wiping the eyelashes and eyelids with a soft cotton ball soaked with water. After the crusts have been allowed to soak a few seconds, gently wipe them away with another cotton ball. Use an outward motion from the inner canthus toward the outer aspect of the eye. Use a tissue to wipe away excess tears and secre-tions around the eye.

3. When looking into the client's eye with a light, shine the light at an angle rather than directly into the client's eye.

4. To irrigate the eye, turn the client to the side-lying position. Remove the eye pad if present. Prop the client's head with a pillow and place a basin or container beneath the client's eye to catch the irri-gation solution. Gently separate the eyelids with the thumb and forefinger. Slight pressure may be placed on the bony prominences around the eye to secure separa-tion of the eyelids, but pressure must *never* be placed on the eye-ball itself. Flush the eye with the irrigation solution using low pres-sure. The solution should be in-stilled into the inner canthus and

RATIONALE/AMPLIFICATION

Eye infections are spread by direct contact. Most microorganisms are re-moved by handwashing.

Crusts on the eye can cause trauma to the delicate eye tissue if not removed gently. Wiping from the inner toward the outer aspect of the eye helps pre-vent the crusts from entering the lac-rimal glands.

Direct light onto the cornea causes ex-cessive tearing and may interfere with the eye examination.

Irrigation solution is not instilled di-rectly onto the cornea because of the great sensitivity of the cornea to any type of pressure. The eyelids are sepa-rated and must be held apart since the normal blink reflex will be activated by the instillation of the fluid into the eye. The fluid runs from the inner to the outer canthus to prevent infection or debris from entering the lacrimal duct, which is located in the inner eye area. Drying the eye will reduce the urge to rub or wipe the eye after irrigation.

ACTION

RATIONALE/AMPLIFICATION

allowed to run toward the outer canthus (Fig. 31-1). Dry the area with a clean cotton ball or gauze pad.

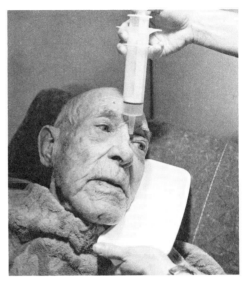

Figure 31.1

5. Before administering eye drops, be sure that the proper medication is being used at the proper time. Always administer medication into the right eye first if both are to be medicated. Have the client sit or lie with head tilted backward. Hold the eyedropper or squeeze bottle in one hand and pull the client's lower eyelid downward with the other hand to form a small pocket with the lid. Tell the client to look up. Without touching the tip of the applicator to the client's eye, squeeze a single drop of medication onto the lining of the lower lid. Do not place the drops directly onto the cornea (Fig. 31-2). Allow the client to blink slowly a few times and instill another drop, if prescribed. Gently blot away any excess medication from the client's face.

The eye is extremely sensitive to medications. It is essential that the proper medication be administered according to the prescribed regimen. They eye applicator is never allowed to touch the eyelid because of the chance of contamination. Having the client look upward helps form the pocket to catch the medication and reduces the urge to blink. By blinking slowly, the client may avoid expelling the medication from the eye. Excess medication should be blotted away so that it will not be absorbed by the body through the lacrimal duct and cause systemic reactions. The medication is always administered into the right eye first so that if distractions occur, the care provider will not have to wonder which eye has already been medicated.

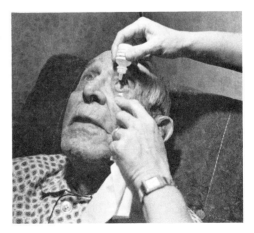

Figure 31.2

ACTION

RATIONALE/AMPLIFICATION

6. Instill eye ointments and salves in the same manner as the eye drops. Hold the lower lid downward and place a small ribbon of ointment along the lower edge, taking care not to touch the applicator to the eye (Fig. 31-3). Ask the client to blink to disperse the ointment. Remove excess ointment with a soft tissue or a cotton ball.

The ointment does not have to cover the entire length of the lower lid since the blinking will disperse it throughout the eye.

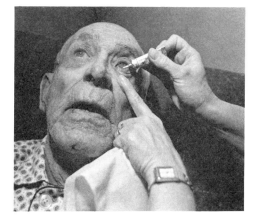

Figure 31.3

7. Compresses may be placed on the eye by soaking a gauze pad in hot water or in ice water (Fig. 31-4). Wring the pad out and fold it into a flat compress. Apply it to the eye. Be sure that the hot compress is allowed to cool somewhat before application. An ice cube may be used for the cool compress if it is wrapped in a gauze pad or cloth before being placed over the eye.

Hot compresses may be used to treat surface eye infections, relieve pain, and help clean the eye. Cold compresses are used to relieve itching, swelling, and irritation. (Hot compresses should not be used on an open, penetrating wound; cold compresses should not be used in eye infection.) The eye is closed during compress treatment so that infection will not be introduced into the eye from the surrounding skin or from the compress itself.

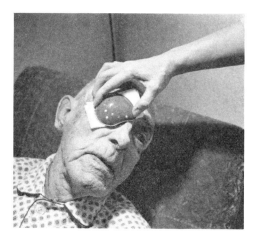

Figure 31.4

ACTION	RATIONALE/AMPLIFICATION
8. Apply an eye patch using tape and a gauze pad. Before applying the patch, ask the client to close both eyes. Place the patch over the affected eye and secure it with two pieces of paper tape (household cellophane tape may be used) that run from mid forehead to the earlobe (Fig. 31-5). When both eyes must be patched, place a separate patch over each eye rather than wrapping a bandage around the client's head.	Eye patches are used to absorb secretions and to immobilize the eye. An eye patch should not be used to treat infections since the dark, moist environment provided by the patch is highly conducive to bacterial proliferation. Patching each eye separately rather than using a circular bandage is more comfortable and less frightening for the client.

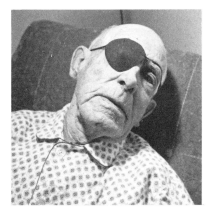

Figure 31.5

9. If the client wears glasses, conditions of the eye may cause abnormal distortions. This may lead to trauma to the eyes as eyeglasses are put on in the usual manner. Show the client how to hold the glasses by the tips of the ear pieces and to guide the glasses over the ears into place (Fig. 31-6).	Distortions in perception may cause the client to poke the ear pieces into one or both eyes when putting them on.

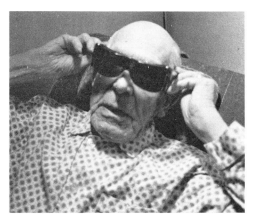

Figure 31.6

ACTION	RATIONALE/AMPLIFICATION

Related Care

See Technique 29 for care of contact lenses and Technique 26 for care of an eye prosthesis.

Age-Specific Modifications

If a child struggles when receiving eye drops, assist the child into a position with the head tilted backward. Instill the eye drop into the inner canthus of the affected eye. Ask the child to blink a few times. When the eye blinks, the drop will roll into the eye and be dispersed throughout the eye surface.	A calm, gentle approach will usually calm the child enough to get the eye drop into the inner canthus area.

Education/Communication

- Teach the client and family to

  Care for the eyes in a safe and efficient manner. Discourage rubbing the eyes. Recommend compresses to relieve irritation.

  Keep the environment free of obstacles that might cause the client to fall during ambulation. Make every effort to keep items in the room in the same place to help the visually impaired client feel more secure.

  Irrigate the eye with the prescribed solution. A pad may be placed under the client's face and under the basin to prevent wetting the pillow. A hand towel with a piece of plastic bag under it will preserve the dryness of the pillow and bed linen. Any clean plastic container may be used to catch the excess irrigation fluid. However, if the client has a contagious condition, all eye care equipment must be kept separate from items used by other family members.

  Administer eye medications correctly. Stress the importance of preventing the applicator from touching the client's skin because it is then contaminated.

  Apply compresses of the proper type for specific problems. Be sure that hot compresses are allowed to cool slightly before being placed on the client's eye. The compress should feel warm, not hot, to the inner aspect of the wrist. To test this, the back of the compress should be tested, not the portion that will be applied to the client's eye.

  Apply eye patches so that they are comfortable and secure. Small amounts of tape are usually adequate. Be sure that the client's eye is closed under the patch.

  Understand the hazards of self-prescription of eye medications. Some over-the-counter drugs can mask serious symptoms that should be reported to a physician. Over-the-counter eye medications, just as all easily available drugs, should be used with caution and restraint.

Referrals and Consultations

Eye problems should be referred to an ophthalmologist or optometrist for resolution. Foreign objects that cannot be removed by normal tearing or irrigation should be removed by an eye specialist to prevent irreversible trauma to the eye.

Evaluation of Health Promotion Activities

Quality Assurance/ Reassessment

- Observe the condition of the client's eyes. Determine if they are clean and free from trauma. Observe the compresses or patches to assess proper application and success of treatment.
- Observe the family member irrigating the client's eye. Note particularly attention to infection-control measures such as direction of irrigation within the eye and use of clean materials.
- Observe the instillation of eye drops or ointments. Note the condition for which the medication is being administered to assess if it is improving.

DOCUMENTATION

Charting for the Home Health Nurse
- Note the condition of the client's eyes in relation to appropriateness and effectiveness of the treatment.

Records Kept by the Client/Family
Records may be kept on a calendar regarding when specific treatments were done. Eye medications may be kept on schedule by placing reminders near the bed. These reminders are placed in a drawer each time the medication is administered. They may be poker chips or buttons that are used to indicate each dose of medicine.

Health Teaching Checklist

Name of Care Provider _____

Relationship to Client _____ Telephone #_____

Taught by _____ Date _____

	EXPLAINED	DEMONSTRATED
Importance of handwashing	_____	
Cleansing of the eyes	_____	_____
Inspection of the eyes with light	_____	_____
Irrigation technique	_____	_____
Administering medications		
Eye drops	_____	_____
Eye ointments and salves	_____	_____
Special methods for children	_____	_____
Compresses		
Indications for	_____	_____
Hot	_____	_____
Cold	_____	_____
Patches	_____	_____
Application of glasses	_____	_____
Environmental adjustments for the visually impaired	_____	_____

Product Availability

Eye patches, medications, and irrigation fluids may be obtained from most drug stores and pharmacies. Gauze pads and cotton balls are available at drug and grocery stores. If sterile solutions are needed for some eye treatments, these may be obtained in various-size containers in drug stores and pharmacies.

32   Ear Care

Background

The ear is not only important for hearing, it is also involved in balance and equilibrium. The glands lining the auditory canal secrete a waxy substance called *cerumen*. Excessive amounts of this wax may block the ear canal and exert pressure on the eardrum. This pressure can cause earache and temporary deafness. The mucous membrane that lines the middle ear is continuous with that of the pharynx. Thus, it is possible for infection to travel along the mucous membrane from the nose or the throat to the middle ear (otitis media).

Assessment of Self-Care Potential

Client/Family Assessment

- Assess the family for any history of ear problems and deafness.
- Assess the understanding of the care provider regarding the instillation of ear drops and the safety precautions involved.

Physical Assessment

- Assess the condition for which the client is being seen in the home. If the ear condition is unrelated, assess the ear problems being experienced to determine if referral is necessary.
- Assess the ability of the client to assume the side-lying position, which will facilitate ear treatments.
- Assess the presence of any hearing loss. Determine how long this has been a problem and the client's degree of adaptation to the loss.
- Assess any history of hearing problems such as ear infections, tubes in the ears, previous surgery, use of hearing aids, or irrigation to remove wax.

Environmental Assessment

- Assess the lighting in the client's room to facilitate administration of ear treatment.

Planning Strategies

Potential Nursing Diagnoses

Alteration in comfort due to pain

Potential for injury to delicate ear tissue

Knowledge deficit regarding care of the ears

Expected Outcomes

Reduction of pain

Resolution of the ear condition

Prevention of infection or trauma to the ears

Education of client and family regarding ear care

Health Promotion Goals
- The client and family will
  Care for the ears competently and confidently
  Instill the ear medications as prescribed
  Understand which symptoms should be reported
  Assist with ear irrigation
  Understand the importance of keeping sharp objects out of the ears

Equipment

Otoscope with proper-size speculum

Extra batteries

Irrigation syringe or bulb syringe and irrigation solution

Basin

Medication and cotton ball

Soft cloth

Interventions/Health Promotion

ACTION

1. Before inspecting the ear with the otoscope, wipe the external ear with a soft cloth. Do not use a cotton-tipped applicator and do not press the cloth forcefully into the ear canal.

2. Inspect the ear with the otoscope by gently inserting the rounded speculum into the ear canal. Pull the upper ear (pinna) gently upward and outward with the fingertips while the base of the hand rests against the client's head. Tilt the otoscope to get a clear view of the entire auditory canal; ask the client to remain motionless.

Ear Drop Instillation

1. Warm the medication by placing the bottle inside a plastic bag and setting the bag and bottle in a pan of warm water for a few minutes. *Never put cold drops in a person's ear.*

RATIONALE/AMPLIFICATION

Use this time to explain to the client and family why a cotton-tipped applicator should not be used to clean the ear. Stress the fact that small items in the ear can cause trauma and infection. Stress that this is particularly important with small children. Demonstrate how to wipe the external ear with the cloth without placing pressure on the ear canal.

Unnecessary roughness or pulling can traumatize the auditory canal. Use the base of the hand to ensure that the client does not move suddenly while the otoscope is in the ear.

Placing the bottle in a plastic bag will preserve the label. Instillation of cold ear drops can cause dizziness and pain. Test the temperature by placing a drop on your wrist; it should feel warm, not hot.

ACTION	RATIONALE/AMPLIFICATION
2. Place the client in a side-lying position with the affected ear uppermost. Clean the external ear with a soft cloth. Grasp the upper ear and gently pull upward and outward.	Pulling the outer ear upward and outward straightens the auditory canal and facilitates insertion of the ear drops (Fig. 32-1).

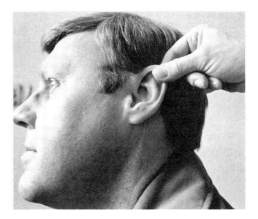

Figure 32.1

3. Insert the dropper just inside the external ear and administer the prescribed amount of medication.	
4. Apply a clean, dry cotton ball over the opening of the auditory canal to contain the medication. Remind the client to remain in the side-lying position for 5 minutes after instillation of the ear drops.	Do not push the cotton ball into the ear canal. If the client remains in the side-lying position for 5 minutes, the medication will have time to disperse to the appropriate areas.
5. Wipe the dropper with a clean cotton ball. Store the medication in the refrigerator, if indicated.	Some medications are unstable at room temperature.

Ear Irrigation

Using an irrigation syringe, flush the auditory canal with warm water, saline, or solution as prescribed. Allow the irrigation solution to return by turning the client to the other side and placing the ear over a basin or soft towel.	The solution should be warm, but not hot. Test the solution by placing a small amount on the inner wrist.

Age-Specific Modifications

When administering ear drops to a child, the top of the ear should not be pulled outward as in the adult. Instead, gently pull the earlobe downward and backward (Fig. 32-2).	The auditory canal in a child is shorter than in an adult. Pulling the earlobe downward and backward straightens the canal and facilitates insertion of the ear drops.

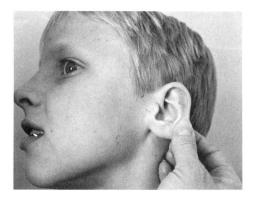

Figure 32.2

**Education/
Communication**

- Teach the client and family to

    Notify the physician at once if pain occurs after instillation of ear drops

    Observe safety precautions when cleaning the client's ears. Urge the family to avoid placing any small or sharp objects (such as cotton-tipped swabs, keys, hair pins) into the ear. Trauma to the delicate lining of the ear can easily result in infection.

    Understand that wax formation in the ears serves a purpose and is not dangerous unless it becomes hardened and occludes the ear canal. Stress the fact that the wax is present to filter impurities that might enter the ear. Its sticky substance traps foreign particles, which might cause infection if allowed to enter the inner ear.

    Chew gum or drink large amounts of fluid if they feel fluid building up in the middle ear

**Referrals and
Consultations**

Continuing hearing loss and pain in the ears are indications that the client should see a physician.

Hearing loss may be progressive. Even if the client has a hearing aid, follow-up visits should be made to the audiologist or otologist to ensure that the hearing correction is sufficient.

Evaluation of Health Promotion Activities

**Quality Assurance/
Reassessment**

- Observe the family during ear drop administration. Check to see that the ear drops are the proper temperature and that the client remains immobile long enough for the medicine to disperse properly.

- Observe the inner canal of the ear for trauma, which may indicate that sharp objects have been used for cleaning the ear.

- If the family will do the ear irrigation, observe their technique and offer suggestions, if needed.

DOCUMENTATION

Charting for the Home Health Nurse

The condition and appearance of the ear should be noted regularly. Any ear treatments, such as irrigation, should be noted on the client record along with assessment of response and outcomes.

Records Kept by the Client/Family

Ask the family to keep track of ear drop administration. They should also keep a record of the frequency of ear irrigation and the results.

Health Teaching Checklist

Name of Care Provider _____

Relationship to Client _____ Telephone # _____

Taught by _____ Date _____

	EXPLAINED	DEMONSTRATED
Cleaning the ear	_____	_____
Inspecting the ear	_____	_____
Ear drop procedure		
Heating the drops	_____	_____
Straightening the ear canal—adult	_____	_____
Straightening the ear canal—child	_____	_____
Ear irrigation procedure	_____	_____
Safety precautions involving ear care	_____	_____

Product Availability

Irrigation bulbs or syringes may be obtained at most pharmacies and drug stores.

33   Foot Care

Background

The feet of ill and bedridden clients are especially susceptible to infection and other problems. Because the feet are farther from the heart than any other body part, they are the most compromised by vascular conditions that interfere with normal circulation. Those conditions that generally affect bedridden clients include footdrop, intermittent claudication, ulcers, and gangrene. Footdrop is a deformity in which the foot is extended abnormally at the ankle in the direction of the sole of the foot. Intermittent claudication is a severe pain in the calf muscles caused by inadequate circulation. It usually occurs during walking but subsides with rest. Ulcers and gangrene are common side-effects of diabetes. They occur because of inadequate circulation to the feet, which retards the natural healing process.

Assessment of Self-Care Potential

Client/Family Assessment

- Assess the family for any history of diabetes. Determine if any of the family members have foot problems and the extent and duration of the problems.
- Assess the condition of the client's and family's footwear. Determine if they wear clean socks. Assess the condition of their shoes and the financial resources to purchase new shoes. Determine if the family members wear used shoes and the priority they give to well-fitting shoes. Many mothers buy shoes that are too large for their children so that shoes will not have to be purchased so frequently.

Physical Assessment

- Assess the condition of the client's feet and lower extremities. Palpate the dorsal and pedal pulses as an indication of the status of circulation to the feet. Check for wounds, blisters, lesions, calluses, ingrown toenails, and unnatural foot position.
- Assess the mobility of the ankles and toes. Assess the client's shoes for abnormal wear, which may indicate that the client walks in an unnatural position.
- Assess the cleanliness of the feet and toes. Check the toenails for proper pedicure.

Environmental Assessment

- Assess the furniture to determine if there is a chair in which the client can comfortably sit while soaking the feet. Determine if the client and family have a basin suitable for soaking the feet.
- Assess the condition of the floors to determine the best place to perform foot care. If the bathroom floor is waterproof, the feet can be soaked there. If the bathroom is carpeted, the procedure may take place in the tub or shower. If the client cannot get out of bed, foot care will have to be done at the bedside.
- Assess the presence of heating capabilities in the room which the client's feet are to be soaked and foot care done. The room should be warm and free of drafts.
- Assess the lighting in the client's room. The feet should be inspected in adequate lighting so that color and potential vascular problems can be detected.

Planning Strategies

Potential Nursing Diagnoses

Potential for impairment of skin integrity

Impaired physical mobility

Knowledge deficit concerning care of the feet

Expected Outcomes

Maintenance of skin integrity of the feet

Promotion or restoration of adequate peripheral circulation

Prevention of foot deformities and infections

Education of the family regarding foot care

Health Promotion Goals

- The client and family will
  Perform foot care in a safe and efficient manner
  Understand the possible side-effects of such conditions as diabetes and peripheral vascular disease, especially as these conditions affect the feet
  Learn how to prevent complications associated with prolonged bed rest
  Obtain the needed equipment to provide a therapeutic environment for proper foot care
  Place the proper priority on caring for the client's feet in relation to overall physical condition and potential for recuperation

Equipment

Footboard

Basin and toenail clippers

Lanolin or petrolatum-based cream

Powder

Cotton stockings

Interventions/Health Promotion

ACTION	*RATIONALE/AMPLIFICATION*
1. Inspect the client's feet thoroughly. Examine both feet for injury such as blisters, cuts, bruises, or infection. Inspect the bottom of the feet as well as the top. Be sure the room is well lighted during the examination.	Due to compromised circulation, many ill clients develop foot problems, which, if found early enough, may be corrected before irreversible damage is done.

ACTION	RATIONALE/AMPLIFICATION
2. Bathe the feet in warm water only; *never use hot water.* Immerse the client's feet in a basin of water for cleaning, even when a bed bath is given (Fig. 33-1).	Due to poor circulation, some clients are not sensitive to temperature extremes in their feet. For this reason, they may receive burns without being aware of it. It is essential to use only warm water in bathing the client's feet. Immersing the feet in warm water gives a sense of comfort and refreshment to the bedridden client.

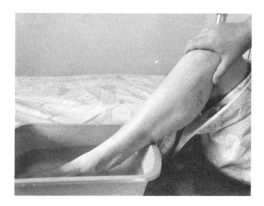

Figure 33.1

3. Dry the feet thoroughly after they have been bathed. Dry carefully, especially between the toes (Fig. 33-2). Brisk but gentle rubbing may enhance circulation, but be careful not to cause trauma to the skin.	The feet should be kept dry in order to preserve the integrity of the skin and to decrease the chance of infection from microorganisms, which grow best in a warm, moist environment.
4. Apply powder to the feet if they tend to perspire (Fig. 33-3). Cotton stockings may be worn while the client is confined to bed. These should be changed if they become soaked with perspiration. Lanolin or a petrolatum-based cream may be applied to the feet if the skin is dry, flaky, or crusted.	Powder will absorb some of the moisture from perspiration and will help keep the feet dry. Creams will help moisturize and soften the skin of the foot.

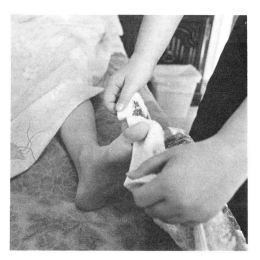

Figure 33.2

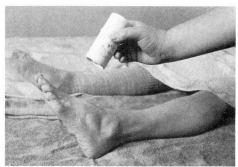

Figure 33.3

ACTION	*RATIONALE/AMPLIFICATION*

Related Care

1. Toenails can be a source of foot problems. To trim the toenails, soak the feet in warm water for about 4 to 5 minutes. Trim each nail carefully, straight across and above the line of attachment to the toe. Do not trim the toenails too short.

   If the toenails are allowed to grow excessively long, they may become ingrown or catch on hosiery, causing trauma. A straight cut across the toe will help eliminate trauma.

2. If the client is confined to bed for extended periods, the feet tend to hyperextend. This condition is known as footdrop. To prevent this condition, place a footboard at the end of the bed. Range-of-motion exercises to the ankles and feet as well as loosening the top covers over the feet may help prevent footdrop.

   Prolonged bed rest places a severe strain on all body parts, especially the feet. The footboard facilitates keeping the feet in the natural position and keeps the bed linens from pushing the tops of the feet downward (Fig. 33-4).

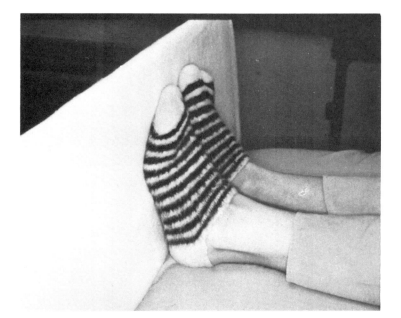

Figure 33.4

Education/ Communication

- Teach the client and family to
  Wash the feet thoroughly and carefully, taking care to clean them completely without trauma. Explain the need to dry the feet thoroughly with special emphasis to the areas between the toes.
  Trim the toenails straight across. Advise them to soak the feet before trimming the nails. Explain that if the toenails become too long, they may traumatize the feet. However, if the toenails are trimmed too short, trauma may also occur. Explain the need to soften the nails by soaking them in warm water before trimming.
  Recognize the signs and symptoms of infection and deformity. Advise them to inspect the client's feet daily for signs of redness, whiteness, scratches, or lesions. Explain about keeping the covers loosely over the top of the feet. Explain what footdrop is and how to prevent it.

Understand how they can best avoid problems when the client's circulation is impaired, such as in diabetes and peripheral vascular disease. Advise the client to check all surfaces of the feet daily using a hand mirror to inspect the bottoms of the feet. Further advise the client that walking is the best exercise for the feet. Emphasize the importance of wearing socks that fit well and are clean. Shoes should be comfortable when they are purchased and should be worn only for short periods at first. Trimming toenails and caring for corns and calluses should be left to a physician or podiatrist. If this is not practical, encourage the client to trim the nails carefully and to avoid trauma to the skin of the foot. These clients should not go barefoot inside or outside of the home. Remind the client to avoid extremes in temperature, either hot or cold. Hot water bottles or ice packs should never be applied to the lower extremities of those with impaired circulation.

Referrals and Consultations

If trauma to the skin of the foot is noted in the client who has compromised circulation, referral to a physician or podiatrist may be in order.

Evaluation of Health Promotion Activities

Quality Assurance/ Reassessment

- Check the condition and progress of healing of the feet. If scratches or trauma are noted, reevaluate the method of administering foot care. Ask the family questions and determine if there are any knowledge deficits. Allow and encourage the family to ask questions and feel comfortable about giving foot care.
- Demonstrate how to trim the client's toenails. Allow the family members to return the demonstration. During each visit, the client's nails may be checked for proper technique and to assess if the frequency of foot care is adequate.
- Check the position and condition of the footboard. It should be secure with a smooth, polished surface that will not allow the client to get splinters. The client's feet should be flat against the board in the natural position.

DOCUMENTATION

Charting for the Home Health Nurse
A progressive record of the condition of the feet and resolution of any problems should be kept by the home health nurse.

Health Teaching Checklist

Name of Care Provider _____

Relationship to Client _____ Telephone #_____

Taught by _____ Date _____

	EXPLAINED	DEMONSTRATED
Foot care in the bathroom	_____	_____
Foot care in the bed	_____	_____
Correct technique for trimming toenails	_____	_____
Precautions to prevent footdrop		
Loosening covers over feet	_____	_____
Footboard	_____	_____
Range-of-motion exercises to feet and ankles	_____	_____

	EXPLAINED	DEMONSTRATED
Precautions for clients with impaired vascular circulation		
Daily inspection of the feet	_____	_____
Gentle cleaning of the feet	_____	_____
Thorough drying of feet	_____	_____
Proper footwear	_____	_____
Trimming toenails, special precautions	_____	_____

Product Availability

A footboard may be purchased at some hospital-supply firms or may be made by placing a sanded and polished piece of plywood at the foot of the bed, extending up to a level of about 1 foot above the bed. If the board will not stand upright at a right-degree angle to the mattress, it may be constructed as a box that will wedge into the foot of the bed (Fig. 33-5).

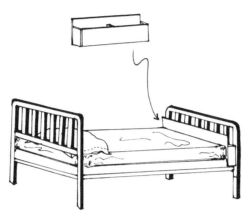

Figure 33.5

34   Hair, Daily Care and Shampoo

Background

Care of the hair includes daily grooming and periodic cleaning of the client's hair and scalp. Failure to keep the hair clean may result in dandruff, a scaly material on the client's scalp resulting from seborrheic dermatitis. The hair is formed in a pouchlike depression in the skin called a *hair follicle*. The hair shaft is the visible part of the hair. The root of the hair is that part embedded in the follicle. Two or more sebaceous glands are associated with each follicle. Secretions from these glands are responsible for the oiliness of the hair when it is not cleaned frequently. There is a constant loss of hair throughout life. The hair is replaced by the continued division of epidermal cells in the germinal area. Cutting or shaving the hair has no effect on its growth; the maximal rate of growth is about 10 mm per month.

Assessment of Self-Care Potential

Client/Family Assessment

- Assess the ability of the care provider to assist the client as needed during the procedure. If the client will need additional assistance to get to the bath or shower, assess the availability of that assistance. If the safety of the client cannot be ensured, recommend that the shampoo be done with the client in bed.

- Assess the understanding and past experience of the care provider in shampooing the hair of a person who cannot get out of bed. Assess knowledge deficits and determine how much information is needed and how and when it may best be offered.

Physical Assessment

- Assess the physical condition of the client to determine if the shampoo must be done in bed or if transport to the bath or shower is possible. Determine how much of the procedure the client can do safely. Assess the condition of the client's hair and scalp. Identify the presence of pediculosis. The eggs (nits) appear as white flakes on the hair shaft that will not shake loose as does dandruff.

Environmental Assessment

- Assess the physical layout of the bathroom to determine if the client may safely be shampooed in the bath or shower. If a wheelchair will be used for transport, determine if it will fit in the bathroom. If the client cannot be safely placed in the bathtub or shower, assess the possibility of using a sink that would allow the client to stay in the sitting position in the wheelchair.

- Assess the bedroom in which the client will be shampooed to determine if running water is present and the nearest water source. Determine whether or not hot and cold running water is available. Experiment with positioning of the bed to allow access to the client's head. Determine how long it takes to heat the client's room in deciding when to wash the hair.

Planning Strategies

Potential Nursing Diagnoses

Potential impairment of skin integrity

Knowledge deficit: family giving shampoo with client in bed

Self-care deficit (grooming)

Expected Outcomes

Prevention of the development or spread of scalp infections

Understanding of how to give a shampoo to a person in bed

Maintenance of cleanliness of client's hair and scalp

Health Promotion Goals

- The client and family will
  Understand how to prevent tangling and matting of the hair due to prolonged bed rest
  Promote the mental and physical comfort of the client by attention to general hygiene measures
  Understand and practice the principles of body mechanics and safety during hair care

Equipment

For daily care
  Comb and brush
  Towel

For shampoo
  Shampoo basin (a curved basin with a spout on one side for draining the water)
  Basin, tub, or bowl that will hold about 7.5 liters (2 gallons) (Two basins are needed if a shampoo basin is not available.)
  Pitcher or water container and cup
  Dryer (optional)
  Plastic sheet (the size of a bathtowel or larger)
  3 bathtowels and a small pad to protect the bed
  2 washcloths

Interventions/Health Promotion

ACTION	RATIONALE/AMPLIFICATION
Daily Care	
1. Encourage the client and care provider to brush the hair vigorously every day. If the client has a scalp condition or sensitivity, use lighter strokes; however, daily hair brushing is still important.	Brushing the hair stimulates the scalp and increases the blood supply. This encourages tissue healing and prevention of tissue breakdown.
2. Place a towel under the client's head and over the client's chest when in bed. If the client can sit up, place a towel over the shoulders.	Brushing causes healthy hair to become dislodged from the scalp. The bed linen and the client's clothing may be protected by a towel.

ACTION

RATIONALE/AMPLIFICATION

3. Divide the hair into sections and brush or comb each section starting near the scalp and pulling in an upward direction. If a comb is used, the teeth should be dull.

Brushing small sections at a time will prevent tangling. An upward motion is used so that the hair shaft is not split or strained during the procedure. The teeth on the comb should not scratch the client's scalp.

4. When brushing or combing tangled or matted hair, keep the hair between the fingers and the brush or comb (Fig. 34-1).

Holding the hair between the scalp and the comb will provide a counter-force and prevent scalp trauma from pulling of the hair.

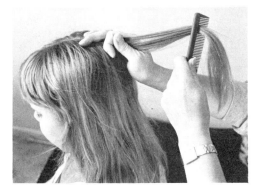

Figure 34.1

5. If the hair is badly tangled, shampoo and rinse well. If the hair is matted due to dried blood, apply undiluted hydrogen peroxide to remove the blood. If the hair is severely matted due to lack of cleansing, apply undiluted cream rinse, allow it to remain on the hair for 5 or 10 minutes, then rinse with clear water and comb small sections at a time. If the tangles cannot be removed, the tangled or matted areas may have to be cut. However, this should be done with the client's permission after a thorough explanation of why it is necessary.

If the underlying cause of the tangled hair cannot be washed away, cutting may be the only way to remove the tangles in order to provide adequate hair care.

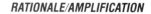

ACTION	RATIONALE/AMPLIFICATION

Shampooing the Hair

1. Place the client in a comfortable position with a pillow under the shoulders. Place a plastic sheet between two towels (Fig. 34-2) and slide it under the client's head. Place another pad on the edge of the shampoo basin (Fig. 34-3).

2. A shampoo basin has a spout on one side. Place the shampoo basin under the client's neck with the spout off the edge of the bed (Fig. 34-4).

A properly positioned pillow will elevate and hyperextend the neck, allowing easier access to the scalp area while maintaining comfort. Placing the plastic between towels prevents discomfort from the client's skin being in contact with the plastic and decreases the natural slipperiness.

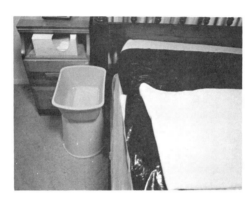

Figure 34.2

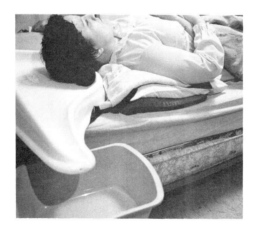

Figure 34.3

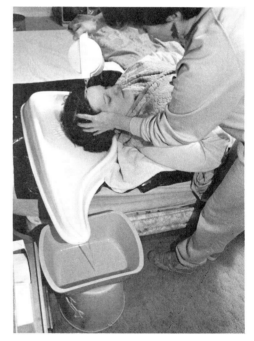

Figure 34.4

3. If a shampoo basin is not available, use a regular basin with additional pillows to prop the client to a sufficient height to allow the rinse water to run into the basin.

Be sure the client is propped to a sufficient height so that discomfort of the neck is avoided.

ACTION	*RATIONALE/AMPLIFICATION*
4. Tuck a piece of plastic under the edge of the basin and allow the plastic to fall over the side of the bed into a second basin, which is used to catch overflow rinse water. Do not leave the client unattended with a plastic bag in bed. Suffocation could result.	The plastic will keep the client and the bed linen dry. Capability of catching the overflow enables clean water to be used for rinsing. Attention to safety precautions is essential.
5. Elevate one side of the basin in the bed so that it tilts toward the overflow receptacle.	Using the principle of gravity, the water may be funneled from the basin on the bed into the basin at a lower level.
6. Brush the client's hair thoroughly and wet it with warm, not hot, water. The water may be obtained from a water source and poured by the cupful over the client's hair. The water may also be brought to the bedside in a pitcher and poured over the client's head.	Brushing will remove the tangles from the hair. The water should feel warm to the inner aspect of the forearm. Hot water may injure the scalp.
7. Apply a small amount of shampoo and lather the hair well. Rinse the hair and shampoo again. Rinse thoroughly after the second shampoo. Work quickly so the client will not tire.	Shampoo left on the hair may cause itching and discomfort. The position of hyperextension of the neck places a strain on the bedridden client. Therefore, it is important that the procedure be accomplished as quickly as possible to prevent fatigue and strain.
8. Test for adequacy of rinsing by pulling a strand of hair between the index finger and the thumb. Anchor the strand next to the scalp before pulling. A squeaking sound indicates the hair is clean and the shampoo has been thoroughly removed.	Anchoring the hair will prevent pulling, which is uncomfortable.
9. Dry the client's hair, neck, and shoulders. If able, the hair may be blown dry. *Remove all standing water before using an electrical instrument to prevent the chance of electrocution.* If not, use a towel to gently rub the hair to remove the excess moisture.	It is important to ensure the client's safety by removing standing water.
10. Arrange the hair in an attractive manner.	Bolster the client's self-esteem by attention to personal appearance.

Related Care

1. If the client is bedfast, consider the possibility of cutting the hair to a short length. Secure the consent of the client before cutting the hair.	Shorter hair is easier to care for and keep clean. It also resists tangling more easily than longer hair.

ACTION	*RATIONALE/AMPLIFICATION*
2. Observe the scalp for broken areas, which are potential sources of infection, and pressure areas over the cranial prominences. Especially notice the mastoid and the occipital areas. Observe the folds behind the ear for redness and tissue breakdown.	Skin areas that receive prolonged pressure due to positioning are susceptible to skin breakdown.

**Education/
Communication**

- Teach the client and family to

  Consider the physiology of hair growth when caring for the client's hygienic needs. Explain how the secretions of the sebaceous glands produce an oily feeling to the hair if it is not cleaned often. Also, explain how stimulation of the scalp is beneficial to the tissue and the hair follicles.

  Understand the importance of nutrition in hair growth and maintenance. Poor diet deprives the hair, as well as the rest of the body, of needed nutrients.

  Use proper technique when shampooing the client's hair in the bed or by whatever method is allowed within the environmental limitations of the client's home. Assist the care provider to experiment with different methods of cleaning the hair to discover which is the easiest and most effective.

Evaluation of Health Promotion Activities

**Quality Assurance/
Reassessment**

- Perform periodic visitations during hair shampooing in order to assess the technique and possibly offer suggestions to the care provider regarding easier methods for completing the task. Occasional demonstration of the proper technique may reinforce the importance of safety precautions. It is particularly important that the water not be too hot for the tender skin of the head and that the client not be exposed to potential hazards, such as suffocation or electrocution.

DOCUMENTATION

Charting for the Home Health Nurse
- Encourage the client/family to keep a record of the days when they shampoo the client's hair and to try to do it regularly.

**Health Teaching
Checklist**

Name of Care Provider _____

Relationship to Client _____ Telephone #_____

Taught by _____ Date _____

	EXPLAINED	DEMONSTRATED
Need for procedure	_____	
Physiology of hair growth	_____	
Importance of nutrition	_____	
Safety precautions	_____	_____
Sectioning hair	_____	_____
Combing the hair without pulling	_____	_____
Bed shampoo set-up	_____	_____
Propping and positioning the client	_____	_____

	EXPLAINED	DEMONSTRATED
Testing the temperature of the water	_____	_____
Shampooing the client's hair	_____	_____
Drying the hair	_____	_____

Product Availability

Commercial shampoo basins are available at many pharmacies and hospital-supply houses.

Commercial preparations are available for cleaning the hair without getting it wet. Although these may be an acceptable alternative when the client is unable to have the hair wash completed at the regular time, these preparations should not be considered a permanent alternative to hair washing with shampoo and water.

35   Handwashing

Background

The mechanical removal of pathogenic organisms from the hands using soap and water should be a part of daily life for everyone. Those times most frequently associated with handwashing are after toileting and before eating. However, when a person who is ill or susceptible to infection is introduced into the home setting, handwashing takes on greater significance. The goal is to prevent contaminating susceptible persons with pathogens that may cause disease. Skin on the fingers and palms contains ridges and grooves in which reside normal flora that may become pathogenic if introduced to the susceptible host.

Assessment of Self-Care Potential

Client/Family Assessment

- Assess the level of understanding the client and family exhibit regarding the transmission of microorganisms. Assess their understanding of the needs and condition of the client. Determine if they understand what the client's condition is and how it is affected by contact with other persons. Assess their motivation to protect themselves and the rest of the family from cross-contamination.

- Assess the usual handwashing regimen in this family. Determine when they customarily wash their hands. Assess their understanding of the need to wash before eating and after toileting.

Physical Assessment

- Assess the hands of the care provider and the client. Assess for breaks in the skin or extreme dryness. Determine if the client or care provider has any dermatologic condition that would be affected by frequent handwashing. Ask if they routinely use a lotion after handwashing.

- Assess the condition of the client. Determine if the goal of handwashing will be to protect the client from cross-infection or to protect the rest of the family from direct contact with contamination from the client.

Environmental Assessment

- Assess the handwashing facilities. Determine if the house has hot and cold running water. Assess the handwashing area for soap. Assess the type and condition of towels in the handwashing area. If the possibility of contamination exists, paper towels are preferable to cloth towels.

- Assess the proximity of the handwashing facilities to the client. If the client has limited mobility, the location of the handwashing area will be very important. If the client is bedfast, handwashing will have to be done in the bed with a basin of warm water and soap.

Planning Strategies

Potential Nursing Diagnoses

Knowledge deficit, technique and importance of handwashing in preventing the spread of infection

Skin integrity, potential impairment

Expected Outcomes

Understanding of technique and importance of handwashing

Prevention of cross-infection

Cleanliness of hands while maintaining skin integrity

Health Promotion Goals

- The client and family will
  Learn the mechanics of proper handwashing
  Understand and follow through on the desired handwashing regimen
  Prevent cross-contamination or self-contamination by direct contact with the hands

Equipment

Soap

Running water

Paper towels

Lotion

Orange stick or nail file

Receptacle for soiled towels with plastic liner

Interventions/Health Promotion

ACTION

1. Explain to the client and the family the rationale behind the handwashing regimen. Be sure that the handwashing area has all of the necessary equipment. For the duration of the client's illness, it is probably preferable to use paper towels, which may themselves harbor pathogenic microorganisms. Lining the waste basket already present in the handwashing area with a plastic liner will facilitate disposal of the soiled towels (Fig. 35-1).

RATIONALE/AMPLIFICATION

Proper handwashing is very important to prevent contamination of a susceptible host. If the family understands who is being protected and is able to see proper handwashing as one of the means of protection, they are more likely to participate actively in the plan. The use of paper towels not only provides an added source of infection control, but their presence serves to remind the family that handwashing should be done properly and consistently. The waste basket liner provides an easy means of disposing of used towels and helps to prevent cross-contamination.

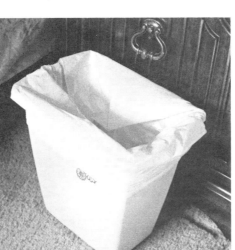

Figure 35.1

ACTION	RATIONALE/AMPLIFICATION
2. Remove all jewelry. Do not put it back on until contact with the client is finished and hands have been washed again.	Bacteria may become lodged within the cracks and crevices of jewelry. In addition, jewelry should not be worn during direct care due to the chance of scratching or injuring the client.
3. Stand in front of the sink with the soap and water controls within easy reach. Bend the knees slightly to accommodate for the height of the sink (Fig. 35-2). The water should be lukewarm.	Adherence to proper body mechanics eases the strain on the back and leg muscles. If the sink is high, a step-stool may be needed. Warm water is used because it removes fewer of the protective oils from the skin than hot water and results in less drying.

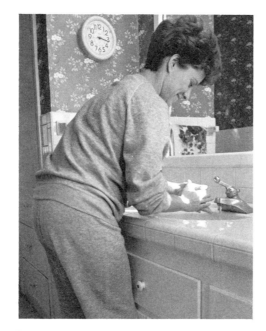

Figure 35.2

4. Wet the hands with water before adding soap. Hold the hands lower than the elbows during the washing procedure (Fig. 35-3). Use a soap that will not change the pH of the skin.	Water should be allowed to drain from the wrists down to the fingertips to allow the removed bacteria to flow with the water into the sink. Normal skin acidity is a factor in controlling bacterial growth and in preventing irritation. It is important to maintain the normal pH of the skin.

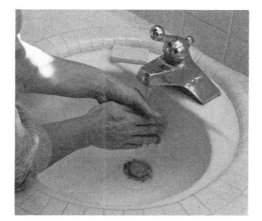

Figure 35.3

ACTION

5. To wash the hands, interlace the fingers and thumbs of both hands and move them back and forth. Wash the hands well for 30 seconds using a rotary motion. Apply this scrubbing motion to all surfaces of the hand (Figs. 35-4 and 35-5).

6. Rinse the hands and wrists under running warm water, allowing the rinse water to flow from the elbows to the fingertips. The fingernails may be cleaned at this time under the running water with an orange stick or nail brush (Fig. 35-6).

RATIONALE/AMPLIFICATION

It is important to clean all aspects of the hand including the interdigital areas. Microorganism counts are lower on the smooth surfaces of the hands and higher in the folds and under the fingernails. Friction aids in the mechanical removal of bacteria and has been found to be more important in the removal of microorganisms than the type of detergent used.

Surface bacteria should run into the sink rather than back up the arm. Clean, well-trimmed nails discourage the accumulation and growth of bacteria under the nails.

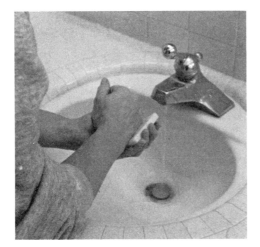

Figure 35.4

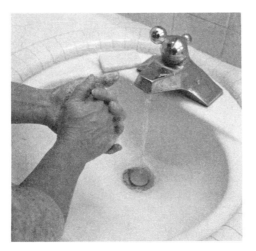

Figure 35.5

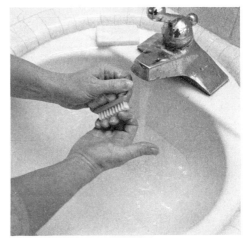

Figure 35.6

ACTION	RATIONALE/AMPLIFICATION
7. Dry the hands from the fingers toward the forearm with a clean paper towel. Turn off the handles of the faucet with the paper towel after drying is complete.	Drying should proceed from the clean hand area toward the unwashed elbow area (*i.e., from clean to dirty*). Since the faucets were turned on while the hands were dirty, they are considered contaminated. Turning the handles off using the paper towel is an excellent habit for family members to cultivate, especially when using public restrooms.
8. Apply lotion as needed and desired to the hands.	Lotion helps restore some of the natural oils lost during washing. It also helps prevent cracking of the skin of the hands, which offers an entry point for bacterial invasion.
9. Return all equipment to the proper place. Clean up spills on the floor and sink. Return any stools or benches to their proper place.	Leaving the handwashing area in a neat condition may prevent accidental falls and tripping when the area is used by others.

Age-Specific Modifications

1. Proper handwashing should be taught to children of all ages. A stool or small bench may be used by the small child to reach faucets and soap (Fig. 35-7).	Children who are too small to wash their own hands should have this process performed for them, using a warm wet cloth and a dry towel, before eating and after toileting. If they are to come in contact with the client, they should have their hands washed or should wash their own hands just as the adults in the family. The keys to infection control are diligence and consistency.

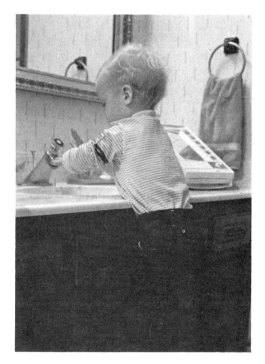

Figure 35.7

2. All persons feeding the newborn should first wash their hands.	The newborn lacks the sophistication of the immune system to provide adequate protection against cross-infection. Handwashing helps prevent the possibility of infection.

**Education/
Communication**

- Teach the client and family

The proper method of handwashing. Be sure that they understand the importance of knowing the goal of the handwashing regimen (i.e., who is being protected). Regardless of the goal, hands should be washed before and after administering direct care to the client. Explain the need to clean all of the surfaces of the hands, including the areas between the fingers. Ask the family members to inspect their jewelry with a critical eye so that they can appreciate how essential it is that jewelry be removed before handwashing to reduce the incidence of harbored bacteria.

The desired frequency of handwashing. Use this opportunity to stress that general hygiene should include washing the hands before eating and after any contact with the anogenital area, such as in toileting, changing a diaper, and sexual activity. In addition, hands should be washed before and after any contact with the ill client or the person susceptible to infection.

Safety precautions involved in handwashing. Explain the need to restore the natural oils and moisture of the skin by using a lotion after handwashing. Explain safety precautions in the handwashing area relating to falls. Emphasize that handwashing should not be done when electrical appliances are plugged in and within reach. These items should be unplugged before the water is turned on.

Evaluation of Health Promotion Activities

**Quality Assurance/
Reassessment**

- Watch the members of the family wash their hands to determine if they understand proper technique. Inspect the hands afterward to determine the effectiveness of washing efforts.

- Discuss with the client and family the reasons for washing their hands to determine if they have a firm grasp of the goals of handwashing. From responses to questions about when they wash their hands and why, it may be determined if they understand what is contaminated and who should be protected.

**Health Teaching
Checklist**

Name of Care Provider _____

Relationship to Client _____ Telephone #_____

Taught by _____ Date _____

	EXPLAINED	DEMONSTRATED
Technique for handwashing	_____	_____
Type of soap to use	_____	
Desired temperature of water	_____	_____
Mechanical friction	_____	_____
Interlacing fingers	_____	_____
Cleaning of fingernails	_____	_____
Proper rinse technique	_____	_____
Proper use of paper towels to dry	_____	_____
Use of paper towels to turn off faucet	_____	_____
Importance of restoring natural oils	_____	_____
Safety precautions	_____	_____

Selected Reference

Larson E: Effects of handwashing agent, handwashing frequency, and clinical area on hand flora. Am J Infect Control 12(2):76–82, April, 1984

36   Oral Care

Background

Cleansing of the mouth, teeth, and gums is important to maintain the client's sense of well-being as well as to prevent tooth decay and infection. Saliva is an important mechanical and chemical cleanser of the mouth. It combines with food particles to aid in digestion. Dental caries are areas of localized destruction of tooth tissue by bacterial action. Demineralization of the surface enamel ultimately causes destruction of the dentin and pulp of the tooth. Caries are actually caused by the acid produced by the bacteria, which form a colony on the tooth surface. The major cause of tooth loss in adults over 35 years of age is gum disease.

Assessment of Self-Care Potential

Client/Family Assessment

- Assess the state of dental health of the family members. Determine the priority placed on dental care by the various members. Ask if the younger children have ever been to see a dentist. Determine if the family practices preventive dentistry or if they see a dentist only when there is a problem.
- Assess the presence of oral hygiene accessories in the home. Determine if all members of the family have their own toothbrushes. Assess the presence of toothpaste, dental floss, and mouthwash.
- Assess the ability and willingness of the client to participate in oral hygiene measures.

Physical Assessment

- Assess the condition of the client's mouth and teeth. Certain medications affect the oral cavity, such as chemotherapeutic agents and some antibiotics. Assess the presence of missing or loose teeth as a result of recent trauma. If the client is unable to eat normally, the mouth will not benefit from the cleansing effects of normal salivation and oral hygiene efforts must be practiced diligently.
- Assess the client's current physical condition. Determine if the condition has contributed to mouth and teeth problems. Assess if the client is able to take fluids. Determine previous treatments that may have an effect on the teeth and gums, such as radiation treatments.
- Assess the presence of artificial dentures. Determine when the client wears the dentures and if the dentures fit well. Inspect the gums to see if there are sores or reddened areas, which may indicate poorly fitting dentures. Sometimes when a person is ill or suffers facial trauma, dentures that have fit will suddenly become loose or uncomfortable. Ask the client when the dentures were obtained and if there have been any problems.

| **Environmental Assessment** | • Assess the presence of running water in the household.
• Assess the physical situation of the home. Determine where the family members brush their teeth to see if there are separate facilities for each person's toothbrush. Determine if the family members rinse their teeth from the same cup and how often the cups are washed. This is particularly important if a communicable disease is known or suspected. |

Planning Strategies

Potential Nursing Diagnoses	Alteration in oral mucous membranes Self-care deficit, hygiene
Expected Outcomes	Maintenance of integrity of oral membranes Maintenance of adequate oral hygiene Prevention or alleviation of oral problems

Health Promotion Goals	• The client and family will
	    Understand the mechanics and safety precautions of administering proper oral hygiene to the client
	    Appreciate the importance of preventive dentistry and daily dental hygiene
	    Observe the teeth, gums, and mucous membranes carefully for early signs of soreness and infection
	    Actively participate in oral care
	    Understand the importance of oral care for the person with artificial dentures

Equipment	Toothbrush and toothpaste
	Small basin
	Dental floss
	Towel
	Cool water and cup
	Mouthwash or hydrogen peroxide
	Lip lubricant
	Swabs, if needed
	Bulb syringe, if needed
	Gloves, if needed
	Tongue blades, if needed
	Additional equipment for dentures
	    Container for dentures
	    Dentifrice or denture cleaner

Interventions/Health Promotion

ACTION

RATIONALE/AMPLIFICATION

Conscious Client

1. Wash hands before giving oral care. Turn the client to a side-lying position with a towel and curved basin under the chin.

The side-lying position will allow the rinse water to return by the flow of gravity and will lessen the chance of accidental choking from the water flowing down the throat.

2. Use a toothbrush with soft bristles. Rinse the toothbrush with cool water and apply a strip of tooth-paste.

Firm bristles may cause abrasions of the sensitive gums. Water softens the bristles.

3. Brush in the direction of tooth growth. Do one section at a time. Place the bristles parallel to the tooth surface, free edge up and extending beyond the gum line (Fig. 36-1). Turn the bristles toward the teeth with one sweeping stroke and bring the tips of the bristles firmly over the gum tissue and the tooth surface. Repeat this stroke 5 times over each section of the mouth, on the outer surfaces, inner surfaces, and biting surfaces (Fig. 36-2).

Brushing in the direction of the tooth will facilitate removal of food particles as well as stimulate the gums. The oral cavity contains a balanced biological system of microorganisms. Oral care should be designed to remove retained food debris, rather than to remove all microorganisms from the mouth. Do not exert force over the gum surface because gum tissue is sensitive and will bleed if traumatized.

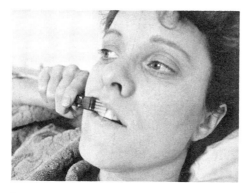

Figure 36.1

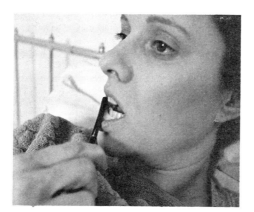

Figure 36.2

ACTION

RATIONALE/AMPLIFICATION

4. Assist with flossing of the teeth if the client is unable to do so (Fig. 36-3). Place the client in semi-Fowler's position. Wrap the dental floss around the middle finger of each hand and loop several times to stabilize. Use the index fingers to stretch the floss. Insert the floss between each of the client's teeth and move in a sawing manner to clean the sides, back, and front of each tooth. To remove the floss, release it from the backmost finger and pull it through the teeth.

Plaque is a buildup on the teeth that forms continually. If left in place, plaque can lead to gum and tooth disease. Flossing helps remove plaque. Care must be taken not to floss too vigorously, which may cause the gums to bleed.

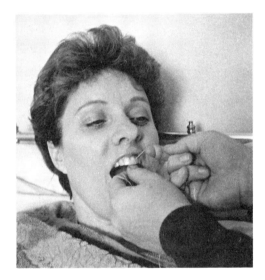

Figure 36.3

5. Allow the client to rinse the mouth and gums with cool water and mouthwash (Fig. 36-4). If the mouthwash is too astringent and causes discomfort, prepare a solution of equal parts of hydrogen peroxide and water.

Thorough rinsing after flossing will rinse the dislodged bacteria and plaque from the mouth. If the client has open lesions in the mouth, commercial mouthwashes may cause burning and discomfort.

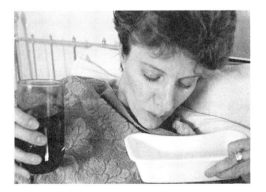

Figure 36.4

ACTION	RATIONALE/AMPLIFICATION

Unconscious Client

1. Turn the client's head well to the side. Place a linen protector under the chin.

Aspiration may occur if the head is not turned to facilitate drainage.

2. Brush the client's teeth gently in the aforementioned manner. Use a padded tongue blade to gently separate the upper and lower teeth.

The oral cavity of an unconscious person is not exposed to the normal stimulation and cleaning from eating. Meticulous oral hygiene is essential.

3. Carefully irrigate the client's mouth with a bulb syringe and a small amount of water. Rinse the teeth and gums, being careful that none of the water enters the throat and trachea. Use a prepared swab dipped in mouthwash to freshen the client's mouth.

Irrigation will remove the debris that was loosened during brushing. However, if the water is allowed to enter the trachea, choking or aspiration may result. The swab may leave the client's mouth feeling fresh, but it should not be used as a substitute for brushing.

4. Repeat the brushing procedure at least twice a day. If the client is breathing through the mouth, refreshing with swabs may be done every hour or two to keep the mouth moist and fresh. Lubricate the client's lips with some type of lubricant after oral care.

Mucous membranes will dry out quickly when oral food and fluids are not being consumed, when the client is mouth-breathing, or when the client is receiving inhalation gases. Frequent mouth care is vital for these clients.

Related Care

Chemotherapy Clients

1. Substitute a saltwater rinse for teeth brushing. Place ½ tsp of salt in 1 cup of warm tap water or sterile water if client has open lesions in the mouth. Encourage the client to thoroughly rinse the teeth and gums before evacuating the water into a basin or the sink.

Chemotherapy predisposes the client to hematologic complications such as bleeding gums. Although brushing may cause trauma to the sensitive gums, oral care is still important to reduce pathogens and add to a sense of comfort and well-being.

2. Check the chemotherapy client frequently for open sores in the mouth. Use a softly padded tongue blade and light. Be careful not to traumatize the tongue and gums while examining the mouth.

The mucosal surfaces of the chemotherapy client become extremely sensitive and will bleed easily.

ACTION	RATIONALE/AMPLIFICATION

Artificial-Denture Clients

1. Wash hands before assisting with denture care. If the client cannot remove the dentures, assist with removal by grasping the upper denture with the thumb and index finger of each hand (Fig. 36-5). Move the upper denture up and down gently to break the vacuum seal between the denture and the roof of the mouth. Once the seal is broken, remove the denture from the mouth. To remove the lower denture, grasp it firmly with the thumb and index finger of each hand and lift gently out of the mouth. During actual removal, rotate the lower denture slightly to prevent stretching the mouth (Fig. 36-6).

The upper denture is held in place by a vacuum seal. Releasing the seal at any break point breaks the vacuum and allows release of the entire surface. The lower denture, on the other hand, does not adhere by vacuum and may be lifted out of the mouth by gentle pressure.

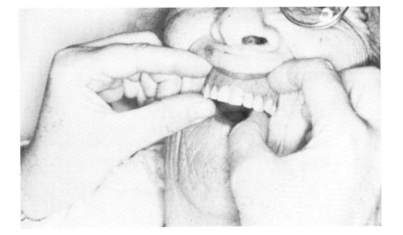

Figure 36.5

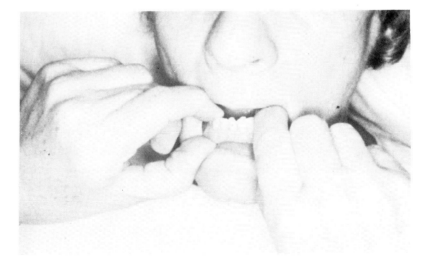

Figure 36.6

ACTION	RATIONALE/AMPLIFICATION
2. Place the artificial dentures in a basin (Fig. 36-7). Remove the basin to the sink to wash the dentures. Warm water is used to wash dentures.	Carrying the dentures in a basin decreases the chance of accidental dropping and breaking. Hot water may damage artificial denture material.

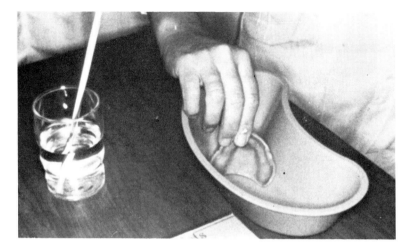

Figure 36.7

3. The dentures may be soaked in an effervescent dentifrice before cleaning. To clean, use a brush and denture-cleansing powder. Apply an upward brushing motion to the lower denture and a downward motion to the upper denture just as is done for the teeth. While the dentures are being cleaned, hold them over a soft towel or a basin of water with a washcloth in the bottom. Rinse the dentures in warm running water (Fig. 36-8).	The effervescent action may remove some of the debris from the dentures. The brushing action will remove accumulated debris, which is harmful and unpleasant if left in the mouth. If the dentures are cleaned over a soft surface, the chance of breakage is decreased if the dentures are accidentally dropped.

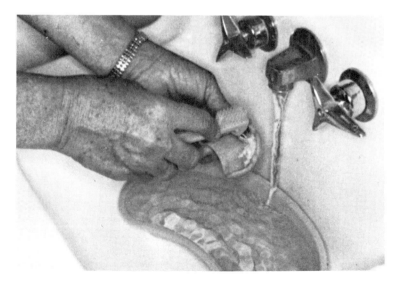

Figure 36.8

ACTION

4. Administer oral hygiene to clean the client's mouth. Replace the dentures by elevating the client's upper lip with one hand while inserting the denture with the other (Fig. 36-9). Insert the upper plate first and press it gently against the roof of the mouth to ensure that the vacuum seal has been made (Fig. 36-10). A commercial adhesive may be used to secure the denture. The lower denture is inserted in a slightly rotated position until it is in place. Press it onto the lower gums with a gentle motion (Fig. 36-11).

RATIONALE/AMPLIFICATION

Securing the client's lips away from the insertion site will decrease the chance of pinching the lip against the teeth and will allow easier access for the dentures. The vacuum seal is the mechanism by which the top denture is held in place.

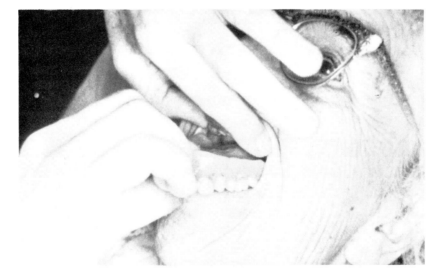

Figure 36.9

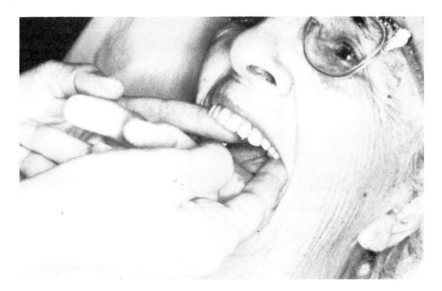

Figure 36.10

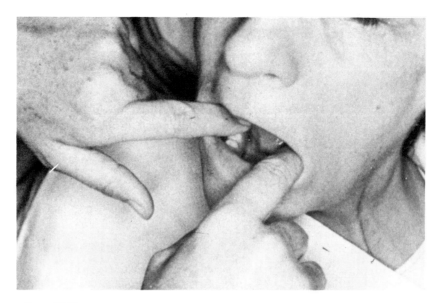

Figure 36.11

**Education/
Communication**

- Teach the client and family to

  Care for the client's teeth in a safe and thorough manner. Explain safety factors, such as using a brush with soft bristles and avoiding excessive pressure on the gums.

  Care for the client's dentures. Explain how to avoid accidents by holding the teeth with a towel or cloth and washing the teeth over a basin of water. Demonstrate the proper method of removing and placing the teeth so that the gums are not injured and the teeth are placed correctly and sealed. Explain the importance of properly fitting dentures. Stress that nutrition may be compromised by dentures that do not fit or are not worn. Further explain to the client and family that if the dentures are left out of the mouth for extended periods, the gum line may change, resulting in poorly fitting dentures.

  Note the condition of the teeth and gums in assessing the effectiveness of oral hygiene. Explain signs and symptoms of infection or irritation such as reddened or whitened areas, bleeding, and lesions.

  Perform oral hygiene in the client receiving radiation to the head and neck. Explain that salivation may be decreased after the first week or two of treatment. Dryness of the mouth may be permanent. Further explain that gum swelling may occur, resulting in improperly fitting dentures. Since dental decay is common after radiation, the client should start on an active dental hygiene program before treatment begins. Brushing with a high-fluoride toothpaste may help decrease decay. When lesions are present, a diluted hydrogen peroxide mouthwash is preferable to commercial preparations.

**Referrals and
Consultations**

If the client's mouth is in obvious need of immediate attention, recommend that a dentist be consulted. Stress the importance of regular dental care.

If the client's dentures are cracked, broken, or ill-fitting, recommend that the client see a dentist to have a new set made. If the financial burden is too great for the family, explore the possibility of social assistance.

Evaluation of Health Promotion Activities

Quality Assurance/ Reassessment

- Document the condition of the client's mouth, teeth, and gums for comparison at a later time. If there are problems, assess and reassess the status to determine if care has been sought and if prescribed therapy is being followed.

- Demonstrate the proper method of adminstering oral hygiene. Allow the client or family to administer the care and evaluate their technique and outcomes. If they show deficits in knowledge or action, explain or demonstrate so that oral hygiene is done correctly and safely.

- Small dye tablets are available from the American Dental Association that will allow the client and family to see for themselves how effectively they are brushing their teeth. After brushing, the person chews the tablet and rinses with cool water. Areas on the teeth where plaque is building up or where debris was missed during brushing will stain red and demonstrate where brushing should be concentrated.

DOCUMENTATION

Charting for the Home Health Nurse
Documentation should include the client's dental status and any recommendations made to the client and family regarding follow-up care. Documentation may include the frequency of visits to the dentist and recommendations made. If problems are found with the gums or teeth, a progressive record of their resolution should be kept.

Health Teaching Checklist

Name of Care Provider _____

Relationship to Client _____ Telephone #_____

Taught by _____ Date _____

	EXPLAINED	DEMONSTRATED
Normal tooth growth	_____	
Toothbrushing technique	_____	_____
Type of toothbrush (soft bristle)	_____	_____
Plaque buildup and removal	_____	_____
Flossing of teeth	_____	_____
Denture cleaning	_____	_____
Care of dentures when out of mouth	_____	_____
Rinse with bulb syringe	_____	_____
Need for regular dental check-ups	_____	
Special precautions for chemotherapy clients	_____	_____
Special precautions for radiation clients	_____	_____
Special precautions for unconscious clients	_____	_____

Product Availability

Toothbrushes are available at most drug stores, pharmacies, and department stores. The types of toothbrushes vary. They may have a long head or a short head, a straight handle or a curved handle, and soft, medium, or firm bristles. Denture cleansers and dentifrices are also available in most pharmacies and grocery stores. Bulb syringes may be found in baby supplies in most grocery stores and pharmacies.

37 Pediculosis, Treatment of

Background

Pediculosis is an infestation of lice on the human body. It is highly contagious by direct contact with the infested person or with an article, such as a hairbrush, which has been in contact with the infested site. Lice do not hop or fly from person to person. They are wingless, gray-brown, hairy, flat insects, less than 6 mm in length, that are capable of crawling over rough surfaces at great speeds. They have special mouth parts for piercing and sucking. Lice live on human blood that is obtained by biting the skin. The body louse often clings to the seams of undergarments. Its bite causes characteristic minute hemorrhagic points that result in a great deal of itching. There are three varieties of lice that infest the human body. They are identified by the area of potential infestation: the head louse (*Pediculus humanis capitis*); the body louse or "cootie" (*Pediculus humanis corporis*); and the pubic or "crab" louse (*Phthirus pubis*). Pediculosis is found at all levels of society without regard to cleanliness. Animal lice are not transmissible to humans nor are human lice able to live on animals.

Nits are the eggs of lice. They are often found on hair shafts to which they adhere by a sticky jellylike substance that is secreted when the eggs are laid. Because the eggs cannot hatch below 22° C (71.6° F), they are deposited very close to the skin where they can remain dormant for as long as 35 days if conditions are favorable. The egg is usually about 4 mm from the scalp when it hatches. Nits are enclosed in white or brown ovoid envelopes, which give them the appearance of dandruff; however, they cannot be brushed or shaken from the hair like dandruff.

Assessment of Self-Care Potential

Client/Family Assessment

- Assess the extent of the lice infestation. If lice are found on one member of the family, it is expected that other members will be affected also.
- Assess the motivation of the family to be rid of the lice infestation. Determine if the family views the problem as serious enough to warrant the time and energy necessary to get rid of the lice.
- Assess the knowledge level of the family regarding the transmission and treatment of lice infestation.
- Assess the financial status of the family in relation to their ability to afford commercial pediculicide preparations. Also, assess the need for child care arrangements if the children must be kept out of school until the pediculosis is under control.

Physical Assessment	• Assess the condition of the skin on the affected individuals. Pay particular attention to the areas where garment seams are found, such as the waist and upper thighs. Note the scalp. Determine if the skin is scratched or infected.
	• Assess the fingernails of the client and family. Since the bite of the louse causes itching, it is important that the fingernails be short and clean to avoid infection.
Environmental Assessment	• Assess the hygiene arrangements of the home. Determine if the family members use the same grooming items. Assess the extent of potential for direct contact with lice-infested accessories, such as linen. Determine if siblings sleep in the same bed and wear each other's clothing.
	• Assess the facilities for cleaning and disinfecting infested clothing and surfaces. Determine if the home has laundry facilities.

Planning Strategies

Potential Nursing Diagnoses	Knowledge deficit regarding treatment of pediculosis
	Potential for impairment of skin integrity
	Social isolation
Expected Outcomes	Elimination of pediculosis from the client and family and from any infested surfaces
	Prevention of reinfestation
	Prevention or treatment of secondary infection
	Education of family and friends to reduce social isolation
Health Promotion Goals	• The client and family will Understand the mode of transmission of pediculosis and methods of prevention Understand how to treat themselves with the pediculicide in a safe and thorough manner Have the knowledge and motivation to take measures to prevent reinfestation Resume their usual roles in society without embarrassment or misunderstanding Understand why scratching of irritated areas is a potential source of infection and refrain from traumatizing their skin
Equipment	Commercial pediculicide or one prescribed by physician
	Shampoo
	Comb and brush
	Clean towels

Interventions/Health Promotion

ACTION

RATIONALE/AMPLIFICATION

Treatment of Body Hair

1. Identify any areas of infestation. To hunt for adult lice, repeatedly part the hair with a tongue blade and watch closely for movement on or near the scalp.

Pediculosis is generally found in the hairy areas of the body (Fig. 37-1). The recommended treatment regimen usually is application of the pediculicide to the head, axillae, and pubic region.

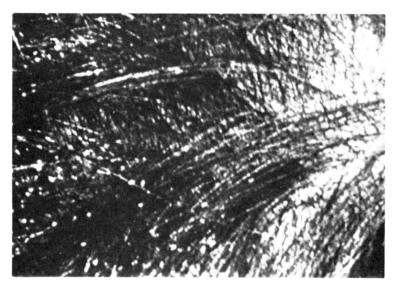

Figure 37.1

2. Explain how to use the pediculicide safely according to directions accompanying the preparation. The solution is usually applied directly to the infested areas. Leave it on the recommended length of time and then rinse well with large amounts of warm water.

Pediculicides may be irritating to delicate tissues, such as the eyes. Care must be taken not to get the solution in the eyes. The lice are destroyed more thoroughly if the preparation is allowed to remain on the hair for about 15 minutes.

3. Most directions accompanying pediculicides recommend that the hair be washed with shampoo and warm water after treatment.

Shampooing will help wash out the dead lice. The nits take a more concentrated effort for removal.

4. Use clean, freshly laundered towels to dry the client's hair. Clean the comb by boiling or soaking in the pediculicide before using it on the client's clean hair. Advise the client to don clean clothing.

Live lice may be reintroduced onto the client's scalp after treatment by using a contaminated comb.

ACTION	*RATIONALE/AMPLIFICATION*
5. Remove the dead lice and nits from the client's hair by using a fine-toothed comb. About 15 minutes after completion of the treatment, begin combing the hair (Fig. 37-2).	Most commercial pediculicides come with a special fine-toothed comb for this purpose. The pediculicide will kill the lice; however, removal of the dead lice must be done by brushing briskly. Since the nits adhere to the hair shaft, they must be removed mechanically by using an extremely fine comb. Axillary and pubic hair may have to be combed if nits are present.

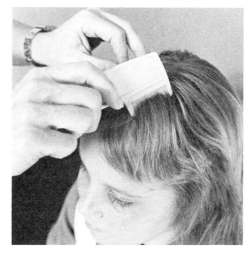

Figure 37.2

6. Gather all towels and clothing in a plastic bag during the treatment. Wash these items in hot water (see Related Care).	Any item that comes in contact with the client's hair before treatment is considered contaminated.
7. Repeat the treatment in 7 to 10 days.	Initial application of the pediculicide kills all of the adult lice, but it does not kill the nits. Reapplication after a week will ensure that the newly hatched lice are also killed.

Related Care

Treatment of the Environment

1. Machine wash all washable clothing and linen that have come into contact with infested person(s) in the past 2 days.	The water in the washer should be hot (125° F). Time should be taken between loads of laundry to allow the water to reheat adequately. An alternative is to run the articles through the hottest dryer setting for at least 20 minutes. Bed linen is removed carefully to avoid fanning it in the air, which would result in spread of the infestation (Figs. 37-3 and 37-4).

ACTION	*RATIONALE/AMPLIFICATION*

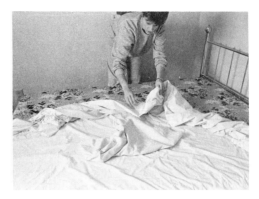

Figure 37.3

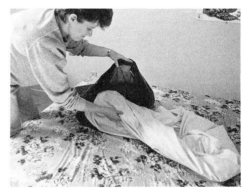

Figure 37.4

2. Personal items of clothing or bedding that cannot be washed or dried should be dry-cleaned or placed in a plastic bag and sealed for 10 days.

Dry heat or absence of a host will kill the adult lice.

3. Disinfect any toiletry items that have been used by the client by soaking them in the pediculicide shampoo or in a pan of water heated to 150° F (Fig. 37-5).

Lice and nits may adhere to combs, caps, hats, scarves, and collars and may survive on these areas for several days until they are able to reach a human body.

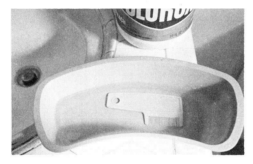

Figure 37.5

4. Rugs and upholstery in the home should be disinfected by vacuuming.

The lice cannot live without a susceptible host.

Age-Specific Modifications

1. Young children are usually susceptible to head lice. Treatment with the pediculicide will have to be done carefully to prevent contamination of the child's eyes.

It is common for young children to come into contact with pediculosis when they begin socialization, such as when they start school or attend a day-care center. If an outbreak of pediculosis occurs, it is essential that all children be checked immediately and consistently until the pediculosis is controlled.

ACTION	RATIONALE/AMPLIFICATION
2. In those confined to bed, treatment must be done by a care provider. Show the family how to treat the client. Place gauze pads over the client's eyes if the treatment must be done in bed. See Technique 34, Hair, Daily Care and Shampooing, for specifics of shampooing a person in bed.	In the infirm or elderly, pediculosis may be a problem due to the discomfort it causes and the chance of spreading the contamination to others. Treatment must include cleansing of the hair and disinfection of the linen.

Education/ Communication

• Teach the client and family to

Recognize the signs and symptoms of lice infestation. Be sure that they can identify lice and distinguish nits from dandruff.

Safely and thoroughly treat pediculosis. Explain the importance of keeping the preparation out of the eyes. If the client or family member has particularly sensitive skin, it may be necessary to test a small amount of the preparation on the skin before treatment to ensure that the person will not suffer from a skin reaction. It may be necessary to consult a physician about alternative medications.

Refrain from sharing toiletry and apparel items with other people, even in the same family. It is important to teach children not to try on hats and scarves in stores. In most states, it is a law that underwear must be kept on while trying on intimate apparel, such as lingerie and swim suits. Emphasize to the family the importance of this measure in preventing lice infestation.

Understand that the lice infestation is a treatable situation and should not cause undue anxiety among family members. It is especially important that parents be discouraged against taking drastic measures, such as cutting the child's hair or shaving the child's head. These measures are unnecessary and have no effect on the treatment of lice infestation. These measures tend to embarrass the child and may cause further social isolation.

Referrals and Consultations

Referral to the state department of public health may assist in tracing contacts who may be participating in the spread of the infestation. In addition, public health personnel may be able to provide follow-up surveillance and monitoring to ensure that the infestation is contained and eradicated.

Evaluation of Health Promotion Activities

Quality Assurance/ Reassessment

Periodic follow-up is essential to ensure that the infestation has been eliminated. The client should be checked two days after initial treatment. It is important to ensure that the infested persons have follow-up treatment in 7 to 10 days.

Observation of the client during treatments may offer insight into understanding of transmission modes and acceptance of the importance of adequate treatment to eliminate the problem.

DOCUMENTATION

Charting for the Home Health Nurse

A record should be kept of which family members were checked for the infestation and which ones received treatment. Some states require reporting of contagious infestations to the department of public health. Some states also require clearance of children who have had a pediculosis infestation before they can return to school.

Records Kept by the Client/Family

Since the pediculicidal shampoo may be irritating to the scalp, the family should keep a record of the frequency with which each member receives this type of treatment.

Health Teaching Checklist

Name of Care Provider _____

Relationship to Client _____ Telephone #_____

Taught by _____ Date _____

	EXPLAINED	DEMONSTRATED
Description of lice and nits	_____	
Signs and symptoms of infestation	_____	
Need for pediculicide treatment	_____	
Application of pediculicide	_____	_____
Removal of lice and nits	_____	_____
Safety precautions	_____	_____
Follow-up checking and care	_____	_____
Decontamination of environment	_____	_____

Product Availability

Commercial pediculicides are available at most drug stores. Some commonly used products are Rid and A-200 Pyrinate. Kwell (lindane) is available by prescription.

Selected Reference

McLaury P: Head lice: Pediatric social disease. Am J Nurs 83:1300–1303, September, 1983

38   Shaving

Background

Social custom dictates acceptance or rejection of facial hair. Most men shave all or part of their facial whiskers every day. During illness, maintaining the usual shaving custom and habits promotes a sense of well-being and control.

Shaving other parts of the body is also considered esthetically desirable by some. Many women shave their axillary area and legs. Continuing this habit during illness adds to comfort and a desirable self-concept.

Assessment of Self-Care Potential

Client/Family Assessment

- Assess the feelings about facial hair in the family.
- Assess the client's usual shaving habits. Determine the time of day the client usually shaves, the type of razor used, and type of lotion used. If the client will be shaved by someone else, assess the usual method of shaving, that is, which areas are usually shaved first and how the skin is usually stretched to prevent cuts and reach all areas successfully.

Physical Assessment

- Assess the degree of weakness being experienced by the client. Determine if the client can assist in the shaving or do the entire procedure alone.
- Assess the area to be shaved for any reddened or broken areas. Determine the presence of bony prominences that will require caution when shaving over and around these areas. Assess the presence of moles, small skin lesions, or any skin appendage protruding from the smooth line of the face. Although these areas may not cause problems when the client is healthy, side-effects from the illness or medication may prompt the need for assistance or extra care.

Environmental Assessment

- Assess the proximity of the client's bed to the bathroom. Determine if the client is strong enough to go to the bathroom or if the shaving procedure should be done in bed.
- Assess the heating arrangements of the room in which the shave will take place. Determine what actions will be necessary to prevent chilling the client.

Planning Strategies

Potential Nursing Diagnoses

Self-care deficit related to grooming

Potential for impairment of skin integrity

Disturbance in self-concept: role performance

Expected Outcomes

Promotion of adequate self-image by proper grooming

Prevention of infection or secondary problems due to trauma to the skin

Promotion of comfort during the convalescence period

Health Promotion Goals

- The client and family will

  Perform the shaving procedure in an expeditious and safe manner as often as the client needs or wants it

  Understand the importance of avoiding trauma to the skin integrity in prevention of infection

Equipment

Razor and blade or electric razor

Skin preparation for electric razor

Shaving lather or soap

Basin of hot water

Bath towel, face towels, and washcloth

Powder

Interventions/Health Promotion

ACTION

1. If the client can go to the bathroom and perform the shaving procedure, warm the bathroom and have all of the equipment prepared ahead of time. Encourage the client to use an electric razor. Do not use shaving lotion. Provide a place for the client to sit down if weakness occurs during the shaving procedure. Allow the client to follow the usual pattern for shaving and be ready to assist if needed.

2. If the client is bedfast, the shave may be done in the bed. The procedure is usually done before or after the bath. Allow the client a chance to participate in this decision. Gather all of the needed equipment before beginning. Protect the client's linen by placing a dry towel around the area to be shaved. For the face, place the towel around the client's shoulders (Fig. 38-1). For the axillae and legs, place a towel lengthwise under the portion to be shaved. Wash hands before beginning procedure.

RATIONALE/AMPLIFICATION

If the client can preserve some of the usual daily routine when ill, a sense of normalcy and self-control can be fostered. Since the client may be shaky from the illness, it is best to use an electric razor to perform the shaving procedure. Shaving lotion usually contains alcohol and causes drying of the skin. Even though it is desirable to have the client participate in care to the extent possible, the most important consideration is the safety and well-being of the client.

If the client is weak or prone to falls, the procedure should be done in bed. If the client is allowed to assist in making decisions about care, feelings of helplessness may be prevented.

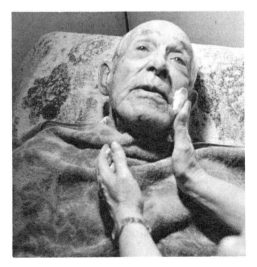

Figure 38.1

ACTION

3. If the shaving is done with an electric razor, shave in both directions across the skin until the hair has been removed. A skin preparation solution may be applied before beginning, if this is the client's habit. Hold the skin over bony prominences or folds of skin taut while shaving.

4. If shaving with a razor and blade, the skin should be prepared before beginning. Apply a warm towel to the area to be shaved. Be careful not to burn the client. Apply soap or lather to the area.

5. To shave the face, shave in the direction in which the hair grows (Fig. 38-2). For facial hair that grows in a downward direction, begin along the sideburns with short downward strokes of about 2½ cm (1 inch). Around irregular surfaces on the face, pull the skin taut and be especially careful, taking very short strokes.

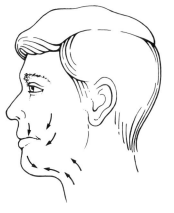

Figure 38.2

6. To shave the axilla, have the client hold the arm alongside the head. Use short strokes, shaving downward. To shave the legs, long strokes are desirable. If the area is marked by curves and contours, such as the knee and ankle, use shorter strokes. A lotion or cream may be applied to the legs after shaving. Wait several minutes before applying deodorant to the client's axillary area.

RATIONALE/AMPLIFICATION

If the bath water is present, be careful to keep the electric razor away from the water to eliminate the chance of electrical shock. Shaving in both directions ensures complete removal of the hair shaft.

Heat, moisture, and lather help to reduce surface tension and soften the beard on the face. Lather and moisture are usually adequate preparation for other body surfaces.

Shaving in the direction that the hair grows prevents nicks and scraping of the skin.

For long, flat surfaces, longer strokes are more comfortable and minimize the chance of nicking or cutting the client.

ACTION	RATIONALE/AMPLIFICATION
7. After washing off the soap or lather and drying the shaved surface, powder may be applied. Observe carefully for any break in skin integrity.	Complete removal of the soap or lather is essential because it may cause skin irritation if left on the skin. Drying the skin will prevent chapping.

Related Care

Inquire if the female client would like to have facial hair removed. If so, shave the hair over the upper lip, on the chin, or other areas requested by the client.	Postmenopausal women sometimes experience a growth of facial hair. Women usually pluck or shave these hairs to produce a well-groomed appearance.

Education/ Communication

- Teach the client and family to

  Perform the shaving procedure in a safe manner. If the family uses a razor and blade, encourage them to be particularly careful when a new blade is placed in the razor or when a new disposable razor is used for the first time. Encourage the family to let the client participate to the extent possible for as long as possible. When the client must be shaved, remind the family to allow the client to make some of the decisions about the procedure. Ability to participate in decisions about care helps bolster the client's self-concept.

  Provide for the comfort and well-being of the client while maintaining a flexible attitude toward shaving. If the client is too tired or disinterested in shaving, the procedure may be delayed until the next day. However, attention to the client's appearance is a way to promote self-confidence and ego.

Evaluation of Health Promotion Activities

Quality Assurance/ Reassessment

- Inspect the client's face for signs of nicks and cuts after shaving. If the client tends to bleed more easily than usual due to medication or illness, a switch to an electric razor may be indicated. The client should be told that this measure is only temporary until the condition causing the bleeding is no longer a problem.

- Inspect the cords on electrical razors to ensure that they are not frayed or loose at connections. Ensure that electrical equipment is not used around water or oxygen sources.

Health Teaching Checklist

Name of Care Provider _____

Relationship to Client _____ Telephone #_____

Taught by _____ Date _____

EXPLAINED   DEMONSTRATED

Safety precautions of

    Electrical razor   _____

    Razor and blade   _____

	EXPLAINED	DEMONSTRATED
Facial shaving technique		
Soaking whiskers before shaving	_____	_____
Lathering facial area	_____	_____
Short strokes with a razor and blade	_____	_____
Aftercare	_____	_____
Axillary shaving technique		
Protecting bed linen	_____	_____
Short strokes with a razor and blade	_____	_____
Aftercare	_____	_____
Leg shaving technique		
Protecting bed linen	_____	_____
Longer strokes with razor and blade	_____	_____
Care around ankles and knees	_____	_____
Aftercare	_____	_____
Shared decision making about shaving	_____	
Frequency of shaving	_____	

Product Availability

Electrical razors are available at most department and retail stores. Razors and blades may be purchased at most discount, grocery, and drug stores. They come in disposable models that can be used until they are dull and thrown away. The razor may be purchased separately, with refills available when the blades become dull.

Monitoring/Surveillance

39   Blood Glucose Monitoring

Background

Blood glucose monitoring is used by selected diabetics at home as a substitute for, or supplement to, urine testing. It is particularly useful in clients who have an altered renal threshold for glucose, where urine testing would not provide accurate results, and for people using an insulin pump. By monitoring their blood glucose, diabetics can administer insulin according to their specific needs, rather than injecting a predetermined amount every day without regard to their individual lifestyle.

Home blood glucose monitoring (HBGM) uses a capillary blood sample to measure the blood glucose. In fasting individuals, venous, capillary, and arterial blood glucose concentrations are essentially identical. The concentrations are higher in capillary blood after ingestion of glucose. The use of reagent strips to test blood glucose should not replace laboratory determinations of blood glucose, but should be used to guide therapy until these tests are available. HBGM is much more accurate than urine testing to monitor the blood glucose. Renal thresholds for spilling glucose can differ from person to person. The results obtained from a urine test reflect the blood sugar prior to the excretion of the glucose and storing it in the bladder. When using urinalysis to monitor blood glucose, it is important to obtain a double voided specimen.

These problems are eliminated with HBGM. Blood is obtained via a finger stick and placed on a reagent strip. The reagent strip may be read against a color chart or placed in a glucose meter for interpretation. Since equipment and reagent strips from each manufacturer are different, it is important to use the correct color chart and glucose meter. The finger stick can be done with a sterile lancet or with an Autolet, a spring-loaded device, which is more comfortable for client use (Fig. 39-1). (See Technique 41, Urine Glucose Testing.)

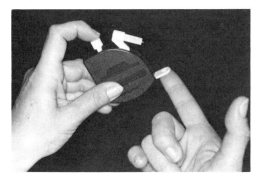

Figure 39.1
Using an Autolet to obtain a capillary blood sample.

Assessment of Self-Care Potential

Client/Family Assessment

- Determine whether the client is usually compliant with medical therapy.
  This is important if the person is to monitor the blood glucose successfully.
- Assess whether the person is motivated to control blood sugar using HBGM.

- Check whether the person will use color chart comparisons to check the reagent strip or whether a glucose meter will be used. Determine that the client does not have visual problems that would prevent using HBGM.
- Check on the availability and price of glucose meters and reagent strips. Assist the client to determine the most suitable meter or reagent.
- Check whether a third-party payor will reimburse the client for HBGM expenses. The expense will be considerably higher than traditional urine testing.

Physical Assessment

- Periodically monitor venous blood glucose levels. Determine whether the capillary blood measurements are comparable.
- Determine whether the person is a candidate for HBGM. Insulin-dependent diabetics will find this technique more beneficial than those who do not require insulin.
- Determine whether the person should use urine testing in conjunction with HBGM.
- Check condition of the skin where the client does finger sticks. Check for signs of infection or peripheral neuropathy.

Environmental Assessment

- Determine that the client will have privacy when away from home to obtain a blood specimen and perform the test. A sink with soap and water is desirable.

Planning Strategies

Potential Nursing Diagnoses

Health maintenance, alteration in: frequent measurements of the blood glucose

Infection, potential for: from frequent finger sticks to obtain blood samples

Knowledge deficit: HBGM program

Expected Outcomes

Maintenance of the blood glucose within a normal range by titrating insulin

Prevention of infection

Increased knowledge of self-management techniques

Health Promotion Goals

- The client and family will
  Incorporate HBGM into the diabetic management program
  Check the blood glucose accurately, 4 times daily or as often as directed by the physician
  Titrate insulin according to the blood glucose measurement

Equipment

Lancets or prepared Autolet

Alcohol sponge (if soap and water not available)

Clean hand towel or paper towel

Reagent test strips

Cotton balls

Paper towel (if using glucose meter)

Wash bottle (if applicable)

Stopwatch or watch with second hand

Color chart or glucose meter and calibration equipment

Interventions/Health Promotion

ACTION	RATIONALE/AMPLIFICATION
1. Warm up and calibrate the glucose meter (if used).	Follow the manufacturer's instructions precisely to calibrate the meter.
2. Remove a reagent strip from the bottle and immediately replace the cap. Check the unreacted reagent strip with the 0 block on the color chart.	If the reagent area is discolored, discard and use another strip to prevent an inaccurate result.
3. Clean the puncture area thoroughly with soap and warm water. Gently manipulate the puncture site.	Warm water promotes peripheral dilation and easier blood flow. This helps ensure a good blood supply. Using alcohol for skin preparation is discouraged because punctures made through wet alcohol can increase peripheral neuropathies.
4. Dry the puncture site with a clean towel or fresh paper towel. Do a finger stick using either a sterile individually wrapped lancet or Autolet. Wait a few seconds to allow blood to begin to flow. Facilitate flow by gently massaging the surrounding tissue toward the puncture site.	The spring-loaded Autolet simplifies self-puncture and is also less painful than the lancets. Do not squeeze directly at the site because this may cause contamination of the sample with tissue fluid.
5. Wipe away the first drop with a cotton ball. Collect a second drop. Apply a large drop of blood sufficient to cover the entire reagent area of the strip. Keep the strip level to avoid spilling the drop.	This prevents contamination of the sample. Using sufficient blood is important. If a small drop is spread over the entire reagent area to give a thin film, color development will be paler than with a large drop, and lower results will be obtained. Also, using a thin layer causes a tendency to overwash the strip, which results in low readings.
6. Stop blood flow by holding manual pressure over the wound with a cotton ball. Clean the puncture site with soap and water after the test is complete.	
7. *Immediately* as the blood is placed on the strip, begin timing for 60 seconds (Dextrostix or Chemstrip bG).	Follow the manufacturer's instructions if a different product is used.

ACTION	RATIONALE/AMPLIFICATION
8. Prepare the strip for comparison with the color chart or interpretation with a glucose meter: *For Dextrostix*	
• Immediately wash the reagent area for 2 seconds with a sharp, constant stream of water using a wash bottle.	Direct the stream across the entire reagent area. It is not necessary to remove every trace of blood from around the edges of the strip. Rinsing under a tap results in overwashing and false low results.
• Immediately compare the color block with the color chart on the package.	Inaccuracies can result if strips from one bottle are compared with a color chart on another bottle. Range is 0 to 250 mg/dl.
• If using a glucose meter, blot the strip on a clean paper towel and insert the strip into the prepared device (Fig. 39-2).	Read the result displayed on the digital readout. Range is 0 to 399 mg/dl.

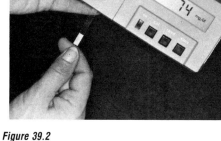

Figure 39.2
Using a glucose meter to measure capillary blood glucose.

For Chemstrip bG	
• Wipe the blood off the reagent strip with a cotton ball.	
• Time for an additional 60 seconds.	
• Compare the color block with the color chart on the package.	Range is 20 to 800 mg/dl.
• Interpolate results that fall between two color blocks on the color chart.	
9. Record the results on a flowsheet (Table 39-1).	

ACTION   *RATIONALE/AMPLIFICATION*

Table 39-1. GLUCOSE MONITORING RECORD

DATE	BEFORE BREAKFAST	BEFORE LUNCH	BEFORE DINNER	BEFORE BED	MEDICATIONS TAKEN	OTHER TESTS

Related Care

Administer insulin according to the
blood glucose reading.

Check blood glucose 4 times daily.   Blood glucose is usually checked be-
                                              fore each meal and at bedtime. Insulin
                                              is administered on a sliding scale as
                                              ordered by physician.

**Education/
Communication**

- Teach the client and family to
  Note the date on the bottle when opening a new bottle of reagent strips. Dis-
    card after 4 months. Do not store in bright light (e.g., on a window sill).
  Select the puncture site that is most comfortable for the client. The earlobe is
    used exclusively in some countries because it is less painful than the fin-
    gers.
  Only use lancets once to prevent infection
  Prepare the skin carefully before doing a finger stick to prevent infection. Use
    soap and water when available. If the client works outside where running
    water is not available, use alcohol swabs.
  Wear a Medic-Alert bracelet to alert emergency personnel of potential prob-
    lems related to diabetes mellitus.

Referrals and Consultations

- Refer a pediatric client to the homeroom teacher or school nurse if problems occur at school.
- Refer the client to the American Diabetes Association, Inc., 600 Fifth Avenue, New York, NY 10020, for self-help information.
- Check whether there are local diabetic group meetings.

Evaluation of Health Promotion Activities

Quality Assurance/ Reassessment

- Periodically recheck the client's technique to ensure accurate results.
- Check the venous blood glucose periodically to compare with the capillary levels for accuracy. Normal fasting specimens will show color development greater than the 45 mg/dl color block. After a high carbohydrate meal or measured challenge, normal results are generally below 130 mg/dl at 2 hours.

DOCUMENTATION

Charting for the Home Health Nurse
Flowsheet of capillary blood glucose measurements and venous blood measurements

Ability of the client to incorporate HBGM into the activities of daily living

Records Kept by the Client/Family
Skin assessment

Flowsheet of capillary blood glucose measurements (see Table 39-1)

Health Teaching Checklist

Name of Care Provider _____

Relationship to Client _____ Telephone #_____

Taught by _____ Date _____

	EXPLAINED	DEMONSTRATED
Finger stick technique	_____	_____
Blood glucose determination	_____	_____
Maintenance of glucose meter (if using)	_____	_____
Obtaining supplies	_____	
Travel arrangements	_____	
Titration of insulin	_____	_____

Product Availability

Glucose meters and reagents are available at medical-supply companies (see the yellow pages of the telephone book) and pharmacies.

Selected References

Plasse NJ: Monitoring blood glucose at home: A comparison of three products. Am J Nurs 81(11):2028–2029, November, 1981

Stevens AD: Monitoring blood glucose at home: Who should do it. Am J Nurs 81(11):2026–2027, November, 1981

40 Neurological Signs

Neurological evaluation of the client may be obtained by objective and subjective data that are gathered through a series of tests and evaluation techniques. The neurological status evaluation may be indicative of a deteriorating condition or as an assessment of the cognitive state. This is particularly important in the home when traumatic injury is being evaluated or when progressive neurological involvement may be a side-effect of medication therapy.

Certain recognizable states of posture are associated with varying degrees of neurological impairment. Decerebrate posturing is assumed because of a brain lesion in the diencephalon, pons, or midbrain; the legs are extended with plantar flexion and the arms are held rigidly at the sides with the palms turned outward (Fig. 40-1). Decorticate posturing is assumed because of a lesion of the corticospinal tract near the cerebral hemisphere; the legs are extended, the feet are extended with plantar flexion, and the arms are internally rotated and flexed on the chest (Fig. 40-2). Flaccid posturing is assumed because of brain damage to the motor area of the brain; there is no muscular control of the body.

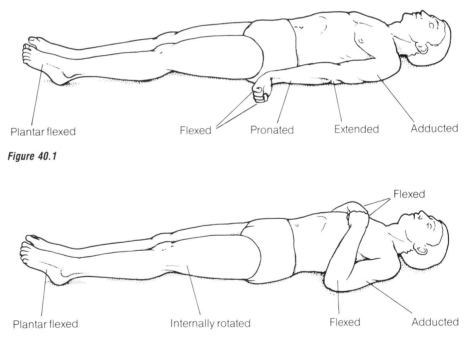

Plantar flexed   Flexed   Pronated   Extended   Adducted

Figure 40.1

Plantar flexed   Internally rotated   Flexed   Adducted   Flexed

Figure 40.2

Disruption of the brain causes a predictable pattern of change in the level of consciousness. Symptoms progress from decreased concentration and lethargy to unresponsiveness. Since the family is usually attuned to subtle changes in the client's response, the ability to check neurological signs is a distinct adjunct to neurological evaluation.

Assessment of Self-Care Potential

Client/Family Assessment

- Assess the willingness and ability of the family to check the neurological signs. If the client is combative or terminal, the family may be reluctant to do the assessment.
- Assess the ability of the family members to read and write if they will be asked to keep a record of the neurological signs on a form such as the Glasgow Coma Scale (see Records Kept by the Client/Family later in this technique).
- Assess the ability of the client to follow simple verbal directions.

Physical Assessment

- Assess the client's neurological signs to establish a baseline against which future neurological examinations may be measured.
- Assess the client's condition. Determine the expected course of progress for the duration of the illness. Assess complications that may arise and prepare the family for them.

Environmental Assessment

- Assess the lighting in the room. For assessment of pupil reaction, the room needs to be slightly darkened. Determine if sunlight can be blocked for the duration of the evaluation.

Planning Strategies

Potential Nursing Diagnoses

Sensory-perceptual alteration due to neurological impairment

Impairment of thought processes due to neurological impairment

Expected Outcomes

Resolution of neurological impairment with restoration to full physical and mental potential

Return to full consciousness

Recovery from or arrest of further paralysis

Health Promotion Goals

- The client and family will
  Learn how to check neurological signs and detect abnormalities
  Understand the need for checking the neurological signs on a regular basis
  Know the symptoms of increased intracranial pressure and what actions to take when signs of this condition arise

Equipment

Flashlight
Stethoscope and blood pressure cuff
Thermometer
Tongue blade or spoon
Cotton-tipped swab
Safety pin
Glasgow Coma Scale

Interventions/Health Promotion

ACTION

RATIONALE/AMPLIFICATION

1. Explain to the client what will occur during the evaluation. Wash hands before touching the client.

Even if the client is unconscious, explain each step including when and why the light is being directed into the client's eyes. It is impossible to determine the exact level of consciousness accurately, and in the event that the client is even slightly aware of the surroundings, an explanation is courteous and anxiety-reducing.

2. Measure the client's eye, motor, and verbal response. Note when the client's eyes open (i.e., spontaneously or in response to some type of stimuli such as speech or pain). Note the client's motor response. Ask the client to move a hand or arm. If this elicits no response, apply a stimulus to the head or trunk, such as a light pin stick, pinching of the inner thighs or inner arms, or a rubbing pressure with the fingertips on the sternum. Determine if the client attempts to remove the source of discomfort or moves in response to it. Ask the client simple questions regarding time, place, and person. If the client is not oriented to time, place, or person, determine if conversation is intelligible or absent. Use the Glasgow Coma Scale to record the client's response.

The Glasgow Coma Scale is a widely accepted means of assessing and recording level of consciousness.

3. Use a safety pin to stroke the skin with first the sharp side, then the dull side to determine the client's ability to distinguish between sharp and dull.

Inability to distinguish between pain sensations is indicative of decreased consciousness.

ACTION

RATIONALE/AMPLIFICATION

4. Assess the pupils by noting their size and reaction to light. Dim the room and shine a light source (such as a penlight or flashlight) directly into the client's open eye. Use the fingertips to hold the eye open since the reflex response to the light will be to close the eyelid (Fig. 40-3).

The pupils are normally equal at about 1.5 cm to 6 cm round and are located in the middle of the eye. In reaction to light, the pupil should constrict promptly. Both pupils should constrict to the same size. Edema of the pupillary muscle may result in abnormal pupil size or in a pupil of a fixed shape and size. Dissimilarity of the pupils may indicate neurologic damage.

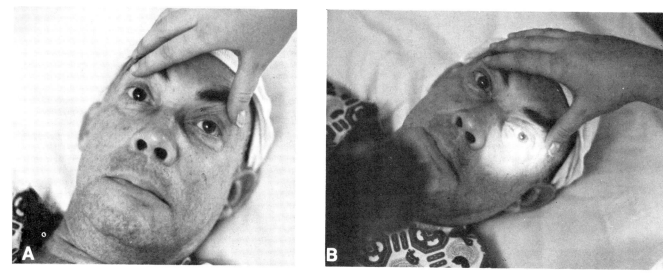

Figure 40.3

5. Assess reflexes to determine possible nerve damage. Assess the blink reflex by lightly brushing the client's eyelashes while holding the client's eyes open. The client should attempt to blink. Test the gag reflex by holding the client's tongue down with a spoon and touching the back of the pharynx with a cotton swab. This should make the client gag. Check the plantar response, or Babinski reflex, by running a spoon handle along the outer lateral aspect of the foot from the heel to the little toe and continuing across the ball of the foot toward the great toe (Fig. 40-4). Flexion of the toes indicates the normal response or a negative Babinski. A positive Babinski is evidenced by fanning of the toes.

Absence of the blinking reflex may indicate damage to the 5th or 7th cranial nerve. Depression of the gag reflex occurs when there is involvement of the 9th or 10th cranial nerve. A positive Babinski may indicate upper motor neuron lesion.

ACTION

RATIONALE/AMPLIFICATION

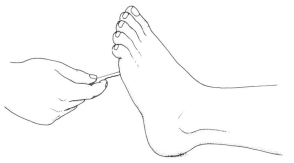
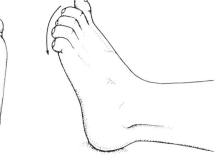

Figure 40.4

Related Care

Vital sign measurement is usually taken in conjunction with neurological signs. Refer to Technique 42, Vital Signs.

Age-Specific Modifications

Questions asked during the neurological assessment must be appropriate to the age and level of understanding of the child. The very young child may be asked questions regarding things that are familiar or in the room at the time. The nonspeaking child will be assessed by the pupillary and motor parameters.

Ask the child what was served for breakfast or lunch, the name of a favorite animal toy, or a sibling's or parent's name.

Education/ Communication

- Teach the family to

  Perform the neurological assessment in a competent manner. Emphasize the type of information that is being sought. Caution the family about the importance of gentleness during the procedure. When checking for response to painful stimuli, care must be taken not to injure the client. A sternal rub or pinching the inner thigh or inner arm is generally considered satisfactory to determine the level of response to pain. Explain the dynamics of pupillary reaction and emphasize the need to darken the environment before checking the pupils.

  Report any noticeable differences observed about the client. The family members know the client well and are more attuned to subtle changes in condition and sensorium.

  Perform the neurological testing on a regular and consistent basis. The neurological signs may be measured several times a day or more frequently depending on the condition of the client and the reason for the measurements. A goal for the family is to set up regular times and to perform the measurements consistently at those times. The importance of having a consistent record should be explained to the family. If the client has a change in reaction at the same time every day, the problem may be related to diet or blood levels of glucose or it may be related to oxygenation deficits. These kinds of trends can be identified if the measurements are checked at the same times each day.

Relate and respond as though the client is fully conscious even though there may be undetermined impairment and apparent unresponsiveness. Explain that the actual level of consciousness is not certain, and the client may be able to hear what is being said. It is therefore important to explain to the client what is happening during the examination.

Recognize signs of progressive neurological impairment. Yawning and sighing are signs of changes in the level of consciousness. Pupils may respond to light briskly. As the coma progresses, respirations increase and then stop momentarily (Cheyne-Stokes breathing). The pupils become fixed at midpoint and are unresponsive to light. Decerebrate posturing becomes more and more pronounced. Apnea and flaccidity occur in the final stages of coma preceding brain death.

Referrals and Consultations

For the client who is neurologically impaired, referral to a speech therapist, an occupational therapist, and a physical therapist may facilitate return to normal activities.

Evaluation of Health Promotion Activities

Quality Assurance/ Reassessment

- Observe the care provider carrying out the neurological assessment. Scrutinize technique and apparent level of understanding about the testing and the results.
- Perform the neurological check after the care provider and compare results.

DOCUMENTATION

Charting for the Home Health Nurse
A progressive record of the client's mental orientation as well as physical manifestations should be kept by the home health nurse during visits. From the record, it should be apparent whether the client is improving, deteriorating, or remaining stable. The record should include a synopsis of neurological examinations as well as subjective and objective data regarding the client.

Records Kept by the Client/Family
- Ask the family to complete the Glasgow Coma Scale as they do regular assessment of the client (Fig. 40-5). They may also make notations about activities that precede and follow periods of neurological change. Encourage the family to write down any questions they may have regarding care or technique.

Health Teaching Checklist

Name of Care Provider _____

Relationship to Client _____ Telephone #_____

Taught by _____ Date _____

	EXPLAINED	DEMONSTRATED
Need for checking neurological signs	_____	
Glasgow Coma Scale	_____	
Eye opening response	_____	_____
Motor response	_____	_____
Verbal response	_____	_____
Pupil assessment	_____	_____

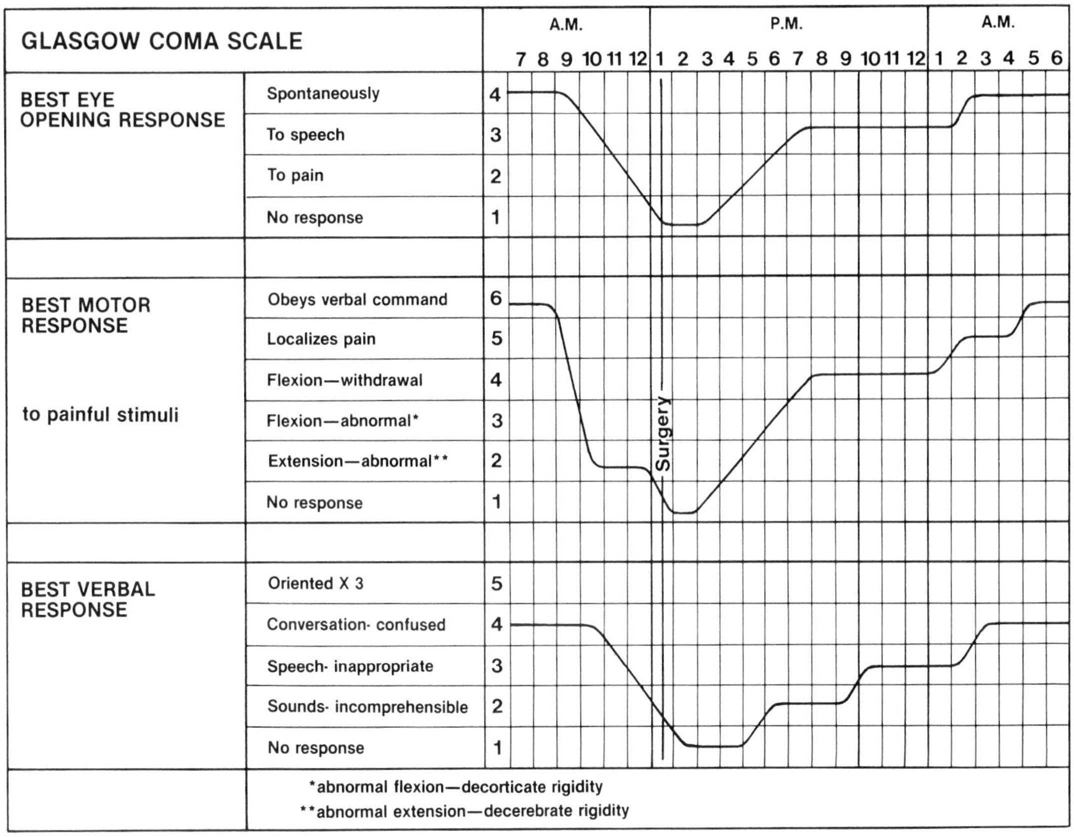

GLASGOW COMA SCALE			A.M. 7 8 9 10 11 12	P.M. 1 2 3 4 5 6 7 8 9 10 11 12	A.M. 1 2 3 4 5 6
BEST EYE OPENING RESPONSE	Spontaneously	4			
	To speech	3			
	To pain	2			
	No response	1			
BEST MOTOR RESPONSE to painful stimuli	Obeys verbal command	6			
	Localizes pain	5			
	Flexion—withdrawal	4			
	Flexion—abnormal*	3			
	Extension—abnormal**	2			
	No response	1			
BEST VERBAL RESPONSE	Oriented X 3	5			
	Conversation- confused	4			
	Speech- inappropriate	3			
	Sounds- incomprehensible	2			
	No response	1			
	*abnormal flexion—decorticate rigidity **abnormal extension—decerebrate rigidity				

Figure 40.5

Glasgow Coma Scale. How to score responses.

Scoring of eye opening: 4 = if the patient opens his eyes spontaneously when the nurse approaches; 3 = if the patient opens his eyes in response to speech (spoken or shouted); 2 = if the patient open his eyes only in response to painful stimuli such as digital squeezing around nail beds of fingers; 1 = if the patient does not open his eyes in response to painful stimuli.

Scoring of best motor response: 6 = if the patient can obey a simple command such as "Lift your left hand off the bed"; 5 = if the patient moves a limb to locate the painful stimuli applied to the head or trunk and attempts to remove the source; 4 = if the patient attempts to withdraw from the source of pain; 3 = if the patient flexes only his arms at the elbows and wrist in response to painful stimuli to the nail beds (decorticate rigidity); 2 = if the patient extends his arms (straightens his elbows) in response to painful stimuli (decerebrate rigidity); 1 = if the patient has no motor response to pain on any limb.

Scoring of best verbal response: 5 = if the patient is oriented to time, place, and person; 4 = if the patient is able to converse although not oriented to time, place, or person (e.g., "Where am I?"); 3 = if the patient speaks only in words or phrases that make little or no sense (e.g., "B—H, N—K."); 2 = if the patient responds with incomprehensible sounds such as groans; 1 = if the patient does not respond verbally at all.

	EXPLAINED	DEMONSTRATED
Reflex assessment		
Blinking	_____	_____
Gag	_____	_____
Babinski	_____	_____
Using a safety pin to differentiate between pain types	_____	_____

Product Availability   The penlight or flashlight may be purchased in any variety store.

41   Urine Glucose Testing

Background

Glucose testing is done to assess the status of a person's diabetic condition. Diabetes results from the body's inability to utilize foods efficiently. When food is digested, it is broken down into glucose, which is stored in the liver and muscle tissue in the form of glycogen. Insulin facilitates this storage process. Diabetics do not produce sufficient insulin; therefore, blood glucose levels rise to abnormally high levels. The normal fasting level of blood glucose is approximately 60 mg to 115 mg/dl blood. Glucose does not appear in the urine until the blood level reaches 180 mg/dl; therefore, urine glucose levels may be interpreted as a "reflection" of the actual blood glucose level.

Blood is not a normal constituent of urine. Certain conditions of the kidney may cause the appearance of blood in the urine (see Related Care, below).

Assessment of Self-Care Potential

Client/Family Assessment

- Assess the level of understanding of the client and family regarding the diabetic condition. Determine if there is a family history of diabetes.
- Assess the motivation of the client and family to follow the health regimen required for successful living with diabetes.
- Assess the ability of the client or family member to perform the glucose testing.
- Assess the eating habits of the family in relation to how they should be altered to compensate for the needs of the diabetic client.
- Assess the daily habits of the family to determine how much exercise the client normally gets.

Physical Assessment

- Assess the client's diabetic condition related to how it was diagnosed, its duration, any complications, and type of treatment regimen. It is particularly important to note the type of medication the client uses to control the diabetes.
- Assess the client's feet and legs for circulatory problems, which are common in diabetic clients.
- Assess the client's eyes with an ophthalmoscope to determine if diabetic retinopathy is present. This will appear as tiny, weblike pouches on the vascular structures in the fundus of the eye.

Environmental Assessment

- Assess the home for an adequate place to perform the testing and to store the equipment.

Planning Strategies

Potential Nursing Diagnoses

Knowledge deficit regarding diabetic care, treatment of crises, and prevention of complications

Alteration in health maintenance

Potential impairment of skin integrity

Alteration in nutrition requirements: potential for more than body requirements as determined by diabetic diet

Disturbance in self-concept: body image and role performance

Expected Outcomes

Understanding of pathology, treatment, and control of the diabetic condition

Adequate monitoring to prevent complications

Prevention of skin breakdown

Understanding and adherence to nutrition regimen

Adjustment and acceptance of new lifestyle

Health Promotion Goals

- The client and family will
  Learn how to perform the glucose testing safely and effectively. They will know when to perform the testing and when to notify the health-care provider of problems.
  Understand the ramifications of a diabetic nutrition regimen and will follow recommended dietary modifications
  Learn to care for the feet and nails so that trauma is avoided, as well as knowing when to report potential complications
  Learn to live in harmony with the diabetic condition

Equipment

Clean specimen container

Reagent materials

Test tube and dropper

Interventions/Health Promotion

ACTION

1. Urine testing for glucose and acetone may be done to determine the success of current treatment modalities. Because the urine reflects the status of the body at a time several hours before the time at which the urine was collected, these tests do not show current blood glucose levels. Advise the client to check the urine levels for ketones whenever the blood sugar levels are high (>240 mg) and whenever the symptoms or illness are present. Ketone determination should not be neglected when the client is doing self-monitoring of glucose.

RATIONALE/AMPLIFICATION

Urine testing may be done to give a more complete analysis of the body's status. Ketones in the blood are an important indicator that the client is at risk for ketoacidosis.

2. *Clinitest (5-drop method):* have the client void into a clean container. Place 5 drops of the urine in a test tube. Rinse the dropper and place 10 drops of water in the same tube. Drop one Clinitest tablet into the mixture of water and urine. Observe the chemical reaction taking place without shaking the test tube. If a rapid series of color changes does not occur, gently shake the tube and compare it with the accompanying color scale.
Clinitest (2-drop method): the 2-drop method is performed in the same manner except 2 drops of urine are mixed with 10 drops of water.

3. Other strips are available that are permeated with reagent. These strips are dipped in the urine and compared with a color chart. Some are combined with ketone determinants.

4. Acetest tablets are used to detect the presence of acetone in the urine. Place the tablet on a paper towel and drop one drop of undiluted urine directly onto the tablet. Color changes in the tablet are compared with a color chart.

Related Care

1. Ensure that the family and the client understand the signs and symptoms of insulin reaction: sweating, pallor, tremors, hunger, altered behavior, anxiety, tachycardia, palpitation, headache, confusion, slurred speech, uncoordination, double vision, drowsiness, convulsions, and coma. At the first sign of any of these symptoms, advise the client to test the serum glucose at once.

Careful observation of the chemical reaction is essential because a "pass-through" reaction can occur when the glucose is very high. This refers to a rapid succession of color changes from orange to dark greenish-brown. This indicates a reading of 4+ or a urine glucose of over 2%. Clinitest involves a chemical reaction. The natural side-effect is heat generation, so advise the client not to touch the bottom of the test tube during the reaction.

The chemical that permeates the strip undergoes a chemical change when coming in contact with the urine. Charts are based on the color that results from the ensuing chemical reaction. Because each strip contains a different type and amount of chemical reagent, it is essential that the strip be compared with the color interpretation chart that has been prepared specifically for it.

The presence of acetone in the urine may be indicative of current or potential problems. The tablet undergoes a color change when coming in contact with the urine. The resulting color is compared with the accompanying color chart.

ACTION	RATIONALE/AMPLIFICATION
2. Ensure that the family and the client understand the signs and symptoms of ketoacidosis: thirst, anorexia, nausea, vomiting, abdominal pain, headache, blurred vision, drowsiness, weakness, shortness of breath or an increase in the rate and depth of respirations, air hunger, fruity-smelling breath, excessive urination, lethargy, stupor, and coma.	
3. Testing for blood in the urine may also be done at the time the specimen is obtained. Dip the reagent strip (such as Hemastix) into the urine and compare with an accompanying color chart.	Blood in the urine may be visible on gross examination with the naked eye. It may also be occult (not visible to the eye). Tests for occult blood will indicate when renal problems may be present.

Education/ Communication

• Teach the client and family to

Recognize when glucose testing should be done in order to prevent complications. If the glucose condition is particularly unstable, it may be necessary to test more frequently. If the condition is well under control, testing daily or even less frequently may be possible. Advise the client and family to be aware of subtle changes indicating the need for glucose testing. It is generally advisable to test more frequently during times of illness or high stress or when symptoms of insulin reaction or ketoacidosis are present.

Understand and comply with dietary restrictions. Emphasize the importance of eating meals at regular times and not skipping meals or prescribed snacks. Advise the client to avoid foods high in sugar content, saturated fat, and cholesterol. Alcohol is not generally considered desirable for consumption by diabetics. Stress that "dietetic" foods are not necessarily compatible with diabetic dietary needs.

Develop a daily exercise plan and adhere to it. Control weight and stress levels.

Adhere to prescribed medication regimen. If insulin is a component of diabetic management, stress the importance of rotation of sites.

Recognize the signs of diabetic emergencies. Report problems to the healthcare provider at once.

Recognize and prevent diabetic complications that arise from prolonged circulatory interference. Stress attention to skin care by daily bathing, protection against minor trauma, and prompt treatment of injuries. Particular emphasis must be given to foot care. Since the feet are especially susceptible to complications from decreased blood circulation, great care must be exercised in trimming the toenails (straight across), checking the feet for trauma, washing the feet daily, and wearing clean, well-fitting socks and shoes.

Understand that it is important to report the presence of occult blood in the urine to the physician.

Referrals and Consultations

Information and assistance may be obtained from the American Diabetes Association, Inc. Diabetics may be referred to a foot specialist for trimming of toenails. Vision screening should be done regularly by a qualified ophthalmology specialist.

Evaluation of Health Promotion Activities

**Quality Assurance/
Reassessment**

- Observe the client and family performing the testing procedure. Note adherence to measures that will help ensure proper results. Determine the presence of symptoms that indicate the need to perform glucose testing.
- Observe the glucose and acetone testing to determine understanding of the dynamics of the procedure. Assess adherence to safety precautions.

DOCUMENTATION

Charting for the Home Health Nurse

- Maintain ongoing records of the urine glucose testing to provide a comprehensive analysis of the client's diabetic condition.
- Record diabetic complications and observations of possible symptoms for future comparisons.

Records Kept by the Client/Family

- Ask the client and family to keep records of the glucose measurements. These records should include the time of day and the method of measurement. The records may be used to predict stability of the diabetic status and the need for more or less frequent testing. See Table 41-1.

Table 41-1. GLUCOSE MONITORING RECORD

DATE	BEFORE BREAKFAST	BEFORE LUNCH	BEFORE DINNER	BEFORE BED	MEDICATIONS TAKEN	OTHER TESTS

**Health Teaching
Checklist**

Name of Care Provider _____

Relationship to Client _____ Telephone #_____

Taught by _____ Date _____

	EXPLAINED	DEMONSTRATED
Urine glucose determination		
Urine glucose testing	_____	_____
Acetone determination		
Acetest tablets	_____	_____
Reagent strips	_____	_____
Potential complications		
Prevention	_____	
Treatment	_____	
Potential emergencies		
Symptoms	_____	
Treatment	_____	

Product Availability

Tablets and reagent strips for testing urine, acetone, and occult blood may be purchased in most pharmacies and drug stores.

Selected References

How to Use Accu-Chek bG and Chemstrip bG for Blood Sugar Testing. Developed in cooperation with the Joslin Clinic Teaching Nurses, Joslin Diabetes Center. Boston, MA, Boehringer Mannheim Diagnostics, Inc.

Nemchik R: The new insulin pumps: Tight control—at a price. RN, May, 1983

Ranch J, McWeeny M: Managing Your Diabetes. Indianapolis, Eli Lilly & Co, 1983

42   Vital Signs

Background

Measurement of vital signs is done to assess the physiologic state of the client in relation to those vital centers of the body that are necessary to sustain life. The vital sign indicators are temperature, pulse, respirations, and blood pressure. The temperature may be taken by the oral, rectal, or axillary route. The pulse may be measured by palpation or by auscultation of the chest area. Palpation is usually done in the radial, brachial, femoral, pedal, temporal, and carotid regions. Respirations may be measured visually or by auscultation. Blood pressure is measured by means of a sphygmomanometer (cuff with pressure gauge) and a stethoscope.

The usual adult temperature range is 96.4° F to 99.4° F (35.8° C to 37.4° C). Temperature regulation may be diminished in the elderly; therefore, temperatures of older adults may be subnormal. Fever is an elevation of body temperature beyond the normal range. Causes may be viral or bacterial infection, drug reaction, brain lesion, or reaction to other body pathology. Fever-producing agents act on the hypothalamus, stimulating heat-production and heat-conservation mechanisms such as vasoconstriction, decreased sweat gland activity, increased muscle tone, and shivering. Body temperature elevation is the consequence. Oral temperatures are usually taken on all adults except those who are unconscious, confused, or subject to seizures; those receiving oxygen by nasal cannula; those with nasogastric tubes; and those who have a pathologic condition of the nose, mouth, or throat. Temperature for these clients is usually measured by the axillary route, although a rectal temperature may be taken.

Pulse rate is governed by the medulla. The elasticity of the vessels also affects the rate. During atherosclerosis, plaque lining the vessels hardens and constricts the diameter. The amount of blood able to be pumped through the vessels is diminished. This causes the right ventricle to exert more force to push the blood into the smaller vessels.

Breathing is regulated by the presence and amount of carbon dioxide, lung inflation, and blood pressure changes. Auscultation involves listening with a stethoscope over the front or back rib cage areas.

Blood pressure is influenced by problems with cardiac output and peripheral resistance. Hypertension occurs when the arterial pressure is significantly above average for the person involved.

Assessment of Self-Care Potential

Client/Family Assessment

- Assess the familiarity of the family with vital sign measurement. Determine if they have ever taken a temperature. Assess their ability to hear through a stethoscope.
- Assess the financial resources of this family to determine if they are able to purchase the needed equipment with which to measure vital signs, such as the stethoscope and sphygmomanometer.
- Assess the priority given by the family and the client to the vital sign measurement. Determine whether or not they anticipate that the effort will be justified in terms of the client's therapeutic progress.

| **Physical Assessment** | • Assess the client's vital signs to establish a baseline against which future measurements may be measured.
| | • Assess the client's condition. From the medical diagnosis and the nursing diagnoses, assess anticipated changes in vital signs so the family may be alerted.
| | • Assess the ability of the client to hold the thermometer in the mouth. Determine if the safety of the client will be compromised by taking an oral temperature because of the possibility of biting the glass thermometer, as could occur in the small child or the client subject to seizures. |

| **Environmental Assessment** | • Assess the noise level of the home. Determine which room will provide the quiet environment in which vital signs should be measured.
| | • Assess the temperature and ventilation of the room in which the client spends the most time. Environmental factors can affect the client's body temperature and respiratory rate. |

Planning Strategies

| **Potential Nursing Diagnoses** | Alteration in health maintenance
| | Knowledge deficit regarding the technique for taking vital signs |

| **Expected Outcomes** | Stability of vital signs
| | Early recognition of complications
| | Proficiency in vital sign measurement |

| **Health Promotion Goals** | • The client and family will
| | Learn the technique for taking the client's temperature by the most appropriate route. They will also learn to assess the pulse and respiratory rate, as well as to measure the blood pressure.
| | Understand the importance of regular measurement of vital signs
| | Understand which variations are acceptable and which warrant reporting to the health-care provider
| | Recognize the interrelationship between vital signs, activity, and change in condition
| | Communicate the vital sign measurements in a consistent and reliable manner to the health-care provider |

| **Equipment** | Thermometer
| | Watch or clock with a second hand
| | Stethoscope and blood pressure cuff
| | Lubricant (for rectal thermometer)
| | Alcohol
| | Tissue |

Interventions/Health Promotion

ACTION	*RATIONALE/AMPLIFICATION*
Wash hands before giving direct care to the client. Be sure that the client is at rest and has not eaten anything hot or cold before beginning.	Cross-contamination can be reduced by proper handwashing. Hot or cold food or beverages may alter vital sign readings.

ACTION

RATIONALE/AMPLIFICATION

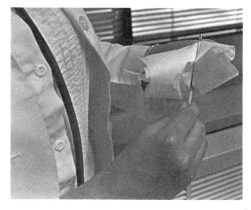
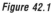

Figure 42.1

Temperature

1. Wipe the thermometer with a tissue and alcohol (Fig. 42-1). Hold the thermometer firmly between the thumb and forefinger and shake the mercury down to the base of the thermometer. Use a repeated flicking motion of the wrist. *Oral:* place the thermometer under the tongue and leave in place for 2 minutes. Remind the client to leave the lips closed around the thermometer. The normal oral temperature reading is around 98.6° F (37° C).
   Rectal: apply a lubricant to the thermometer (Fig. 42-2). Gently insert it into the rectum 2.5 cm to 3.5 cm (1–1½ inches) in the adult (Fig. 42-3). Hold the thermometer in place for 3 to 5 minutes. The normal rectal temperature reading is 99.6° F (37.5° C). Cleanse the client's rectum after completion.

The lips, rather than the teeth, should be closed around the thermometer to prevent breaking it.

A lubricant is used to reduce the friction encountered as the thermometer is introduced into the rectum. The thermometer should be held in place to prevent accidental breakage or trauma to the rectum.

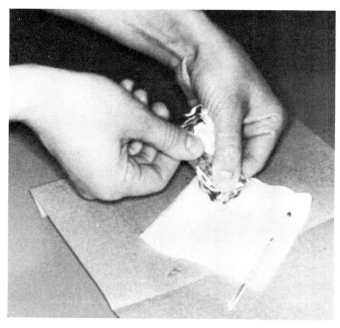

Figure 42.2

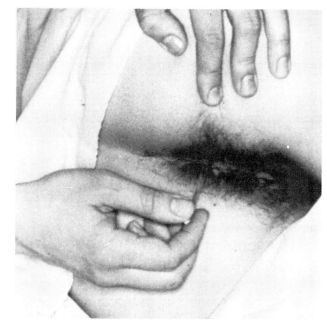

Figure 42.3

ACTION	**RATIONALE/AMPLIFICATION**
Axillary: dry the client's axilla with a soft towel. Hold the thermometer in place, with the bulb against the client's axillary tissue for 7 to 10 minutes. Fold the client's arm across the chest during temperature measurement (Figs. 42-4 and 42-5).	Moisture in the axillary region may interfere with temperature measurement.

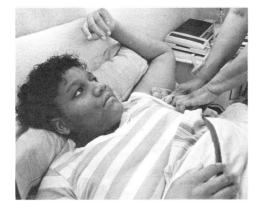

Figure 42.4

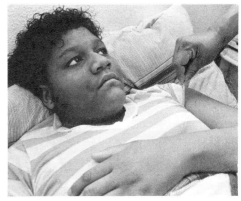

Figure 42.5

2. Read the thermometer. Wipe the thermometer with a rotating motion toward the bulb. Hold the thermometer at eye level and rotate it until the column of mercury comes into view. Read the value at the level of the mercury. If any fecal material remains on the thermometer, remove it with warm water and a tissue.	Mercury expands when heated according to the amount of heat applied. This allows the thermometer to measure the proper temperature consistently.

Pulse

1. Ensure that the client is in a position of comfort. Use the tips of the second and third fingers to measure the pulse. Apply gentle pressure on the appropriate artery until the pulsation can be felt. Support the dependent part, such as the client's hand if the pulse is being taken in the wrist, on a firm surface.	The thumb and index fingers have pulses of their own, which can be mistaken for that of the client; therefore, they should not be used to measure the pulse. Gentle pressure is necessary to allow perception of the pulse without obliterating it.

ACTION

RATIONALE/AMPLIFICATION

2. Count the pulse for 30 to 60 seconds. If it is irregular, count it for at least 60 seconds. Normal ranges are 60 to 72 beats/minute for men and 72 to 84 beats/minute for women. Auscultate the apical pulse by placing the stethoscope over the apex of the heart and counting for 1 minute (Fig. 42-6). Measure the radial pulse on the inner aspect of the wrist (Fig. 42-7). Locate the pedal pulse on the top of the foot, over the instep (Fig. 42-8). The femoral pulse is located in the groin area (Fig. 42-9). The carotid pulse may be felt in the neck area, about 2 to 3 inches below the mastoid process, under the mandible (Fig. 42-10).

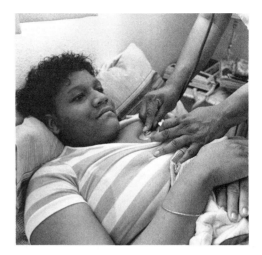

Figure 42.6

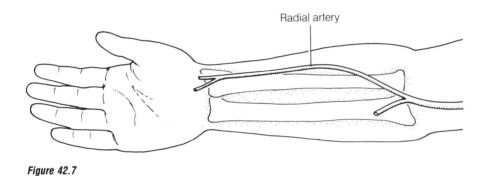

Radial artery

Figure 42.7

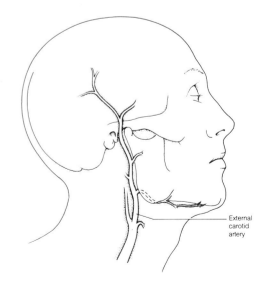

Dorsalis pedis artery

Figure 42.8

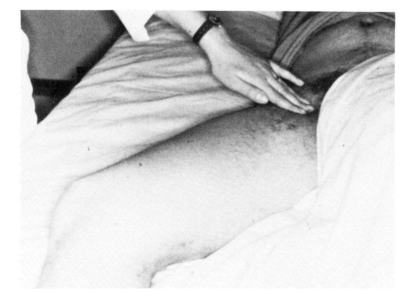

Figure 42.9

External carotid artery

Figure 42.10

ACTION	RATIONALE/AMPLIFICATION

Respirations

Observe the rise and fall of the client's chest. Count the number of breaths the client takes in 30 seconds. The normal adult respiratory rate is 16/minute to 20/minute.

A complete cycle of inspiration and expiration constitutes one respiration. It may be helpful to count the respirations immediately after counting the pulse, with the fingertips still on the client's artery. This way the client will not be aware that the respirations are being counted, and will not consciously or unconsciously alter the respiratory rate.

Blood Pressure

1. Apply the sphygmomanometer cuff to the client's arm above the antecubital fossa or to the leg above the popliteal fossa. The American Heart Association recommends that the limb circumference dictate the cuff size. Use the small adult cuff for the limb that is less than 23 cm. For the limb that is 24 cm to 32 cm, use the standard cuff. For the limb that is 32 cm to 42 cm, use the large arm cuff. For the limb that is 42 cm to 50 cm, use the thigh cuff. Place the bottom edge of the cuff about 1 inch above the antecubital fold with the marked arrows over the artery (Fig. 42-11).

Place the cuff in such a position that the gauge is easily visible and the cuff is not too tight while not inflated. The client should sit or lie comfortably. The arm should be fully supported on a flat surface at heart level. If the position of the arm varies or if the arm is not supported, the readings may not be accurate.

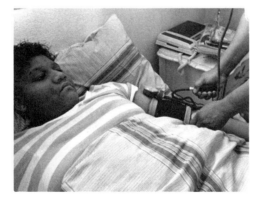

Figure 42.11

ACTION	*RATIONALE/AMPLIFICATION*
2. Place the diaphragm or bell of the stethoscope firmly over the artery so that the sound can be transmitted without distortion. If in doubt about the location of the artery, palpate it with the fingertips and place the diaphragm directly over the area where the pulse is felt.	The edges of the diaphragm should be completely against the skin to limit the amount of extraneous noise, but not with enough pressure to obliterate or modify the pulse. A comparison of the present blood pressure reading with the client's usual or past readings is often more significant than the actual numerical reading at any one time.
3. Inflate the cuff to a point about 20 to 30 mm Hg above the last systolic reading or until the pulsation can no longer be felt on palpation. Do not leave the cuff on any longer than necessary.	Pressure from the cuff interferes with the normal flow of blood through the vessels.
4. Determine the systolic pressure by slowly releasing the pressure valve at a rate of 2 to 3 mm Hg per second. The point at which the first pulse beat is heard is the systolic reading and the point at which the sounds cease is the diastolic reading. Read the level of the mercury or the position of the arrow on the gauge. Wait 2 minutes and measure the blood pressure again. The recorded pressure should be an average of these two readings. If the values are abnormally high, low, or otherwise unexpected, take the reading in the other arm using the same technique.	Systolic pressure is the point at which blood in the artery is first able to force its way through against the pressure exerted by the inflated cuff. The diastolic pressure is the point at which blood flows freely through the artery and is equal to the amount of pressure normally exerted on the wall of the arteries when the heart is at rest.
5. The blood pressure may be measured by the palpation method. Apply the cuff to the upper arm and locate the radial pulse. Inflate the cuff. The radial pulse will be obliterated at this point. As the cuff is slowly deflated, note the point at which the radial pulse is again palpable. The reading at which the first beat is felt is the systolic reading. It is generally 10 mm Hg lower than the auscultated systolic pressure. Diastolic pressure is not measurable by palpation.	If the family member cannot hear adequately auscultate the blood pressure, palpation may afford a mechanism to monitor the general level of the client's pressure. Also, the blood pressure is not audible in some clients, such as those who are near death or those who are extremely obese.

ACTION	RATIONALE/AMPLIFICATION

Age-Specific Modifications

| Temperature readings in children under the age of 6 years are usually taken by the axillary route. Temperature-sensitive strips, which are placed against the skin, may also be used to monitor the child's temperature. | Small children may bite the thermometer placed in their mouths. |

Education/ Communication

- Teach the client and family to

    Take the vital signs when the client is at rest or normally active. Measurement should not occur immediately after the client has had a hot or cold drink, has been smoking, or has undergone unusual exertion. These activities can give false readings.

    Measure the temperature safely. Be sure that they understand the importance of holding the thermometer when a rectal temperature is taken. If there is any chance that the client may bite down on the thermometer, advise the family to take the temperature by the axillary route. Remind the family that there are discrepancies between the client's temperature according to the route used for measurement. The rectal route tends to be a degree higher than the oral route, and the axillary tends to be about a degree lower.

    Explain that the pulse rate is a reflection of the beating of the heart. With each heartbeat, the blood is propelled through the veins. Pressing too hard will block the blood flow and make it impossible to count the number of beats per minute.

    Advise the family member who is measuring the respiratory rate about assessing this measurement when the client is unaware. Explain that it is a natural reaction to alter the rate when a person knows someone is counting.

    Blood pressure is often difficult for the family to assess. There may be extraneous noises during auscultation. They may not be sure when the beating sound stopped. Reassure them that they will become more proficient with practice. The important thing to emphasize is that they will become accustomed to how the blood pressure usually sounds so that when it is higher, lower, or unusual, they may be warned to take appropriate action (i.e., call the health-care provider, take a certain medicine, or cease activity as indicated by the client's particular condition).

Referrals and Consultations

Unexpected or unusual fluctuations in vital signs should be reported to the health-care provider for interpretation.

Evaluation of Health Promotion Activities

Quality Assurance/ Reassessment

- To assess technique, take the vital signs immediately after the family member. This should be done in a positive, nonjudgmental way, such as offering, "Let's see how closely we agree on measuring his blood pressure this morning." Observe the family member taking the vital signs and offer suggestions if needed.

- The record of the vital sign readings should be fairly stable. There should be no great discrepancies without a good explanation, such as unusual exertion or medication administration.

DOCUMENTATION

Charting for the Home Health Nurse
Vital signs should be measured and recorded, either in a narrative or on a graphic form, during each visit.

Records Kept by the Client/Family
If the family members are asked to measure vital signs, they should record the measurements each time they are taken. This may be done in a notebook or tablet. Any pertinent data should be noted as well, such as activity prior to measurement, medications taken, or changes in technique from usual methods.

Health Teaching Checklist

Name of Care Provider _____

Relationship to Client _____ Telephone #_____

Taught by _____ Date _____

	EXPLAINED	DEMONSTRATED
Temperature measurement		
Oral	_____	_____
Axillary	_____	_____
Rectal	_____	_____
Skin strips	_____	_____
Safety precautions	_____	_____
Pulse measurement		
Radial	_____	_____
Carotid	_____	_____
Pedal	_____	_____
Femoral	_____	_____
Respiratory measurement	_____	_____
Blood pressure measurement		
Auscultation	_____	_____
Palpation	_____	_____
Cuff application and fit	_____	_____

Product Availability

Glass thermometers are available at most discount stores, pharmacies, and drug stores. Temperature-measurement skin strips are also available at most drug stores and pharmacies. Blood pressure cuffs and stethoscopes are now available in many all-purpose stores that sell beauty and health aids. They are also available at pharmacies, drug stores, and hospital-supply houses. If the blood pressure will only be monitored for a short time, this equipment may be rented from some hospital-supply rental outlets. Digital blood pressure equipment is available; however, the accuracy of this equipment seems to depend a great deal on the adequacy of technique.

Selected Reference

Birdsall C: How accurate are your blood pressures? Am J Nurs 84(11):1414, November, 1984

Safety

43   Antiembolus Stockings

Background

Antiembolus stockings prevent blood clot formation by exerting pressure on the small veins and capillaries of the legs. This forces blood into the larger veins, thus accelerating the blood flow and preventing pooling and clotting of blood. A proper fit of the stockings is essential. Stocking measurement methods vary slightly with different stocking brands, although general measuring guidelines can be followed.

Assessment of Self-Care Potential

Client/Family Assessment

- If the client is unable to apply the stockings, determine that a family member is available and willing to perform the procedure.

Physical Assessment

- Assess both legs for the presence of sensation and movement.
- Assess both legs for skin integrity, infections, sores, or edema.
- Assess both feet for adequacy of venous return.
- Note excessive obesity, height, or thinness. These body types will require special stocking sizes.

Environmental Assessment

- Note height of chairs used by client in relation to client body build. The height of the chair must be such that pressure is not exerted on the popliteal space while sitting. Feet should rest flat on the floor without popliteal pressure while sitting. Use of a footstool can add height to the feet in relation to the chair seat.
- Assess the height of the bed. It should be low enough to prevent popliteal pressure if the client dangles or sits on the side of the bed.

Planning Strategies

Potential Nursing Diagnoses

Health management deficit: inability to apply stockings

Potential for skin impairment due to improperly applied or fitted stockings

Expected Outcomes

Understanding of the proper method of stocking application

Prevention of thrombi by the wearing of properly fitting antiembolus stockings

Health Promotion Goals

- The client and family will
  Purchase the appropriate size of stockings
  Properly apply the hose
  Conduct periodic assessment measures as taught

Equipment

Tape measure

Stockings of the appropriate size

Interventions/Health Promotion

ACTION	RATIONALE/AMPLIFICATION
1. Measure the client's legs to obtain a good stocking fit.	The client lies on the back or side for 5 to 10 minutes. For knee-length stockings, measure the largest part of the calf. Then, with the client lying on the side, measure from the back of the knee to the bottom of the heel. For waist-length or thigh-length stockings, measure the largest part of the calf, measure the largest part of the thigh, and measure the distance from the gluteal furrow to the heel.
2. Record measurements for use as baseline data as well as for use in future purchase of stockings.	These measurements can assist in future assessments by comparing measurements.
3. Compare measurements to manufacturer's scale to determine required size.	Purchase a minimum of two pairs to allow for laundering and change.
4. If the client is excessively obese, thin, tall, or short, special sizes will have to be obtained.	If regular sizes are applied to clients of unusual sizes, the fit will be too tight or too loose.
5. Apply the hose: • Elevate legs 5 to 10 minutes and assess for circulatory problems. • If no problems exist, clean and dry the legs. • Turn the stocking inside out. • Insert hand into the stocking, grasping the heel and turning the foot part right side out. • Place the heel band onto the client's heel; pull the stocking foot over the client's foot.	Powder or lotion may be applied sparingly, being cautious not to rub the leg vigorously. *Note:* be cautious not to leave pressure-inducing wrinkles. Never roll or fold stocking over.
6. Allow one hour to elapse after removing the hose before applying another pair of hose.	Assess for proper fit: 　Insert finger freely between top of hose and leg. 　Assess toes for skin color and skin temperature. Assess for venous return.

Related Care

If the client is also on anticoagulant therapy

1. Obtain a Medic-Alert bracelet.	In the event of injury, the bracelet serves as a guide to appropriate therapy.
2. Instruct the client to avoid aspirin and alcohol.	Aspirin and alcohol alter blood clotting times.

ACTION	RATIONALE/AMPLIFICATION
3. Take precautions against cutting or bruising by arranging furniture to avoid accidents.	Observe any indicated safety features.
4. Avoid walking barefoot.	
5. Inform the dentist or podiatrist of the use of anticoagulant therapy.	
6. Use an electric razor rather than a razorblade.	
7. Do not use over-the-counter drugs without physician approval.	

Education/ Communication

- Teach the client and family to
  Measure for hose fit, following the general guidelines above plus manufacturer's directions
  Purchase a minimum of two pairs of hose
  Apply hose correctly
  Wear hose no more than 8 hours consecutively
  Apply only clean hose. Wash stockings according to manufacturer's directions
  Refrain from vigorously rubbing the leg with lotion
  Periodically reassess for proper fit and application
  Adhere to prescribed medical regimen

Referrals and Consultations

- Refer to a podiatrist for corn paring, callus care, and care of ingrown toenails.

Evaluation of Health Promotion Activities

Quality Assurance/ Reassessment

- Observe the family assistant applying the hose.
- Make periodic home visits to assess the proper application of the hose. Assess the sensation, integrity, and circulation of the lower legs, the skin temperature, stasis, and skin color of toes.
- Periodically measure leg and compare that measurement with original baseline measurement, particularly if the leg is edematous.

DOCUMENTATION

Charting for the Home Health Nurse
- Document reassessment data related to skin temperature, stasis, and skin color of toes, any changes in measurement of leg, and preventive measures adhered to.

Records Kept by the Client
Any questions or concerns
Any complications noted

Health Teaching Checklist

Name of Care Provider _____

Relationship to Client _____ Telephone #_____

Taught by _____ Date _____

	EXPLAINED	DEMONSTRATED
Application of stockings	_____	_____
Care of stockings	_____	
Checking for appropriate fit	_____	_____
Adherence to related medical regimen	_____	
Assessment for complications (venous return, skin color of toes, changes in leg measurement)	_____	_____

Product Availability

Antiembolus stockings are available through most pharmacies. If the client is excessively obese, thin, tall, or short, special sizes are available from orthopedic-supply firms.

44 Arm Sling

Background

The purpose of applying an arm sling is to relatively immobilize and support an arm. The sling is made of a cloth material and suspends the arm from the neck or shoulders.

Assessment of Self-Care Potential

Client/Family Assessment

- Determine the availability and willingness of a family member to assist the client as needed.
- Assess the client's daily activities and employment requirements to determine any areas in which the client/family will require assistance during the rehabilitation phase.

Physical Assessment

- If the immobilized arm is the dominant one, assess the capabilities of the nondominant hand/arm in performing required activities during rehabilitation (e.g., eating, dressing, writing, combing, bathing, driving, etc.).
- Assess the adequacy of circulation in the injured arm (if casted or tightly bandaged). Observe for venous return by depressing the fingernail beds. Assess the fingers for edema. Feel the skin of the hand to determine any changes in temperature (coldness or heat to the touch). Assess the skin under the edges of the cast to determine the presence of skin irritation or breakdown. Note the presence of any unusual odor from the injured arm, as well as expressions of pain in the area of the injury.

Environmental Assessment

- Determine if a family member or friend can alter clothing to accommodate cast, sling, or large dressings if needed (enlarging sleeves or armholes of shirts, blouses, and dresses).

Planning Strategies

Potential Nursing Diagnoses

Skin integrity, potential impairment of

Self-care deficit

Comfort, alteration in, pain

Expected Outcomes

Proper application of the sling to maintain proper alignment

Adjustment to the altered physical status with compensation by using the other arm

Prevention or control of pain and discomfort

Health Promotion Goals

The arm, hand, and wrist will be supported in a functional position.

The hand will be supported above or level with the elbow.

The sling will be applied in such a manner as to reduce strain on the neck.

Circulation of the injured arm will be maintained.

Activities of daily living and employment will be resumed in their usual pattern.

Equipment   Sling (commercial or hand made; see directions, Fig. 44-3.)

Interventions/Health Promotion

ACTION

1. Place the sling in such a position that the center of the long side of the triangle is placed under the wrist and the free point of the triangle under the elbow. One strap of the sling is placed under the arm to the shoulder. The other strap is placed over the arm and up to the other shoulder.

2. Cross the straps at the client's back, bring them around to the front, threading them through the client's belt loops, cross in front, and bring to the back waist to be tied (Figs. 44-1 and 44-2).

RATIONALE/AMPLIFICATION

Securing the sling in this manner reduces the pressure on the neck and shoulders. Threading through the belt loops keeps the sling from "riding up."

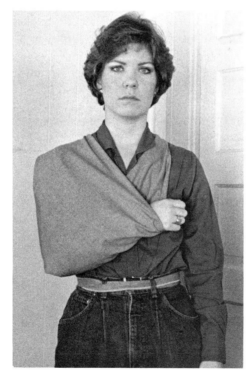

Figure 44.1
An example of a properly applied sling.

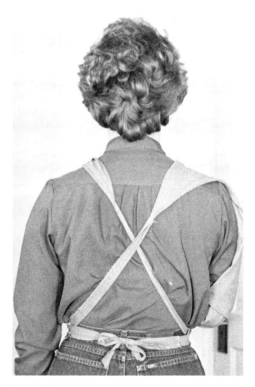

Figure 44.2
A method of sling application that removes the weight of the immobilized arm from the neck.

3. Secure the sling so that the hand is level to or above the elbow.

Support the hand and wrist in a functional position, using washcloths, rubber balls, or other devices as needed.

ACTION	RATIONALE/AMPLIFICATION
Related Care	
1. If requirements of daily living are disrupted significantly, make arrangements for assistance through church, family, or community resources.	Activities such as driving to work and child-care requirements may require outside assistance.
2. If a cravat is used for a sling, position the knot so it does not rub the cervical vertebrae.	Tie the knot to the side of the neck.
3. Slings are also available commercially that use Velcro for adherence.	These reduce the need for a knot at the neck.

Age-Specific Modifications

Slings are available for children in varied sizes and in bright colors.

Education/ Communication

- Teach the client and family to
  Properly apply the sling without excess pressure on the neck
  Maintain a functional position of the wrist and hand with the hand positioned above the level of the elbow
  Properly construct a sling if desired
  Periodically consistently assess the hand for circulation impairment, infection, and skin breakdown if a cast or bandage is applied to the arm or hand

Referrals and Consultations

- Refer to the state rehabilitation commission if job retraining is necessary.
- Obtain homemaker services if the disability causes serious deficits in home maintenance.
- If home confinement results from the injury, refer to Meals-on-Wheels.

Evaluation of Health Promotion Activities

Quality Assurance/ Reassessment

- Reassess on a periodic basis the application of the sling with attention to the position of the hand relative to the elbow and the functional positioning of the wrist and hand.
- Evaluate for presence of complications such as edema of the hand, venous return to the fingers, and skin irritation and breakdown.
- Evaluate the home situation for accomplishment of activities of daily living.

DOCUMENTATION

Charting for the Home Health Nurse
- Note presence of complications to the injured arm.
- Document positioning of the hand and wrist.
- Note progression of rehabilitation.
- Note any deficits in activities of daily living with provisions made for alleviating the deficits.

Records Kept by the Client/Family
- Monitor for the presence or absence of complications by checking the following several times daily on a scheduled basis:
  Venous return to hand of injured arm
  Edema in the hand of the injured arm
  Skin breakdown on the edge of the cast or bandage
  Presence of foul odor from the injured arm

Health Teaching Checklist

Name of Care Provider _____

Relationship to Client _____ Telephone # _____

Taught by _____ Date _____

	EXPLAINED	DEMONSTRATED
Construction of sling, if desired	_____	_____
Application of sling	_____	_____
Positioning of hand and wrist	_____	_____
Assessing for complications	_____	_____

Product Availability

The sling will usually be sent home with the client from the emergency room or physician's office where it was applied. However, if another sling is desired, it can be purchased from any hospital-supply firm, or it can be constructed with very elementary sewing skills, as shown in Figure 44-3.

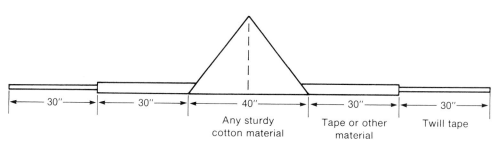

←— 30″ —→ ←— 30″ —→ ←— 40″ —→ ←— 30″ —→ ←— 30″ —→
Any sturdy cotton material   Tape or other material   Twill tape

Figure 44.3

45   Bandaging

Background

Bandages are continuous strips of woven material that are applied to a body part. There are several types of bandage material. Ace bandages are commercially prepared bandages made of woven elastic material that is capable of giving strong support. Gauze is a soft, porous, woven, light-weight cotton material that molds easily to body parts and is used frequently to retain dressings. Kling and Kerlix are types of woven, porous, self-adhesive gauze that stretch and mold to body parts.

Bandages may be used for a variety of purposes. They are used to limit the motion in an affected part. They may also be used to secure a dressing, traction, or splint. Dressings are used to provide support to an area and to apply pressure to body parts. They may also be used to aid in return of venous circulation from the extremities to the heart.

Assessment of Self-Care Potential

Client/Family Assessment

- Assess the ability of the family members to participate in bandaging. Some persons are unable to tolerate wounds, bleeding, or pain.
- Assess the financial resources of the family in regard to procuring bandage material. Some of the bandages are reusable, such as the Ace bandage. However, if an open wound is draining, replacement of bandages may be necessary. Assess the resources available to the family regarding purchase of needed bandage material.

Physical Assessment

- Assess the area to be bandaged. Determine if any cuts or breaks in the skin are present. Assess the color and condition of the area for later comparisons.
- Assess the feelings of the client regarding the bandage. Assess willingness to keep the bandage on securely and to have the bandage rewrapped when needed.

Environmental Assessment

- Assess the general cleanliness of the home. If cleanliness is not a priority, added emphasis on the importance of keeping wounds and bandages clean may be needed.
- Assess the layout of the house. Determine how close the client will be to areas such as the bathroom. If the client is very mobile and must travel a long way to needed areas, additional bandage support may be needed.

Planning Strategies

Potential Nursing Diagnoses

Impaired physical mobility

Actual or potential impairment of skin integrity

Potential for injury

Knowledge deficit regarding proper application of bandages

Expected Outcomes

Maintenance of mobility potential

Prevention of complications from bandaging

Prevention of injury by application of the bandage using proper technique

Understanding of bandaging procedure

Health Promotion Goals

- The client and family will
  Learn how to apply the bandage properly and will do so in a manner to accomplish the intended purpose of the bandage
  Understand the importance of keeping the bandage in the proper position. They will also understand the need for consistent and comfortable bandage application.
  Understand the reason for the bandage
  Report any complications resulting from bandaging

Equipment

Specified bandage

Medications, dressings, equipment, as needed

Tape, clamps, pins, or clips

Interventions/Health Promotion

ACTION	*RATIONALE/AMPLIFICATION*
1. Wash hands before beginning the bandaging procedure.	Handwashing has been shown to be effective in reducing the incidence of cross-contamination.
2. Place the part to be bandaged in normal anatomical position. Help the client to get into a comfortable position before applying the bandage. Be sure that the body part is supported.	Placing the part in the normal functioning position helps to prevent deformities and discomfort. It also enhances circulation to the affected part and facilitates rehabilitation.
3. Apply padding to separate adjacent skin areas and to protect bony prominences (Fig. 45-1).	Friction and pressure from the bandage can cause mechanical trauma to the skin.

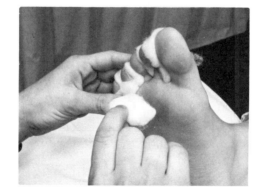

Figure 45.1

4. Apply bandages from the distal to the proximal parts.	The distal area is the farthest away from the midline of the body. Proximal is nearest the midline. Application of the bandage toward the midline encourages return of venous blood to the heart.

ACTION

RATIONALE/AMPLIFICATION

5. Anchor the beginning of the bandage by making several turns at the start. Secure the end of the bandage. Apply even pressure throughout the length of the bandage. Secure the bandage with pins, clamps, clips, or tape.

Securing the bandage at the beginning and end will add stability and help the bandage last longer. Uneven pressure can interfere with blood circulation and cell nourishment. It may also slow the healing process.

6. If possible, leave a small area of the bandaged extremity exposed, such as a finger or toe (Fig. 45-2).

An exposed area allows for direct visualization of the affected limb for checking circulation.

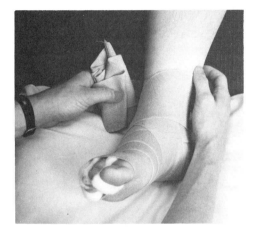

Figure 45.2

7. Basic bandage patterns are the following:
   Circular: each round of bandage slightly overlaps the entire previous round, thus creating a bandage that is the width of the material itself (Figs. 45-3 to 45-6).

A circular bandage is used primarily to anchor a bandage at the beginning and termination points. It may also be used to anchor a dressing.

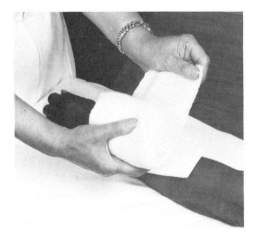

Figure 45.3

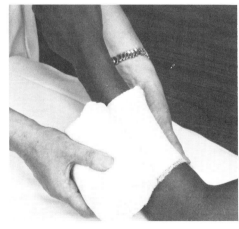

Figure 45.4

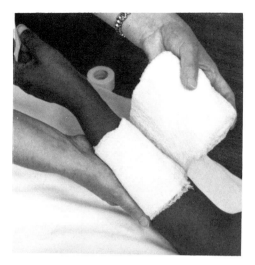

Figure 45.5

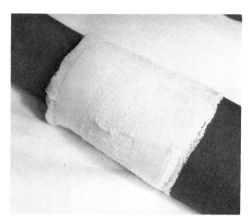

Figure 45.6

ACTION

Spiral: each round of the bandage slightly overlaps the previous round to create a progression up the part (Figs. 45-7 to 45-10).

RATIONALE/AMPLIFICATION

A spiral bandage is useful for a cylindrical body part such as the finger, wrist, or trunk.

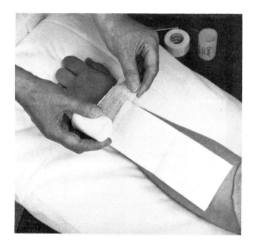

Figure 45.7

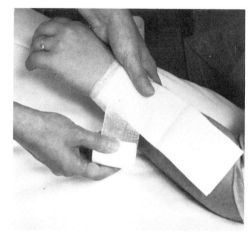

Figure 45.8

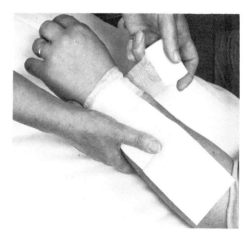

Figure 45.9

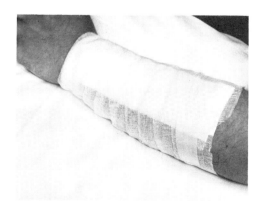

Figure 45.10

ACTION

Spiral reverse: this bandage is anchored by several rounds of spiral bandage. Then, with each succeeding round, the top of the bandage is turned under (Figs. 45-11 to 45-14).

RATIONALE/AMPLIFICATION

A spiral reverse is used for bandaging a cone-shaped body part, such as the thigh, leg, or forearm.

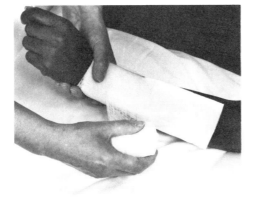

Figure 45.11

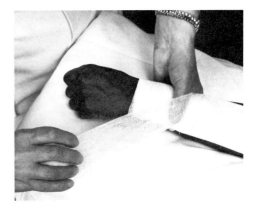

Figure 45.12

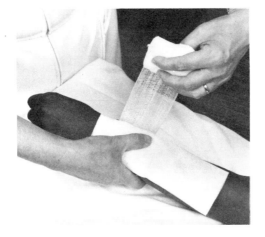

Figure 45.13

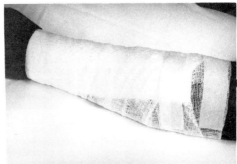

Figure 45.14

Figure-8: a figure-8 bandage is anchored by several rounds of spiral below a body joint. A round is then made above the joint and alternately below and above until the entire joint is covered (Figs. 45-15 to 45-18).

A figure-8 bandage provides a snug fit and is generally used for immobilization of joints such as the knee, wrist, elbow, and ankle.

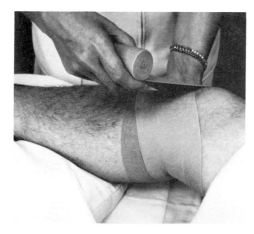

Figure 45.15

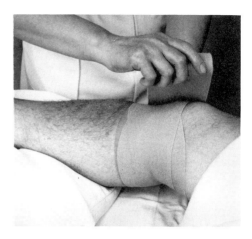

Figure 45.16

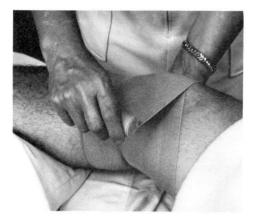

Figure 45.17

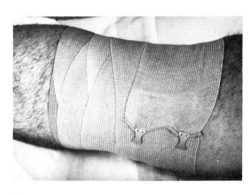

Figure 45.18

ACTION

Spica: this is the same bandage technique as the figure-8 except that it generally covers a much larger body area, such as the hip (Fig. 45-19).

RATIONALE/AMPLIFICATION

The spica bandage is useful in bandaging the breast, shoulder, groin, or thigh.

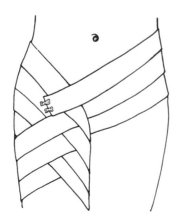

Figure 45.19

ACTION	RATIONALE/AMPLIFICATION
Recurrent: the bandage is first positioned by two circular turns. The roll is then turned perpendicular to the circular turns and passed back to front and front to back, overlapping each time until the area is covered. It is secured by making two circular turns over the initial circular turns (Fig. 45-20).	A recurrent bandage is used for anchoring a dressing on the head, a stump, or a finger.

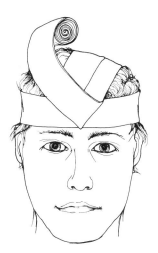

Figure 45.20

Education/ Communication

- Teach the client and family to
  Properly apply the bandage. Teach them the method of application as well as indications that signify the bandage should be changed.
  Care for the bandages. Explain where to purchase bandages and how to wash them, if washable. Ace bandages are to be washed in mild detergent, rinsed thoroughly, and allowed to drip dry. If a healing wound is located under the bandage, explain the technique and importance of first applying a sterile dressing to the wound before bandaging.
  Watch for possible complications of bandage application. Tell them to leave a distal portion of the bandaged part exposed so that they can observe for complications such as discoloration, loss of sensation, and swelling. Elevation of body parts may help relieve swelling due to trauma. However, swelling may also be an indication that the bandage has been applied too tightly.
  Be sure that the part to be bandaged is in normal anatomical position before proceeding. It is important that the bandaged part retain as much function as possible.

Evaluation of Health Promotion Activities

Quality Assurance/ Reassessment

- Observe the bandage to see that it is secure and is accomplishing the purpose for which it is intended.
- Observe the bandaging process to see that infection-control precautions are taken. Watch technique and offer suggestions if needed.
- Inspect the bandaging materials to see if they are still in proper condition. Ace bandages may become stretched after much use. Note whether the material being used is the best one for this particular bandage.

DOCUMENTATION

Charting for the Home Health Nurse

A notation describing the part to be bandaged should be made. Describe the part and the condition of the skin. Any unusual characteristics, such as bruises, cuts, or swelling, should be noted so that these will not be mistaken for sequelae of the bandage therapy.

Records Kept by the Client/Family

Ask the family to keep a record of how often they change the bandage. They may also write down any questions that they wish to ask the home health nurse during the next visit.

Health Teaching Checklist

Name of Care Provider _____

Relationship to Client _____ Telephone #_____

Taught by _____ Date _____

	EXPLAINED	DEMONSTRATED
Importance of handwashing	_____	
Placement of part to be bandaged	_____	_____
Padding between adjacent skin areas	_____	_____
Leaving a small skin area for observation	_____	_____
Bandage methods		
Circular	_____	_____
Spiral	_____	_____
Spiral reverse	_____	_____
Figure-8	_____	_____
Spica	_____	_____
Recurrent	_____	_____

Product Availability

Ace bandages, Kerlix, Kling, and gauze bandages may be obtained at most pharmacies and drug stores.

46   Burn Care

Background

Burns may be caused by chemical, thermal, or electrical sources. The first-degree burn features a reddened skin area without blisters or areas of induration. With the second-degree burn there is blistering and peeling of the skin with some induration and pain on being touched. A third-degree burn produces skin that has a leathery appearance with induration; no pain is evidenced when the skin is lightly touched because the nerve ends have been damaged.

Assessment of Self-Care Potential

Client/Family Assessment

- Assess the amount and type of support system the client has at home to provide care during recuperation and rehabilitation after a burn.
- Assess the financial resources of the family. If the client is the breadwinner, will time off from work cause financial hardships? If the client is a child, will a working parent have to remain home to provide care?

Physical Assessment

- Assess the extent of the client's burns. Determine the amount of activity limitation and the potential for rehabilitation.
- Assess the amount of pain the client is experiencing. Assess current and alternative pain-relief methods.

Environmental Assessment

- Assess the client's access to bathing facilities. Determine if the client will be able to cleanse the wound twice daily without problem.
- Assess the distance between the client's home and the areas of therapy and rehabilitation. Assess modes of transportation.

Planning Strategies

Potential Nursing Diagnoses

Alteration in comfort due to pain (acute and chronic)

Potential for injury from infection

Impaired physical mobility

Anxiety

Self-concept, disturbance in body image

Expected Outcomes

Reduction or control of pain

Reduction of infection and prevention of reinfection

Promotion of new tissue growth with minimal disfigurement and maximal range of motion

Emotional stability

Promotion of a positive self-image

Health Promotion Goals

- The client and family will
  Provide safe care designed to assist the client to reach full potential with minimal discomfort and disfigurement
  Care for the burns without causing cross-contamination
  Perform rehabilitation therapy consistently

Learn to stress what the client can do instead of dwelling on what the client cannot do

Provide a satisfactory psychological climate

Equipment

Dressings

Pain medication

Bandages (for pressure dressings)

Workout equipment for rehabilitation

Interventions/Health Promotion

ACTION	*RATIONALE/AMPLIFICATION*
1. Careful handwashing should precede and follow any care for the burned client.	The great problem with burns is the ready access into the circulatory system for microorganisms. Handwashing reduces the number of microorganisms present on the hands.
2. For a minor burn, clean the wound and remove foreign matter by scrubbing the area with cool water and a mild soap. Rinse the wound with sterile saline, if available, or with water that has been boiled and then cooled by placing the pan in an ice bath. Apply an antiseptic cream to the site and cover it with a sterile dressing.	Cool water relieves some of the discomfort and may help reduce edema. Soap helps to remove microorganisms that may cause infection. The sterile dressing will help keep the site clean and prevent infection.
3. For the client with a major burn, home care should emphasize a positive future. A major concern is wound care, which includes changing dressings on grafted and nongrafted sites using sterile technique (see Technique 65, Wound Care). Other areas may blister and break down after discharge from the hospital. These areas must be dressed and monitored.	Focusing on the future helps the client make the psychological adjustment to future orientation and provides optimism and a point of positive reference. Sterile dressings help prevent reinfection.
4. Pain relief is another major concern. Pain and itching remain a problem for many months. Plan the client's pain medication around periods of greatest physical activity. Explore other avenues of pain control.	Since pain control is a long-term problem with burned clients, the problem of addiction is very real. Use of imagery and self-hypnosis may help the client control pain.
5. Exercise therapy will help prevent scarring and will enhance return of full range of motion. Splinting and wearing pressure garments may help reduce scar formation.	Exercise is essential not only for the client's physical return to function, but it also gives the client an active part in rehabilitation.

**Education/
Communication**

- Teach the client and family to

  Expect the pain and itching to last for many months. Even after the burn is healed, the stretching of the skin during rehabilitation causes pain and itching. Pain and tingling, such as that associated with vascular insufficiency, may be present in the limbs. Medication to control itching may be given throughout the day rather than waiting until the itching has already become unbearable. Pain medication should be given 20 minutes before activities that are likely to increase discomfort, such as stretching or exercise periods. Explore alternative ways of dealing with pain in an effort to curb drug dependence.

  Understand how essential exercise is to recovery from the burns. Help the client and family accept the fact that exercise therapy may be needed for 1 or 2 years. Assist in the formulation of an exercise program and encourage the client to adhere to it. Daily therapy sessions may be needed for a time. Assist the client to arrange transportation to these sessions by contacting local service organizations or church groups.

  Counteract boredom, which may cause an upset of the client's sleep/wake pattern. If the client sleeps during the day and cannot sleep at night, both client and family may become frustrated. Advise the family and client to provide diversion and activity to keep the client awake from 14 to 16 hours per day so that the client will sleep well at night. A medication to help the client sleep may be needed.

  Understand the mechanism for scar maturation. It is essential that the client be told early in the recovery period that the scar will get worse before it gets better. The client who leaves the hospital expecting to look normal in a few weeks will have a great shock when the scars continue to look the same or worse. Explain to the client and family that a person who has survived burns over 50% of the body surface may expect that the scars will take from 6 months to 2 years to mature completely. However, point out that eventually the scars will fade and soften. Reconstructive surgery is an alternative that may be explored with a plastic surgeon.

- Consider vocational counseling if the client will be unable to return to a former occupation.

**Referrals and
Consultations**

A physical therapy referral may be needed to help the client work out a satisfactory exercise program to reach full potential functioning. Sessions at the physical therapy gym may be necessary for a time. Later the client may be able to perform the therapy in the home with follow-up visits to the therapist.

Occupational therapy may benefit the client who will have to seek an alternative occupation during or after rehabilitation.

Reconstructive surgery may be recommended. A referral to a plastic surgeon should be made early in the rehabilitative process so the physician will be familiar with all aspects of the case.

Evaluation of Health Promotion Activities

**Quality Assurance/
Reassessment**

Continuing reassessment of the amount of pain medication needed by the client will help to determine the effectiveness of alternative modes of pain control.

Observation of the burn area will determine if healing is occurring as it should. It should be remembered that scar maturation may take as long as several years.

Talking to and listening to the client will give insight into the client's level of anxiety and optimism. The healing process is one of highs and lows; however, continuing reassessment of the client's outlook is necessary in order to determine if depression or psychoses may be developing.

DOCUMENTATION

Charting for the Home Health Nurse
Keep records of the appearance of the scar as well as aspects of the rehabilitative process. Pain control should be documented so that a progressive picture of the rehabilitation process may be seen.

Records Kept by the Client/Family
Ask the family to keep track of how much pain medication the client uses. They also should set up a written time schedule for exercises and document deviations from the schedule. If dressings are needed, the family may keep a record of the frequency of dressing changes in order to assess the progress of healing.

Health Teaching Checklist

Name of Care Provider _____

Relationship to Client _____ Telephone #_____

Taught by _____ Date _____

	EXPLAINED	DEMONSTRATED
Wound management	_____	_____
Pain relief	_____	_____
Exercise therapy	_____	_____
Scar maturation process	_____	
Vocational counseling	_____	

Selected Reference

Marvin J: Planning home care for burn patients. Nursing '83 13:65–67, August, 1983

47 Cane Walking

Background

Persons with limited mobility deficits benefit from the use of a cane to increase their independence and their confidence in their own mobility skills. Canes are the assistive device of choice for persons having one-sided weakness or disability of a limited nature.

Assessment of Self-Care Potential

Client/Family Assessment

- Assess the willingness and ability of the care provider to provide support and assistance to the client during the initial use of the cane until competence in cane walking is achieved.
- Assess the willingness and ability of the family to make desired environmental alterations to provide safe and convenient use of the cane.

Physical Assessment

- Assess the client's strength and grip in the hand to be used with the cane. Assess the tightness of the grip to determine the appropriate diameter of cane handle.
- Assess the client's balance and coordination to determine selection of type of cane. If balance is poor, the appropriate cane is one with a broad base, such as a tripod or quadripod.
- Determine the overall strength of the client on the side to be used with the cane.
- Assess the client's visual acuity to determine if it is sufficient to be able to detect obstacles that could cause a fall.

Environmental Assessment

- Determine the frequency of need for climbing stairs or steps and the height of the steps. Note if stable bannisters or handrails are present beside stairs and steps.
- Inspect the bathroom to determine if assistive armrests are available or can be installed on the commode. Assess the shower to determine ease of entry and the feasibility of renting or purchasing a shower stool with rubber suction cups on the legs. Inspect the shower floor to determine if non-skid devices can be applied or are present.
- Determine if a sturdy, comfortable chair with strong armrests is present in the home to provide support to the client while in the process of sitting or rising from a sitting position.
- Inspect the floors of the environment to determine if they are slippery and waxed and to determine if wax can be eliminated or if soft-pile carpet is present or can be installed. In addition, observe if scatter rugs or other hazardous items are lying on the floor.
- Assess the furniture arrangement to determine if the furniture can be arranged near the walls to eliminate obstacles to mobility.

Planning Strategies

Potential Nursing Diagnoses

Mobility, impaired physical

Body-image disturbance

Expected Outcomes

Safe and independent ambulation using the appropriate cane

Resumption of former lifestyle without appreciable alteration

Health Promotion Goals

- The client and family will
  Climb and descend steps and stairs safely and independently
  Sit and rise from a sitting position safely and independently
  Develop safe independent use of the cane while walking
  Be supportive of the client's progress toward independence

Equipment

Appropriate cane

The single straight-legged cane with a half-circle handle is simple to use and inexpensive. It is available in lightweight metal or plastic or in the traditional wood. The metal and plastic types are adjustable in height, usually from 34 inches to 42 inches. This cane is especially appropriate for the person needing to use stairs frequently. The half-circle allows it to be hung on the person's arm or on a chair arm when not in use. This cane is selected if the client has a good grip in the hand using the cane and has good balance and coordination.

The straight-legged, straight-handled cane differs from the cane described above in the construction of its handle. It is indicated for persons whose disability prevents good grip of the hand using the cane. The handle is larger than the curved handles, thus allowing for a better grip. The negative feature of this cane is that it cannot be hung on the arm or chair when not in use and is thus less convenient. It is also adjustable in height.

The tripod (having three prongs) and quadripod (having four prongs) canes have a broad base, providing good support for persons with poor balance. In addition, they are free-standing, thus allowing for convenience in eliminating the problem of "dropped canes." A negative factor exists in that with the base being a broad one, it also provides a source of "tripping" for other persons in the environment. These canes, too, are adjustable.

Note: apply rubber tip(s) to the selected cane to prevent slipping.

Interventions/Health Promotion

ACTION	*RATIONALE/AMPLIFICATION*
1. Adjust the height of the cane. (See Fig. 47-1.)	The cane should extend from the floor to the client's hip joint. When holding the cane approximately 4 inches beside the unaffected foot, the arm should be slightly bent at the elbow.
2. Until the client walks independently, apply a strong belt around the client's waist.	This provides a means for the assisting person to hold, thus providing support to the client without obstructing movement.
3. Advise the client to wear non-skid, low-heeled shoes.	Comfortable broad-based shoes assist in preventing falls.

ACTION	RATIONALE/AMPLIFICATION
Walking With the Cane	
1. Instruct the client to stand erect and look straight ahead rather than at the feet.	This encourages good posture and body alignment.
2. Ask the client to hold the cane in the hand of the unaffected side.	This allows the strength of the client's unaffected side to be used to support the weakened side.
3. Instruct the client to hold the cane approximately 4 inches out from the unaffected foot, bearing weight on the unaffected foot while bringing the cane and affected foot forward simultaneously (Fig. 47-1).	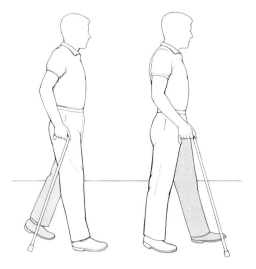

Figure 47.1
Appropriate gait while walking with a cane. Note that the recommended height of the cane is to the hip joint, with the arm slightly bent. The shaded area indicates the affected leg.

ACTION	RATIONALE/AMPLIFICATION
4. Ask the client to then transfer weight to the affected foot and the cane simultaneously while the unaffected foot is brought forward.	
5. Advise the client to take small steps until confidence is achieved in walking independently.	Small steps increase a sense of balance.
Sitting From a Standing Position	
1. Select a sturdy chair with strong armrests.	A straight-backed chair that is strong and well balanced will provide necessary support for the client.
2. Ask the client to stand in front of the chair with backs of legs touching the chair seat.	This provides a sense of exact location of the chair seat.
3. Have the client reach down with both hands (holding the cane out and in one hand) and firmly grasp both armrests, lowering the body into the chair.	The strength of the arms is thus used to support the body weight into a sitting position.
4. Instruct the client to hang the cane on the armrest.	Forming a habit of securing the cane on the armrest prevents the cane from falling and/or becoming misplaced.

ACTION	*RATIONALE/AMPLIFICATION*

Rising From a Sitting Position

1. Instruct the client to take the cane into the unaffected hand to be ready for ambulation when the standing position is assumed. Have the client place the unaffected foot slightly forward of the other and, grasping both armrests, lean slightly forward, applying pressure on the armrests and rising to a standing position.

   Using both hands on both armrests and using maneuvers designed to increase balance reduce the possibility of falling.

2. Allow a few seconds to become completely balanced prior to beginning to walk.

   Ensuring balance prior to walking increases stability.

Climbing Stairs

1. Instruct the client to transfer the cane to the weak side.

   This frees the stronger hand to assist in climbing the stairs.

2. Have the client grasp the handrail with the unaffected hand and shift the body weight to the affected side.

   This frees the strong leg to negotiate the step.

3. Then tell the client to lift the strong foot to the next step, transfer the body weight to that leg, and bring the affected leg up to the step.

   This allows maximum use of the strength present in the unaffected side to achieve safe negotiation of stairs.

Descending Stairs

1. Have the client hold the cane on the affected side.

   The strong arm is thus freed to be used on the handrail to assist in descending the stairs.

2. Instruct the client to lower the weak leg to the next step. The unaffected foot is then brought to the step while balancing with the unaffected hand on the handrail.

   The full use of the strong side is available for supporting and balancing the weak side.

Related Care

1. If the client has poor vision or if the home environment is poorly lighted, a light-weight flashlight can be mounted on the cane with the light beam focused directly in front of the cane.

   A cane can be purchased with a light on it (see Product Availability) or the light can be mounted by a family member.

2. Advise the client to use special caution when ice is present on walkways or outside steps.

   The combination of limited mobility and the use of a cane creates an especially hazardous condition in icy weather.

Education/ Communication	• Teach the client and family to Focus on the client's strengths rather than weaknesses Walk independently, ascend and descend steps independently, and rise and sit independently. Focus on independence in activities of daily living will promote a positive self-image. The former lifestyle should be resumed with little or no alteration.
Referrals and Consultations	• Consult the State Rehabilitation Agency if marked changes in employment or lifestyle are required. • Refer to Meals-on-Wheels if the client is homebound or if the weather is especially hazardous. • Consult the Social Security Office if food stamps are deemed necessary and the client qualifies.

Evaluation of Health Promotion Activities

Quality Assurance/ Reassessment	• Periodically reassess the client's independent functioning and safe use of the cane. • Note correction of environmental hazards or addition of unsafe aspects of the environment.
DOCUMENTATION	*Charting for the Home Health Nurse* • Note client progress in independent ambulation and other functions of daily life. • Document any major family/client adjustments required in lifestyle and progress in making the alterations. *Records Kept by the Client/Family* Major concerns and questions Steps taken to complete referral process

Health Teaching Checklist

Name of Care Provider _____

Relationship to Client _____ Telephone # _____

Taught by _____ Date _____

	EXPLAINED	DEMONSTRATED
Ambulation	_____	_____
Alteration of positions	_____	_____
Negotiating steps, stairs	_____	_____
Safety factors in the environment	_____	

Product Availability

The cane of choice can be rented or purchased from any hospital-equipment firm. The stool with suction tips on the legs (for shower use) can also be purchased or rented from a hospital-equipment firm or improvised by a family member. The cane with flashlight mounted on it can be purchased from Green Mountain Products, Inc., Muller Park, Norwalk, CT 06852, or can be improvised by a family member.

Selected Reference

Nursing Photobook: Providing Early Mobility. Springhouse, PA, Springhouse Corporation, 1984

48   Cast Care

Background

Casts are applied to provide immobilization of an extremity and/or joint following injuries causing fractures or sprains or to correct structural defects. Casts can be applied to only one part of an extremity or can be as extensive as a body cast. Traditionally casts were made of plaster of Paris. Current developments allow casting to be done using synthetic materials such as fiberglass and polyester or cotton.

Assessment of Self-Care Potential

Client/Family Assessment

- Assess the family to determine if a member is willing and capable of assisting the client as needed with activities of daily living.
- Assess the client and family to determine if they are oriented toward full independent functioning (within the limits of safety) for the client.

Physical Assessment

- Assess the casted extremity every 3 to 4 hours for the first two days following casting and daily thereafter for the following:
  Skin color distal to the cast
  Edema distal and proximal to the cast
  Sensation in the digits
  Venous return in the digits
  Skin temperature distal to the cast
- Assess the cast for
  Roughness around the edges. These cause skin irritation and should be filed and/or covered with moleskin or another padding substance to create a smooth edge.
  Signs of drainage or bleeding from under the cast, indicating infection or bleeding. If noted, circle the spot and write the date and time it was first noted.
  Cracking of the cast. In addition to being unsafe, cracks reduce the immobilization function. The cracked cast requires replacement or repair.
  Moisture on the cast. If the cast is applied near the perineal area, it should be waterproofed by wrapping plastic or other waterproof substance around it.
- Assess pain in the casted extremity. Severe pain over a bony prominence under the cast may indicate a pressure area (Fig. 48-1). Sites most susceptible in the lower extremities are the heel, malleoli, dorsum of the foot, head of the fibula, and anterior surface of the patella. On the upper extremities, susceptible sites are the medial epicondyle of the humerus and the ulnar styloid.

Environmental Assessment

- If the cast is applied to the leg or foot and crutches are used, assess the environment for objects such as throw rugs on the floor.
- A cast applied to an extremity causes an initial sense of imbalance. Assess the environment to determine if the furniture can be arranged so that the client can counter imbalance by holding on to furniture or handrails while walking.
- If the cast is applied to the dominant arm, assess the environment to determine if alterations can be made to assist with eating, writing, dressing, toileting, and driving. If environmental manipulation alone is not sufficient to attain client independence of functioning, assess the availability of homemaker services.

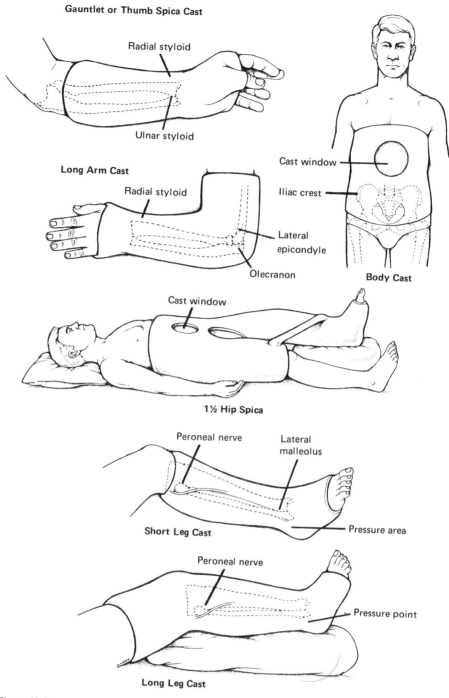

Figure 48.1
Commonly applied casts.

Planning Strategies

Potential Nursing Diagnoses

Mobility, impaired physical

Comfort, alteration in: pain

Skin integrity, potential impairment of

Expected Outcomes

Healing and rehabilitation of the casted body part while promoting mobility

Alleviation of pain

Prevention of skin irritation and breakdown

Health Promotion Goals

- The client and family will
  Properly maintain the cast
  Frequently assess the cast and the skin under the edges of the cast to determine skin condition
  Periodically assess the casted parts for circulatory and neurological deficits

Equipment

Good lighting to facilitate neurological and circulatory assessments

If synthetic cast, blow dryer to dry the cast after it becomes wet

Cast, applied in hospital, clinic, or physician's office (Table 48-1)

Table 48-1. COMPARISON OF CASTING MATERIALS

MATERIAL	DRYING TIME	TIME UNTIL WEIGHT BEARING	ADVANTAGES	DISADVANTAGES
Plaster of Paris	At least 24 hr	48 hr	Inexpensive	Heavy; crumbles, causing skin irritation; must be kept dry; no weight bearing during drying time
Polyester and cotton knit casting tape	7 min	15 min	Light-weight; less restrictive; less likely to become indented while drying due to short drying time; resists crumbling; less bulky; with nonabsorbent lining can immerse in water	More costly; more difficult to mold; less effective for immobilizing severe displacement; rougher surface often snags clothing and furniture
Fiberglass	15 min	30 min	Same advantages as polyester and cotton knit casting	In addition to the disadvantages listed for polyester and cotton above, a special blade is required to remove a fiberglass cast
Plastic casting tape	5 min	20 min	Same as listed for polyester and cotton knit casting	Same as listed for polyester and cotton knit casting

Interventions/Health Promotion

ACTION

1. Reassess the extremity for circulatory complications on a frequent basis, initially every 2 hours.

2. If the edges of the cast are rough, pad them with foam rubber or strips of adhesive tape.

3. If the cast is plaster do not allow the cast to get wet. Waterproofing allows showering.

RATIONALE/AMPLIFICATION

As the casting material dries, it shrinks, causing inhibition of circulation. Detection of numbness, absence or weakening of pulses in the extremity, change in skin color of the extremity, or edema signal a need to reevaluate the cast for appropriate fit.

Rubbing of the skin by rough cast edges for long periods of time causes the skin to break down.

Moisture causes crumbling of the plaster, and the cast becomes soft and misshapen.

ACTION	RATIONALE/AMPLIFICATION
4. If the cast is synthetic and the cast can be moistened, it should be flushed with water and dried thoroughly after showering, swimming, or bathing.	Dry by first blotting with a towel, and completing the procedure with a blow dryer on cool or warm setting, moving it in a sweeping movement over the entire cast.
5. If sand, dirt, or small articles get under the cast, irritation and infection can occur. Remove all irritants from under the cast.	For plaster casts, a well-padded reaching device, such as a coat hanger, can be used to remove the particles. Use care to avoid scratching or cutting the skin. For synthetic casts, flushing with water will remove the particles.

Related Care

ACTION	RATIONALE/AMPLIFICATION
1. Avoid vigorous activity of the casted body part.	Vigorous activity can reduce the alignment of the fracture.
2. If the weight of an arm cast is uncomfortable, wear an arm sling.	See Technique 44, Arm Sling.
3. Perform range-of-motion exercises on all noncasted joints twice daily.	See Technique 1, Active and Passive Range-of-Motion Exercises.
4. Alter clothing as needed.	Since the cast increases the circumference of the body part, arm holes and pantlegs often have to be enlarged. Select clothing in which seams can be ripped and inserts applied to avoid destroying clothing.

Education/ Communication

• Teach the client and family to
  Assess the casted extremity for circulatory and neurological impairment. If
    impairment is found, report it immediately to the nurse.
  Remove sand or other potentially harmful particles from under the cast
  Smooth any rough edges of the cast and apply padding to the edges
  Waterproof the cast (if plaster) prior to showering
  Make necessary environmental adaptations to promote safety, independence,
    and comfort

Referrals and Consultations

• Consult local agencies and client's church to assist in transportation if driving is impossible and family members are unable to assist.
• If confinement to the home is anticipated, refer to Meals-on-Wheels.

Evaluation of Health Promotion Activities

Quality Assurance/ Reassessment

• Periodically assess the circulatory and neurological status of the casted body part.
• Examine the quality of the cast and note any indications of drainage.
• Assess the level of independent functioning of the client.

DOCUMENTATION

Charting for the Home Health Nurse
• Note any alterations in the circulatory status and neurological status of the casted body part in comparison to the other extremity.
• Note any odor, drainage, and structural damage to the cast.
• Note the client/family understanding of limitations imposed by the cast, care of the cast, and ability to assess neurological and circulatory alterations.

Records Kept by the Client/Family
Questions and concerns
Evidence of bleeding or drainage
Alterations of circulatory status or neurological status

Health Teaching Checklist

Name of Care Provider _____

Relationship to Client _____ Telephone #_____

Taught by _____ Date _____

	EXPLAINED	DEMONSTRATED
Circulatory and neurological assessment	_____	_____
Prevention of damage to the cast	_____	
Environmental and clothing adaptations	_____	_____
Range-of-motion exercises to other joints	_____	_____

Selected Reference

Lane P, Lee M: Special care for special casts. Nursing '83 13:50–51, July, 1983

49   Client Transfer Aids

Background

A client may be unable to perform basic transfer maneuvers independently due to weakness or lack of coordination or balance. Devices are available to assist in transferring the client. Most commonly used are the mechanical lift and the transfer board.

Assessment of Self-Care Potential

Client/Family Assessment

- Assess the willingness and ability of the family assistant to support and assist the client in transfer maneuvers as needed.
- Assess the physical strength and coordination of the family assistant, to the extent that it will be required in the selected transfer maneuver.
- Assess the ability of the assistant to follow and remember directions.

Physical Assessment

- Assess the client's readiness for increased physical activity.
- Assess range of motion of all joints that will be needed in the process of completing transfer maneuvers.
- Assess the client's ability to move in bed and to sit independently.
- Assess the client's balance and coordination.
- Determine the client's comprehension, memory, and ability to follow directions.
- Assess the client's strength in the shoulders and arms since most transfers require at least partial lifting of the body using the arms.

Environmental Assessment

- Assess areas of the home where assistive devices will be used to determine if adequate space is available for use of the selected device.
- If a transfer board is to be used, assess the height of the bed and chairs in relation to wheelchair; they should be approximately equal in height.
- If an over-bed trapeze is to be used, assess the style of the headboard of the bed as well as the trapeze to determine if it can be installed. If it cannot be applied, determine if a hospital bed can be rented.

Planning Strategies

Potential Nursing Diagnoses

Physical injury, potential for

Mobility, impaired physical

Disturbance in self-concept, body image

Expected Outcomes

Accomplishment of safe transfer techniques

Increased independence in lifestyle through use of transfer aids

Family support of client independence and safety

Health Promotion Goals

- The client and family will
  Select the appropriate transfer technique
  Rent or purchase the equipment necessary
  Demonstrate safety in transfer maneuvers

Equipment
Appropriate transfer device
  Mechanical lift: for a client whose weight or level of immobility is beyond the strength and abilities of family members
  Transfer board: this device is smaller and less expensive and is appropriate when the client is partially or totally immobile. It can be used if the surfaces involved in the transfer are of approximately equal height. It should be smooth and should be covered with a cloth (pillowcase) prior to use to reduce friction to the skin in the process of sliding across it.
Over-bed trapeze
  This device is attached to the head of the bed and is suspended over the client's head position while lying in the bed. It provides a means of support for movement in bed and while in process of transfer. It can also be used for exercise to strengthen the upper body and arms.
Transfer belt (also called "walking belt")
  The transfer belt has handles that can be grasped by the assistant for ease in assisting clients with crutch walking, use of a walker, or in transfer techniques. It is applied outside the client's clothing and is secured with front buckles (Fig. 49-1). It can be purchased commercially or made in the home. If made in the home, cut a 3- to 4-inch strip of cotton webbing approximately 48 to 52 inches long. Wrap it around the client's waist over the clothing and tie it into a square knot. Use the belt to provide a secure grip of the client while in the process of transfer.

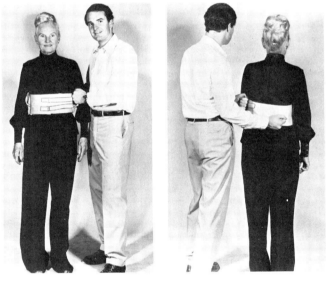

Figure 49.1
Use of a transfer (walking) belt. The handles on the sides and back allow the assistant to support the client until independent mobility is achieved.

Interventions/Health Promotion

ACTION	RATIONALE/AMPLIFICATION
*Mechanical Lift (From Bed to Wheelchair)**	
1. Explain the procedure to the client/family.	Knowledge of what to expect reduces fear for both the client and family.

* The procedure is the same for all transfers.

ACTION	*RATIONALE/AMPLIFICATION*
2. Place the wheelchair parallel to the bed and remove legrests and armrest nearest the bed.	Remove as many obstacles to transfer as possible.
3. Lock the wheelchair wheels.	This secures the wheelchair, preventing unintentional moving.
4. Put the slings (or other device provided by the manufacturer for lifting the client) securely under the client's buttocks and mid-back.	Place the slings centrally to provide a balanced lift.
5. Maneuver the lift in place. Apply brake to wheels of the lift. Secure the sling to the lift by means of chains or straps provided.	Double check the security of the chains to prevent accidental slipping.
6. Raise the client by pumping the hydraulic mechanism.	Advise the client to hold onto the straps or chains as the transfer occurs to increase the feeling of security.
7. Pivot the client to a position directly over the wheelchair.	Place hands under client's knees and use hands to guide the transfer.
8. Lower the client slowly into the wheelchair by releasing the hydraulic mechanism. Disconnect the sling. Remove the sling if desired. Replace armrest and legrests. Position client with respect to body alignment, safety, and comfort.	If the client is to remain in the chair for an extended period of time, remove the sling to prevent skin irritation. If the client is unable to sit independently, a vest or belt restraint can be applied during the sitting phase. Use pillows to improve comfort and alignment.

Note: adaptations for toilet use and shower use are available with the mechanical lift to be used instead of the slings.

Transfer Board

1. Place pajama bottoms on the client or a pillow case (or other cloth) on the board.	Cloth prevents friction during the movement involved in the transfer procedure.
2. Move the wheelchair parallel to the bed, lock wheels, and remove armrest nearest the bed.	Securing the wheelchair and removing the armrest prevents accidental falling.
3. Advise the client to sit up in the bed parallel to the wheelchair and close to the mattress edge on that side.	This places the client in a position to prepare for movement.
4. Instruct the client to shift body weight away from the wheelchair and slide the board securely under the buttocks. Place the other end of the board securely on the wheelchair seat.	The board is placed securely on both the bed and wheelchair to prevent the possibility of falling in the process of transfer.
5. Instruct the client to slide across the board onto the chair. Tilt the body away from the bed and remove the board. Replace armrest. Unlock wheelchair and proceed with movement.	Body alignment is secured by the use of pillows for positioning.

ACTION	*RATIONALE/AMPLIFICATION*
Transfer Belt	
1. Apply the transfer belt over the client's clothing and secure it.	Using the transfer belt to assist with client moves provides an excellent mechanism for gripping and thus providing support.
2. Place arms around the client's waist. Grasp the handles of the transfer belt and assist the client with the transfer.	Use arm and leg strength to assist the client, thus preventing unnecessary strain to the back.
Over-Bed Trapeze	
1. Instruct the client to grasp the trapeze with both hands, using this leverage to assist with movement in bed as well as with transfer maneuvers.	Use of the trapeze allows the client to use arm and upper body strength to assist with the transfer.
Related Care	
1. Provide skin care on a frequent, regular basis. Direct attention specifically to the buttocks and around the waist.	Friction burns and pressure areas develop often with frequent uses of transfer devices.
2. With all position changes, allow the client time to regain balance prior to another movement.	Rushing the client to a new position often causes imbalance, slipping, and falling.
3. Examine functioning of all equipment both before and after each use.	Worn out belts, weakened chains, or improperly functioning lifts can precipitate a fall.

Education/ Communication

- Teach the client and family to
  Use the transfer board if that is the selected method of transfer. It can be used in all transfers if the two surfaces are approximately of equal height. In addition, it is lightweight and easy to carry outside the home.
  Use the mechanical lift if it is the appropriate method of transfer. In addition, maintenance of the lift should be taught, and frequent assessment should be done of all working parts prior to and following each use.
  Frequently assess vulnerable skin areas for pressure areas and friction burns
  Report any falls or other accidents
  Use the transfer belt if it is appropriate for assistance
  Use proper body mechanics and body alignment during the transfer procedure
  Use the over-bed trapeze for leverage during transfers

Referrals and Consultations

- If equipment is not functioning correctly, or if there is a concern about its functioning, return to rental or purchasing agency or call the agency to pick up the device. Most important, *if there is a question about safety, do not use the device.*

Evaluation of Health Promotion Activities

Quality Assurance/ Reassessment

- Observe a return demonstration of the transfer maneuver to determine adherence to safety measures and recommendations.
- Periodically examine vulnerable skin areas for pressure areas and friction burns.
- Periodically reassess the client's level of mobility. If mobility capability increases, reassess for a different mode of transfer.

DOCUMENTATION

Charting for the Home Health Nurse
- Document client/family skill in using the transfer technique.
- Document the skin condition in areas prone to friction burns or pressure.
- Note neuromuscular assessment findings.
- Assess client condition following any accidents.

Records Kept by the Client/Family

Any questions or concerns

Any notice of reddened areas

Any alteration in mobility skills or indications of readiness to adapt to alternate transfer methods

Events surrounding any accident

Health Teaching Checklist

Name of Care Provider _____

Relationship to Client _____ Telephone #_____

Taught by _____ Date _____

	EXPLAINED	DEMONSTRATED
Functioning of transfer aid	_____	_____
Use of transfer aid	_____	_____
Skin assessment	_____	_____
Use of body mechanics	_____	_____

Product Availability

The transfer aid is readily available through a home health rental or purchase agency. If desired, a transfer belt can be made in the home (see under Equipment earlier in this procedure).

Selected References

Klabak L: Getting a grip on the transfer belt. Nursing '78, 8:10, February, 1978

Wolff L, Weitzel MH, Zornow RA, Zsohar H: Fundamentals of Nursing, 7th ed, pp 420–426. Philadelphia, JB Lippincott, 1983

50 Crutch Walking

Background

Crutches are the mobility aid of choice when the client has (1) a leg impairment that prevents full weight-bearing on the leg, (2) sufficient upper body and arm strength to properly use crutches, and (3) a relatively good sense of balance and coordination.

The appropriate gait to be taught depends on the amount of weight-bearing capability the leg can sustain. The appropriate gait will have been recommended by a physical therapist or the physician. It will have been taught by a physical therapist but often needs to be reinforced by the nurse.

Assessment of Self-Care Potential

Client/Family Assessment

- Assess the willingness of the care provider to assist the client during the initial stages of crutch use until competent crutch walking is achieved.
- Assess the ability and strength of the care provider to provide assistance to the client while learning crutch walking.
- Assess the willingness and ability of the family to make necessary environmental changes to assist in the safe and convenient use of the crutches by the client.
- Assess the necessity for role change within the family structure and any need for job alterations because of temporary mobility impairment.

Physical Assessment

- Assess the arm and upper body strength to support the weight of the body while using the crutches.
- Assess the client's coordination and balance to compensate for the loss of the use of the leg.
- Assess the sufficiency of visual acuity to sense obstacles that may cause falls.
- Assess the client's mental alertness and ability to follow directions.

Environmental Assessment

- Determine the presence of steps that must be climbed in the process of everyday living.
- Determine if a sturdy, secure chair with strong armrests is present to reduce the hazard and effort required to get into a sitting position and rise from sitting.
- Assess the doorways, hallways, bathroom, dining room, and kitchen to determine if adequate space exists for use by the crutch-walking client. If adequate space does not exist, determine if furniture can be rearranged within those areas to better accommodate the client's use.
- Examine the floors to determine if they are waxed and slippery or in any way pose a hazard. Check if throw rugs and other obstacles on the floors can be removed during the time of crutch walking.

Planning Strategies

Potential Nursing Diagnoses

Mobility, impaired physical

Skin integrity, impairment, potential

Coping, ineffective, individual, family

Expected Outcomes	Safe mobility skill with the use of crutches
	Prevention of axillary skin breakdown
	Provision of adequate rest of the affected leg to promote healing without permanent impairment
	Maintenance of independence in daily living, school, and/or employment
Health Promotion Goals	• The client and family will Learn safe crutch use techniques with the appropriate gait Independently change from a standing to a sitting position and return to a sitting position Climb and descend stairs unassisted and safely
Equipment	Crutches, made either of light-weight aluminum or wood and of the proper height
	Rubber tips, axillary pads, and hand grips applied to the crutches
	Well-fitting, flat, non-skid, lace shoes

Interventions/Health Promotion

ACTION	RATIONALE/AMPLIFICATION
Adjust crutches for correct height.	
1. Stand and place a crutch under each armpit. Place each crutch 4 to 6 inches in front of and to the side of the feet. Support the upper body weight on the handgrips, holding the back straight and looking straight ahead.	If the crutches are too tall, the crutch pads will rub the client's armpits, causing soreness. If the crutches are too short, they will be awkward to use, adding to imbalance and incoordination. Handgrips that are too low put pressure on the axilla, while handgrips that are too high are awkward.
2. Measure the gap between the axilla and the axillary pad. It should be two fingers wide. If it is more or less than that, adjust the crutches to that height.	
3. Remain in the same position. Grasp the handgrips. Adjust the handgrips so the elbow is flexed 30 degrees (Fig. 50-1).	

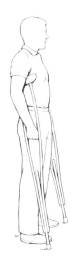

Figure 50.1
Proper stance and height of crutches. Note that the client is looking straight ahead and standing with good body alignment.

ACTION	RATIONALE/AMPLIFICATION
4. Lean against the wall to practice balancing. When balance is achieved in this position, shift the body weight in different positions while standing with the crutches.	Safe crutch use requires balance, coordination, and timing. Practice related to balance prior to attempting walking will promote safety and self-confidence.
5. Select the appropriate gait.	The gait is selected according to the type and severity of disability.
6. Teach a minimum of two gaits.	Changing from one gait to another relieves fatigue. In addition, the client can use one gait for faster speeds and another one in crowded situations where a slower speed is necessary.
7. Bear weight on hands, not the axillae.	Axillary weight-bearing puts pressure on the brachial plexus, producing crutch paralysis. Initial symptoms are tingling in arms, hands, and fingers.

Standing Position

Place crutches approximately 8 inches in front of and to the side of the toes.	Taller persons require a wider base; shorter persons use a narrower base.

Two-Point Gait (Fig. 50-2)

	The two-point gait is for clients who cannot bear full weight on either leg, but who have good balance and coordination. This is a fast gait.

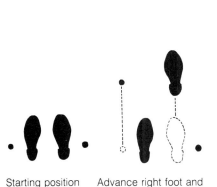

Starting position   Advance right foot and left crutch   Then advance left foot and right crutch simultaneously.

Figure 50.2
Two-point gait.

Three-Point Gait (Fig. 50-3)

	This gait is used if the client has full use of both arms and one leg and has good balance and coordination. It is fairly rapid but requires strength and balance; the arms must be able to support the entire body weight.

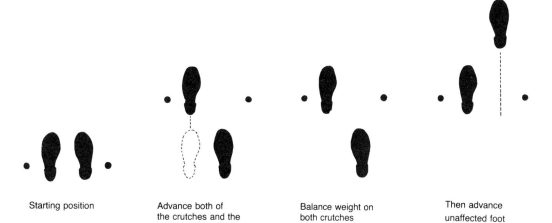

| Starting position | Advance both of the crutches and the weak foot | Balance weight on both crutches | Then advance unaffected foot |

Figure 50.3
Three-point gait.

ACTION

Four-Point Gait (Fig. 50-4)

RATIONALE/AMPLIFICATION

This gait is used if a client cannot support full weight on either leg. It is a slow but stable gait. Each leg must be able to move separately and hold a considerable amount of weight.

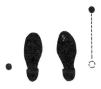

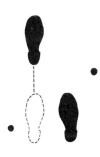

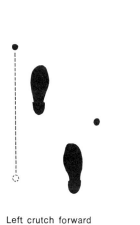

| Right crutch forward | Advance left foot | Left crutch forward | Advance right foot |

Figure 50.4
Four-point gait.

ACTION	RATIONALE/AMPLIFICATION

Tripod Simultaneous Gait (Fig. 50-5)

This gait is slow and labored. A tripod position is constantly maintained.

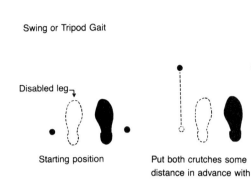

Swing or Tripod Gait

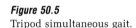

Disabled leg

Starting position

Put both crutches some distance in advance with weight on unaffected leg

Then swing forward with weight on unaffected leg again

Figure 50.5
Tripod simultaneous gait.

Standing

1. Slide forward in the chair, unaffected foot slightly under the chair.

2. Grasp the handpieces of the crutches or the arms of the chair. Bear weight on the unaffected foot and the hands, lifting the body to a standing position.

Make sure both crutches are within reach when the standing position is completed.

Sitting

1. Approach the chair so the backs of the legs are touching the chair seat. Shift the crutches to the hand on the affected side.

Getting a "feel" for the exact location of the chair gives a sense of confidence.

2. Place the hand of the unaffected side on the armrest of the chair while the crutches are placed at the side or back of the chair.

The chair must be close enough to provide support while changing positions. In addition, the chair must be a sturdy one with a broad base so as not to be easily upset. The armrests should be strong enough to support the weight that will be placed on them during position changing.

3. Place the left hand on the left armrest and lower the body into the chair (Fig. 50-6).

Using the arms to assist in weight-bearing reduces the strain on the legs.

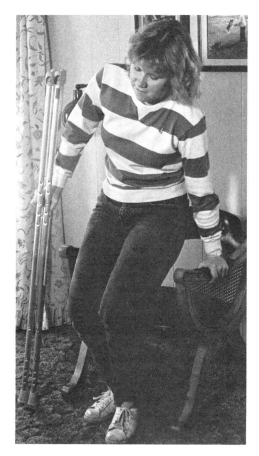

Figure 50.6
Assuming a sitting position with the use of crutches.

ACTION	RATIONALE/AMPLIFICATION
Climbing Stairs	
1. Advance the unaffected leg up to the next step.	If a strong handrail is present, use the handrail for support with the arm on the stronger side, holding both crutches with the hand on the weaker side.
2. Advance the crutches and the weaker leg.	
Descending Stairs	
1. Place feet forward on the step.	
2. Place crutches on the lower step. Advance the weaker leg first, then the stronger one.	The stronger leg shares the work of raising and lowering the body weight with the client's arms. Note: the stronger leg goes up the stairs first and down the stairs last.

Education/ Communication

- Teach the client and family to
  Frequently assess the axilla, palms, and unaffected foot for calluses, redness, and friction blisters, and the arms and hands for tingling and numbness. If these exist, the crutches should be assessed for proper height, the shoes for proper fit, and the use of the crutches in such a manner as to avoid axillary weight-bearing.

Provide assistance with ambulation until the client is fully independent in walking, climbing and descending stairs, and rising and sitting

Encourage independence in all living functions within the limits of safety

Improvise where possible so the former lifestyle is altered as little as possible

Verbalize feelings related to the mobility impairment both to other family members and to the nurse

Achieve any role alterations, necessary employment/school adjustments that may occur during the rehabilitative phase

Referrals and Consultations

- If employment alteration is a permanent or long-term necessity, refer to the state rehabilitation commission for job retraining assistance.
- If the disability is a long-term one and excessive financial strain is placed on the family, consult the department of human resources for possibilities of assistance.
- For some disabilities, support groups exist (multiple sclerosis, quadraplegics, etc.). Knowledge of these can be gained through consultation with a social worker.

Evaluation of Health Promotion Activities

Quality Assurance/ Reassessment

- Observe crutch-walking, rising and sitting, going up and down stairs until the client has mastered the technique.
- Visit the home periodically to assess the achievement of independent mobility and general independence in lifestyle.

DOCUMENTATION

Charting for the Home Health Nurse
Skin condition of feet, axillae, palms of hands, any indication of brachial palsy

Alterations necessary in lifestyle, progress of referrals and consultations

Records Kept by the Client/Family
Any questions or concerns

Skin complications of axillae, palms, feet, tingling of arms and hands

Health Teaching Checklist

Name of Care Provider _____

Relationship to Client _____ Telephone #_____

Taught by _____ Date _____

	EXPLAINED	DEMONSTRATED
Crutch stance	_____	_____
Appropriate gait	_____	_____
Going up and down stairs	_____	_____
Sitting and rising	_____	_____
Assessment for indications of brachial palsy, skin complications	_____	_____
Environmental safety features	_____	

Product Availability

Crutches either of wood or light-weight aluminum can be rented from medical-equipment rental firms or can be purchased from pharmacies or from the hospital where the client was treated. Crutch tips, hand-grip pads, and crutch pads for axillary areas are also available where the crutches were rented or purchased.

Assistive devices for sitting and rising from the toilet and shower safety stools are also available from medical-equipment rental stores.

Selected References

Brunner L, Suddarth D: Lippincott Manual of Nursing Practice, 3rd ed, Philadelphia, JB Lippincott, 1982

Nursing Photobook: Providing Early Mobility, pp 104–109. Springhouse, PA, Springhouse Corporation, 1984

51 Decubitus and Pressure Area Care

Background

A decubitus ulcer, also known as a *pressure sore* or a *bedsore*, is a circumscribed area in which cutaneous tissue has been destroyed. The destruction is caused by a restriction of blood flow to the area from excessive or prolonged pressure. Most common sites of pressure sores are over bony prominences and between folds of flesh in obese clients. Decubitus ulcers are a potential problem of the immobile. Those particularly at risk are the elderly, the obese, the emaciated, and the paralyzed.

The stages of decubitus ulcer formation are the following:

Stage I: reddening of the skin not relieved by massage or by relief of the pressure believed to have caused it

Stage II: superficial tissue damage involving skin breakdown

Stage III: ulceration involving the dermis, which may or may not include the subcutaneous tissue; stage that produces serosanguineous drainage

Stage IV: ulceration into the deep structures with invasion of the deep tissue or structures such as fascia, connective tissue, muscle, or bone

Assessment of Self-Care Potential

Client/Family Assessment

- Assess the understanding of the client and family regarding the cause of decubiti over pressure areas.
- Assess the motivation of the client and family regarding prevention of decubiti. Determine the priority they place on skin care and prevention of skin problems.

Physical Assessment

- Assess the condition of the client's skin. Assess the bony prominences and skin folds for signs of discoloration and tissue breakdown.
- Assess the condition of pressure areas and decubiti that are already present. Note the stage or amount of tissue destruction. Assess the kind of care or treatment the area has received and its apparent effectiveness.
- Assess the general condition of the client. Note nutritional status, ability of the client to eat, incentive for the client to eat, and amount of adipose (fat) tissue on the client. Note the mobility of the client, circulatory status in extremities, urinary and bowel continence, sensory perception in extremities and trunk, and the level of hydration.

Environmental Assessment

- Assess the condition of the client's bed. Determine if the desired number of pillows for adequate positioning is present.
- Assess the proximity of the client's bedroom to the main areas of activity in the home. Determine if the client is far removed from the mainstream of activity, such as upstairs or in an adjoining apartment. This isolation may predispose to longer periods of immobility and lack of adequate repositioning.

Planning Strategies

Potential Nursing Diagnoses

Actual or potential impairment of skin integrity

Alteration in nutrition: less than body requirements

Impaired physical mobility

Knowledge deficit regarding prevention of pressure areas

Expected Outcomes   Prevention or healing of decubitus ulcer

Adequate nutrition and mobility of client

Education of family regarding proper care of the decubitus

Health Promotion Goals
- The client and family will
  - Understand how to prevent decubitus ulcers by proper turning technique and frequent repositioning
  - Learn how to care for the decubitus ulcer to promote healing
  - Understand the importance of proper nutrition to tissue repair and maintenance of skin integrity
  - Learn how to prevent the spread of infection
  - Be able to promote the client's comfort

Equipment   Cleansing solution

Normal saline solution

Heat lamp

Medicated ointment (if prescribed)

Disinfectant solution

Dressing (if necessary)

Irrigation kit (if needed)

Sterile irrigation syringe (50 ml)

Sterile irrigation solution

Sterile basin

Padding for linen

Interventions/Health Promotion

ACTION

1. Wash hands carefully before and after caring for the immobilized client.

2. Turn the immobilized client at least every 2 hours. Each time the client is turned, inspect the skin for signs of pressure areas, which include discoloration (redness or whiteness), lack of sensation, and breaks in the skin. Gently massage bony prominences with lotion (Fig. 51-1). Place the client in a variety of positions, including prone. If a recliner is available, place the client in various positions of reclining to vary the pressure on the skin. The client may be placed in the prone position for variation. Be sure that breathing is not inhibited. Rolled pads may be used to keep body parts in proper align-

RATIONALE/AMPLIFICATION

Handwashing has been shown to remove the majority of pathogenic organisms present on the skin.

Movement and massage will promote the circulation to the area, bringing needed nutrition to the cells and preventing destruction of tissue cells. Each alteration in position causes a shift in the areas receiving pressure. Evenly distributed pressure throughout the body will prevent excess pressure on one area. Padding should be used judiciously. Pillows are the best form of padding.

ACTION	RATIONALE/AMPLIFICATION

ment (Fig. 51-2); however, be sure that the pads themselves do not cause pressure.

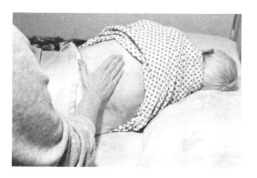

Figure 51.1

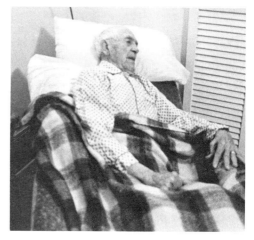

Figure 51.2

3. Cleanse the pressure sore. Agents used in cleansing include hydrogen peroxide and povidone-iodine. These solutions should be rinsed off with saline solution.

Cleansing with an antiseptic helps decrease the number of organisms in the area to prevent colonization in the warm, moist environment.

4. Irrigate the decubitus ulcer if there is a large amount of drainage. Place padding under the ulcer area to catch the irrigation fluid. Open the sterile basin and pour sterile irrigation fluid (usually normal saline) into the basin. Don sterile gloves and draw up the solution into the syringe. Gently irrigate the ulcer, allowing the solution to flow away from the ulcer onto the padding.

Irrigation may help clean the open sore without contaminating it with pathogenic microorganisms.

5. The dry method of treatment includes using heat, such as a heat lamp, to dry the tissue for a period of 20 minutes, with the lamp kept at a distance of 18 to 20 inches (45 cm to 50 cm). The skin must be checked every 5 minutes during treatment. (See Technique 53, Hot and Cold Applications.) The area may then be covered with a bandage or left open to room air. *Never use a sun lamp or infrared lamp for decubitus care.*

A dry, clean environment may decrease the proliferation of microorganisms, thus decreasing the chance of infection. Heat promotes circulation to the area. Infrared lamps and sun lamps focus concentrated heat to an area. The danger of burning the client is too great for these type of lamps to be considered safe. The maximum wattage for a heat lamp is 25 watts for decubitus care.

6. The wet method includes dressings that create a moist environment. After the area is cleaned, a transparent material such as Op-site is placed on the area to seal in the body's normal defensive secretions, such as the leukocytes,

The moist environment is believed to hasten wound healing by acceleration of granulation and epithelialization, which are essential to tissue regeneration.

ACTION	RATIONALE/AMPLIFICATION
plasma, and fibrin. The dressing is left in place until it becomes dislodged; then it is replaced. This type of dressing is transparent so the wound is visible for continuing assessment.	
7. Do not place rubber or plastic next to the client's skin. The more desirable bed coverings are sheepskin, eggcrate mattress, and other coverings designed to decrease pressure and enhance circulation. The use of these devices does not eliminate the need to turn the client regularly or to massage pressure areas.	Rubber and plastic may cause the client to perspire, resulting in a warm, moist environment, which may be conducive to the proliferation of pathogenic microorganisms. Special mattresses are designed to distribute the client's weight evenly and thus reduce localized pressure while promoting comfort.

Related Care

1. Encourage bowel and bladder control if the client is able to cooperate. Offer the bedpan and urinal frequently. Change the linen and clean the client's skin as often as necessary to keep the client dry.	Moisture from incontinence causes maceration of the skin.
2. Encourage the intake of a high-protein diet. Between-meal feedings may help to ensure an adequate intake.	A deficient nutritional status is detrimental to the healing process.

Education/Communication

- Teach the client and family to
  Understand that the desired aspect of treatment of pressure areas and decubitus ulcers is *prevention*. It is much easier to prevent tissue breakdown than it is to treat it. Explain that decubiti are caused by prolonged pressure, which restricts the blood flow to the area, resulting in tissue breakdown. Stress that frequent turning, relief of pressure, and promotion of circulation to the skin over bony prominences are essential to prevention and early detection.
  Turn the client using proper body mechanics and technique. (See Technique 2, Body Mechanics.) Encourage the client to initiate and adhere to a schedule for turning.
  Be able to identify those at risk for the formation of pressure areas and decubitus ulcers. Contributing factors to decubitus ulcer formation are continuous exposure of the skin to moisture, circulatory impairment, a break in the skin, inadequate nutrition, dehydration, inhibited sensory reception, and a lack of natural adipose tissue, which normally pads bony prominences.

Referrals and Consultations

If the tissue breakdown is extensive, surgical intervention may be necessary.

Evaluation of Health Promotion Activities

Quality Assurance/Reassessment

- Observe the family doing decubitus care and assess their technique.
- Teach the family about the turning schedule and the formation of pressure areas. Determine if they understand the role of even distribution of pressure in the prevention of decubiti.

- Inspect the client's skin and decubiti to determine the effectiveness of the prevention or treatment regimen. Keep a progressive record of the condition and suggest alterations as needed.

DOCUMENTATION

Charting for the Home Health Nurse
The home health nurse should keep a record of the appearance, size, and extent of the decubitus ulcer. A record of other pressure areas should be kept, and these areas should be checked on subsequent visits to determine their status.

Records Kept by the Client/Family
The family should have a schedule for turning the client. The form of recording might be writing down the schedule and only making an entry when the schedule cannot be followed, stating the reason. This method will allow them to see if the schedule may need to be altered.

The family may keep a record of the appearance of the pressure area along with measurements to determine if the condition is improving or worsening.

Health Teaching Checklist

Name of Care Provider _____

Relationship to Client _____ Telephone # _____

Taught by _____ Date _____

	EXPLAINED	DEMONSTRATED
Stages of decubitus ulcer formation	_____	
Signs of pressure areas	_____	
Importance of turning the client regularly	_____	
Decubitus care		
Importance of handwashing	_____	
Cleansing of decubitus ulcer	_____	_____
Rinsing of decubitus ulcer	_____	_____
Dressing of decubitus ulcer		
Dry method	_____	_____
Wet method	_____	_____
Selection of a mattress for the bed	_____	
Importance of bowel and bladder control	_____	
Importance of nutrition	_____	
Record keeping regarding turning	_____	_____

Product Availability

Transparent dressings and irrigation kits are available at many pharmacies or drug stores.

Sheepskin and eggcrate mattresses may be purchased through hospital-supply houses.

Selected References

Ahmed M: Op-site for decubitus care. Am J Nurs 82(1):61–64, January, 1982

Byrne N, Feld M: Preventing and treating decubitus ulcers. Nursing '84 14:54–57, April, 1984

Kurzuk-Howare G: Decubitus ulcer care: Moist vs dry healing. Am J Nurs 83(10):1461, October, 1983

52   Hemophiliac Treatment

Background

Modern developments have improved the treatment of hemophilia, so that painful hemorrhages, severe crippling, and the constant threat of death, while still present, are no longer the norm. Hemophiliacs can now lead more useful and less painful lives. Hemophilia is sex-linked and inherited. The antihemophiliac factor (AHF) is an essential intrinsic clotting factor. In the hemophiliac, it is not present at birth nor through the remainder of life. The severity of the condition is determined by the level of AHF present in the circulatory system. The hemophiliac condition ranges from very severe, in which the client may bleed from very minor trauma or spontaneously, to the mild form in which the client bleeds only from operative procedures, dental extractions, or severe trauma.

The AHF can be replaced to control bleeding and achieve and maintain homeostasis successfully. The specific clotting factor is removed from plasma and is available in concentrated form. Although the cost of the factor is prohibitive to many clients, those who receive it can lead relatively normal lives. Most often, therefore, the administration of the AHF concentrate is reserved for severe emergencies.

The genetic pattern of hemophilia is that females are carriers and it is transmitted to the carrier's male offspring. Thus, the sons of hemophiliacs cannot pass the disease on to their children, but the females become carriers. Fifty percent of the carrier's sons will have hemophilia. It is a familial disease although generations may be skipped in the process of transmission.

Assessment of Self-Care Potential

Client/Family Assessment

- Assess the family to determine willingness and ability to perform hemophiliac care in the home.
- Assess the parents (if the client is a child) for feelings of guilt at having transmitted the disease.
- Assess the other male children for the factor.
- Assess the feelings of siblings in relation to feeling neglected in the process of the extensive attention required for the client.
- Assess the family's knowledge of the condition.
- Assess the school/employment place to determine if someone there will learn to perform hemophiliac care.

Physical Assessment

- Assess the client for signs of bruises or bleeding of the gums, in areas where the client has received minor bumps or trauma, or at injection sites.

Environmental Assessment

- Assess the home and school/employment areas used by the client for sharp corners and edges on furniture, doors, walls (toys, if a child).
- Assess the motor vehicle used by the client for potential injurious features. The seatbelt buckle should be padded with foam rubber to prevent unnecessary pressure on the abdomen.
- Assess the shoes and clothing items to determine their safety. They should be snug but not tight; they should not have decorative buttons or buckles with sharp edges.
- Assess the work items used by the client for potential injurious features.

Planning Strategies

Potential Nursing Diagnoses

Physical injury, potential for

Fear related to anticipated serious bleeding

Expected Outcomes

Provision of protection from injuries that could cause bleeding episodes

Compliance with medical regimen and environmental adaptation recommendations

Normal life expectancy with a high quality of life

Development of a sense of independence in the process of dealing with hemophilia

Health Promotion Goals

- The client and family will
  Alter the environment to make it as injury-free as possible
  Demonstrate the procedure of home infusion of AHF concentrate
  Refer the health provider to an appropriate person in the school/workplace who will assist in reducing injury potential, and learn the procedure of infusion of AHF concentrate

Equipment

Padding for corners and sharp edges in the home, school or workplace, motor vehicle

AHF concentrate, alcohol sponges, syringe with filtered needle, double-pointed needle, scalp vein needle, tourniquet, 10 ml of normal saline, 2 × 2 dressing

Interventions/Health Promotion

ACTION	RATIONALE/AMPLIFICATION
Home Infusion of AHF Concentrate	
1. Store vials containing the dehydrated AHF in a cool, dry place in temperature above freezing.	Keep one vial in the home and one in the school/work place in a place easily accessible to the person responsible for administration. Also take a vial on trips or vacations, however short.
2. Reconstitute the AHF: • Cleanse tops of normal saline and concentrate vial with alcohol sponge.	Reconstitute just prior to use. AHF does not remain stable at room temperature. The strength decreases with time following reconstitution.
• Insert one end of the double-pointed needle into the normal saline vial. Hold the normal saline vial upside down and insert the other end of the needle into the concentrate. The vacuum will transfer the normal saline into the concentrate for reconstitution.	Maintaining an inverted position of the vial sustains the vacuum and assists in the subsequent transfer of saline into the concentrate.
• Remove the normal saline vial from the needle. Rotate concentrate in palms of hands until full reconstitution occurs.	Shaking destroys the protein and weakens the activity of the concentrate.

ACTION	*RATIONALE/AMPLIFICATION*
3. Draw the reconstituted solution into the syringe, using a filtered needle.	The filtered needle removes any concentrate particles that may not have dissolved.
4. Draw 10 ml from a second vial of normal saline into a syringe and attach to a scalp vein set-up. Apply a tourniquet and perform a venipuncture. Release the tourniquet and inject 5 ml of normal saline slowly.	Injection of the normal saline prior to the AHF ensures that the needle has entered a vein.
5. Remove the syringe of saline from the scalp vein set-up; attach the syringe containing the AHF and inject it.	The AHF can be injected at any rate.
6. Disconnect the syringe from the scalp vein set-up; reconnect the syringe containing normal saline and inject the remaining 5 ml of normal saline.	Flushing with normal saline ensures that all AHF has been injected.
7. Gently remove the scalp vein needle. Apply a 2 × 2 gauze sponge with gentle pressure for 5 minutes or until bleeding stops. Dispose of needles and syringes safely.	Pressure must not be so harsh as to bruise, yet must be of consistent pressure to stop bleeding.

Related Care

1. Take caution not to prick a finger while preparing the AHF.	AHF is made up of many units of plasma, thus creating a potential for contracting hepatitis with a finger prick.
2. Transport the client immediately to the emergency center if intracranial bleeding or bleeding in the mouth, neck, or mediastinum occurs. Observe while in transport for respiratory distress, and keep the client as calm and quiet as possible.	Compression of the trachea is the major complication.
3. For bleeding in other areas of the body, particularly of a minor nature, initiate local measures to stop bleeding: Pressure for 15 to 20 minutes Immobilization Application of cold measures Application of local anticoagulants	If local measures are unsuccessful in stopping bleeding, initiate infusion of AHF. This can be done by a prepared family member, a teacher, school nurse, or a person in the work environment. These steps, properly performed, give the client increased independence and control over the disease complications.

**Education/
Communication**

• Teach the client and family to
  Make recommended environmental alterations to prevent injury
  Assess all new environments in which the client will be spending much time
    for hazardous elements
  Communicate with school/workplace to initiate environmental protection in
    those areas

Screen new clothing, shoes, and toys to prevent injury

Assess new motor vehicles being bought, as well as the present one being used, for safe seatbelt buckles

Stop bleeding using local measures

Transport client to emergency center when serious bleeding occurs or if bleeding is not responsive to local measures

Administer AHF

  Reconstitute AHF.

  Perform venipuncture.

  Inject AHF.

  Flush with normal saline.

  Stop bleeding.

Encourage client independence within limitations of illness

Referrals and Consultations

Refer the client to the local chapter of the Hemophilia Foundation for information relating to assistance available for hemophiliac clients in the local area: National Hemophilia Foundation, 25 W. 39th Street, New York, New York 10018.

Evaluation of Health Promotion Activities

Quality Assurance/ Reassessment

- To assess the venipuncture technique, obtain a manikin arm and let the client or family member practice the venipuncture. Observe the return demonstration. Periodically bring the manikin arm on home visits and reassess the knowledge of the technique, using the arm.
- Periodically review with the family the method of stopping bleeding using local measures.
- Ascertain if the telephone number of the local emergency center is clearly visible on or near the telephone.
- Visit the school/work place to assess the knowledge of local methods of stopping bleeding and the skill in reconstituting and administering the AHF by the person responsible for administering it.
- Periodically reassess the home/school/work place for safety.

DOCUMENTATION

Charting for the Home Health Nurse
- Note environmental alterations performed in the home/school/work place/car, as well as those needing to be altered.
- Document the names of the persons in the home/school/work place who have been taught to administer the AHF and to provide local measures for stopping bleeding. Document the adequacy of skills related to the techniques and further surveillance or observation needed.
- Note injuries/complications as they occur.

Records Kept by the Client/Family

Incidence and extent of injury/bleeding

Measures taken to stop bleeding

Questions and concerns

**Health Teaching
Checklist**

Name of Care Provider _____

Relationship to Client _____ Telephone #_____

Taught by _____ Date _____

	EXPLAINED	DEMONSTRATED
Need for environmental surveillance and alteration	_____	
Coordination with school/workplace: AHF administration, environmental alterations	_____	
Local methods of stopping bleeding	_____	_____
Administration of AHF	_____	_____
Reporting to emergency center	_____	
Importance of client independence	_____	

Product Availability

AHF is available with a physician's prescription but is extremely expensive. The combination of medical treatment and required AHF administration is financially prohibitive for many families. Therefore, information of available assistance should be sought through the United Hemophilia Association.

Selected References

Brunner L, Suddarth D: Textbook of Medical-Surgical Nursing, 5th ed. Philadelphia, JB Lippincott, 1984

Warren B: Maintaining the hemophiliac at home and school. Nursing '74 4(1):74–76, 1974

53   Hot and Cold Applications

Background

Hot and cold apparatus are applied to the client's body in order to change the tissue temperature, locally or systemically, for a therapeutic purpose. Reactions depend on the mode and duration of application, the degree of heat and cold applied, the condition of the tissue, and the amount of body surface covered by the application. It is vital that therapeutic heat and cold in the home be monitored carefully in order to prevent trauma to the skin.

Therapeutic applications of heat and cold are dependent on proper duration of treatment to achieve desired effects. Prolonged treatment may have the opposite effect than what was intended. Heat should be applied for a short duration, 15 to 30 minutes. The effects of this type of treatment are vasodilation, increased blood flow to the area, increase in local metabolism, healing, and pain relief. Prolonged heat application ($>$1 hr) causes reduction of blood flow to the area with deprivation of nutrients and oxygen to the involved tissue. If the heat is removed for 15 to 30 minutes and reapplied, the vasodilation effect is reestablished. Cold should be applied for 15 to 30 minutes to achieve vasoconstriction, reduction of edema, decrease in local tissue metabolism, an increase in the blood supply available for vital centers, and numbness of the nerve endings, resulting in anesthesia of the tissue. Prolonged application of cold ($>$1 hr) can result in vasodilation, cell dysfunction, and permanent damage to the tissues. People generally become less sensitive to subsequent applications of heat and cold.

The types of hot and cold applications include the following.

Hot Applications

AQUAMATIC PAD

The Aquamatic pad is a rubber pad of tubular construction that can be filled with distilled water. An electrical control unit heats the water and keeps it at an even temperature. The temperature is set by using a plastic key. Another type of pad uses moist heat as a therapeutic aide and contains a heating element and a pad that is located within the unit. The pad may be removed and saturated with water, wrung out, and returned to the unit. The heating unit is applied with the moist side toward the client.

HEAT LAMP

The heat lamp is a gooseneck lamp, containing a 60-watt bulb, and is applied 18 to 24 inches from the body site. The lamp provides therapy by means of dry-heat radiation.

Cold Applications

ICE APPLICATIONS

Ice may be applied in the form of a frozen, flat, rubberized or plastic bag containing a chemical substance that is frozen. It must be covered when applied to the body. Sealable plastic freezer bags may be filled with water and put in the freezer. These bags may be molded over coffee cans or glasses to fit the area to which they will be applied. Ice may also be applied in the form of chips, which are placed in bags, collars, or gloves. These may then be molded to the area to which they will be applied. Any application of ice must be covered with some type of cloth cover before being applied to the body.

COLD SPONGE BATH

A cold sponge bath is a means of reducing body temperature by sponging the skin with cool water. Alcohol used to be added to the water to hasten evaporation; however, this practice is seldom used now because of alcohol's drying effect on the skin.

Applications That May Be Either Hot or Cold

PACKS

Packs are moist applications of heat or cold that may cover extensive body surface areas. Packs may be sterile or nonsterile. The hot pack is sometimes called a *fomentation*. A heating device may be used to keep the pack warm. The cool pack is sometimes moistened in water that has been cooled with some ice chips. Ice packs may be used to keep the temperature of the pack at 75°F. Ice packs may also be placed in the axillae, groin, and head areas in an effort to reduce the body temperature by evaporation.

COMPRESSES

Compresses are hot or cold moist dressings or washcloths that are applied to a smaller body area than packs. Compresses generally require more frequent changing and may be either sterile or nonsterile. Hot compresses hasten the suppurative process and improve circulation. Cold compresses diminish the formation and absorption of bacterial toxins, cause vasoconstriction, decrease tissue metabolism, and cause sensory anesthesia.

SOAKS

A soak is the immersion of a body part, such as a hand or foot, into a cold or hot liquid medium to which medications may be added. Soaks may also refer to wrapping the body part with gauze and saturating it with fluid. This type of soak is usually a sterile procedure.

Assessment of Self-Care Potential

Client/Family Assessment

- Assess the availability of the family when determining the best time for application of heat and cold. If the family will be away from the home, the client should not be left with hot or cold applications in place. Frequent surveillance is necessary.
- Assess the state of coherency of the client. Determine if assistance can be summoned if the application is too hot or too cold or is left on too long.

Physical Assessment

- Assess the client's health history, with particular emphasis on any conditions that might cause impaired circulation or a decrease in skin sensitivity. Determine any mobility limitations afflicting the client that might hinder the client's attempts to remove the hot or cold application. If the client is paralyzed, timing and monitoring will have to be altered to ensure that the client's skin is not traumatized.
- Assess the appearance of the site to which the hot or cold apparatus will be applied. It is essential that a baseline be established so that proper monitoring of the treatment can be done.

Environmental Assessment

- Assess the location of electrical outlets if the unit must be plugged into a socket. If the outlet is not convenient, assess the home for extension cords. Determine if the bed could be moved into a more convenient position or if the client is able to receive the therapy in an alternate location.
- Assess the home for adequate facilities to prepare sterile soaks. Hot and cold running water and heating facilities are usually needed. Assess the general cleanliness of the home in determining if sterile soaks may safely be done in the environment.
- Assess the bed or chair in which the therapeutic agent will be applied. If the application is wet, padding may be necessary to prevent soiling the mattress or cushions.

Planning Strategies

Potential Nursing Diagnoses

Potential impairment of skin integrity

Sensory–perceptual alteration due to temperature fluctuation or systemic alterations

Alteration in comfort: pain

Expected Outcomes

Prevention of untoward side-effects, such as tissue injury

Resolution of the physical problem for which the therapy was ordered

Reduction or elimination of pain

Health Promotion Goals

• The client and family will
  Learn how to perform the hot and cold application safely and efficiently
  Maintain the integrity of the client's skin
  Understand the signs and symptoms that indicate the need for alterations in the treatment
  Be able to assess the effectiveness of the treatment
  Know what factors to report to their primary health-care provider

Equipment

Thermometer

HOT APPLICATIONS

Aquamatic heating pad
  Distilled water
  Key
  Fabric covering
  Thermostatic regulatory unit
Heat lamp
  Gooseneck lamp
  60-watt bulb
Hot pack
  Towels
  Solution (as ordered)
  Basin or sink with hot water
  Bath blanket
  Waterproof covering (such as a large plastic trash bag)
  Dry pack or covering (towels)

COLD APPLICATIONS

Ice treatment
  Frozen bag or collar or plastic glove or plastic bag or ice bag
  Ice chips
  Cover for frozen appliance
  Bath blanket or sheet
Cold sponge bath
  Bath basin
  Bath blanket or sheet
  Cool to tepid water
  Washcloths and towels
  Plastic for lining bed and mattress (if needed)
Cool wet pack
  Bath towels, for moistening
  Basin
  Ice chips
  Towels for dry pack or covering
  Waterproof cover (such as a large plastic trash bag)

APPLICATIONS THAT MAY BE EITHER HOT OR COLD

Compresses (hot or cold), sterile
 Solution, sterile
 Sterile gauze squares or sterile washcloths
 Sterile basin
 Sterile forceps
 Sterile gloves
 Sterile towels for covering gauze
Compresses (hot or cold), clean
 Solution
 Gauze squares or washcloths
 Clean towel for insulation
 Clean gloves for application (if needed)
Soaks (hot or cold)
 Solution as ordered
 Basin and towels

Interventions/Health Promotion

ACTION	*RATIONALE/AMPLIFICATION*
1. Wash hands before doing any treatments for the client.	Handwashing has proven to be the single most effective means of controlling the spread of infection.
2. Measure the client's temperature before beginning a treatment that may alter systemic or local temperature.	A baseline is needed to determine if the results of the treatment are therapeutic or pathogenic.
3. Gather all of the needed equipment at the bedside or in the bathroom before beginning the procedure. Assist the client to assume a position of comfort before beginning the procedure. Provide some type of diversion, if appropriate. If the treatment will be done on a dependent limb, provide some means of support for comfort.	Unnecessary delays can alter the temperature of the application. If the client will be immobilized for a period of time, be sure that interruptions are minimized. Turn on the TV or provide a book for the client, if desired. Place the telephone in a convenient place and take measures to ensure that the doorbell does not disturb the client. The ideal arrangement is to have someone in attendance.

Aquamatic Pad

1. Fill the reservoir of the heating unit two-thirds full with distilled water (Fig. 53-1, A). Allow the water to enter and fill the pad by tilting the pad end to end (Fig. 53-1, B).	Distilled water is used to reduce the buildup of mineral deposits in the mechanical parts of the unit. By tilting the unit, it is possible to disperse the water evenly while eliminating air bubbles that may interfere with even heat conduction.

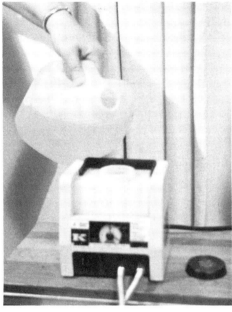

A　　　　　　　　　　　　　　**B**

Figure 53.1

ACTION	*RATIONALE/AMPLIFICATION*
2. Cover the pad with a cloth cover. Place it on the client at the desired location. Watch carefully for the appearance of erythema or undesirable side-effects.	The cover should be thick enough to prevent burning of the client. Local skin reaction is the body's way of warning that tissue damage may be imminent. The heating source must be removed at the first signs of local discoloration before irreparable tissue damage is done.
Heat Lamp	
1. Check the client's skin to be sure that it is dry, clean, and free of exudate.	Liquids conduct heat, so dry skin is less likely to be burned. Exudate may interfere with the treatment and may be a source of burns or discomfort.
2. Place the lamp at a level of 18 to 24 inches away from the treatment area. Place the lamp at an angle rather than directly over the area of skin to be treated (Fig. 53-2). Be certain that the bulb is no greater than 60 watt.	The light should be to the side of the client to prevent it from accidentally falling onto the treatment area. A 60-watt bulb produces enough heat to treat the area without the chance of burning the skin, which would be a greater possibility with a stronger bulb. Never place the lamp under the bed linen or allow it to come in contact with bed linens or the client's clothing because this could cause a fire.

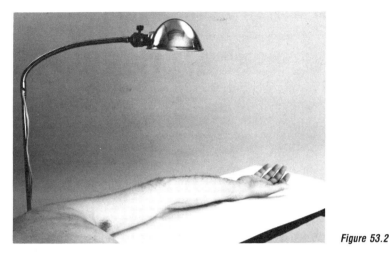

Figure 53.2

ACTION	**RATIONALE/AMPLIFICATION**
3. Check the client frequently during the treatment (q 5 min). The recommended duration of the treatment is 15 to 20 minutes.	Some clients are more sensitive to heat than others. If the skin becomes reddened, the treatment should be discontinued. Check to see that the bulb does not get any closer than 18 inches to the skin.

Ice Applications

1. Remove the frozen application from the freezer or place the ice chips in the container that will best meet the desired outcomes of therapy. Cover the frozen application with a soft cloth cover (Figs. 53-3 and 53-4).	If the area to be treated is very small or irregularly shaped, a plastic glove filled with ice chips is light-weight and can be molded to the area. A small, sealable sandwich bag may be used with success as well. If the area is large and flat, such as along the length of a cast, a long, flat freezer bag may be used. A larger, sealable plastic bag may be filled with water, placed on a cookie sheet, and placed in the freezer and frozen to produce a long, flat surface.

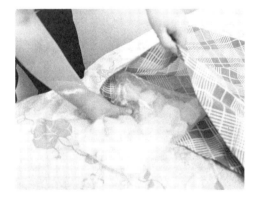

Figure 53.3

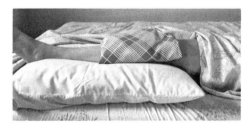

Figure 53.4

2. Check the frozen application frequently during the treatment period (q 5 min) to ensure that skin damage is not occurring. Maximum benefit is usually gained when the application is left in place for 15 to 20 minutes.	Cold produces vasoconstriction and reduces tissue metabolism. Prolonged use of cold may cause tissue damage. Cold has an anesthetic effect on the skin. This effect may inhibit the body's normal defense mechanisms, such as pain, that alert one when damage is taking place.

ACTION	RATIONALE/AMPLIFICATION

Cold Sponge Bath

1. Prepare the bath for the client just as for a bed bath except that cool water should be used (see Technique 27, Baths, Cleansing). Place padding on the bed and a bath blanket over the client.

The client's clothing is removed. The water may be cool tap water or cold water to which ice chips have been added. Chilling of the client is undesirable and is likely due to the presence of the ice packs and the cold water. The blanket over the client will help prevent chilling.

2. Sponge portions of the client's body with the cool water. While one part of the body is being sponged, keep the remainder of the body covered. Sponge by immersing the washcloth, wringing it out, wrapping it around the hand, and rubbing the client's body with long, gentle strokes. The face, trunk, and thighs are usually the primary areas that are sponged.

The goal of the cool sponge bath is to lower the client's body temperature by evaporation through large skin surfaces.

3. Apply ice packs to the groin, axillae, and head areas during the procedure to encourage reduction of body temperature.

Ice packs in strategic areas will help facilitate temperature reduction.

4. Measure the client's temperature every 5 to 7 minutes to assess the effectiveness of the procedure. The procedure should be stopped after 15 to 20 minutes. It may be reinstituted after a 15-minute break or as prescribed.

The major benefits of the treatment will be gained during the initial 15 minutes.

5. After the sponge bath, dry the client's skin gently and assist with the replacement of light clothing, such as light-weight pajamas or a gown. Light covers should be left on the client.

Due to the evaporation from the client's skin, a general feeling of being cold may be present. However, donning large amounts of heavy clothing or using heavy blankets will only cause an elevation in the client's temperature.

Moist Packs or Compresses

1. Wash hands before preparing the pack or compress. If the procedure is sterile, prepare an area on which to place the sterile equipment for application.

If there is danger that the treatment area may rupture or if the area contains open sores, sterile treatments may be prescribed to prevent contamination.

2. Test the solution to see that it is the prescribed temperature by pouring a small amount over the wrist. If hot solution is ordered, place the bottle of sterile solution in the sink and run hot water over it for several minutes. The solution may also be placed in a microwave oven to be warmed if there is no

The solution should be very warm when poured over the inner aspect of the forearm and wrist. This area is very sensitive, so if the solution feels warm here, it will be warm to the sensitive treatment area. Great care must be taken not to heat the solution excessively in order to avoid burning the client or the care provider. Leave

ACTION

RATIONALE/AMPLIFICATION

metal on the container or seal. The solution should not be heated excessively and should never boil. Cold solutions may be kept in the refrigerator with the sterile seal intact or may be placed in a basin of ice for about 30 minutes prior to the treatment.

the solution sealed until ready to test and use. To test, pour a small amount onto the wrist without touching the lip of the sterile container to the skin in order to preserve the sterility of the contents. The test solution is discarded because it is no longer sterile.

3. For the nonsterile soak, immerse the towel or gauze pad in the solution in a basin, wring it out, and wrap it around the site, molding it to the skin. Cover the site with a dry pack (towel) and a piece of plastic, such as a trash can liner or a laundry bag (Fig. 53-5). Secure the plastic with masking tape or tie gauze around it (Fig. 53-6). Leave in place 15 to 30 minutes.

The pack is molded to the skin because air is a poor conductor of heat and would diminish the desired effects of even distribution of heat. Securing the liner will help prevent soiling the linen.

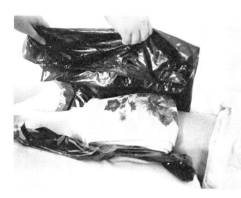

Figure 53.5

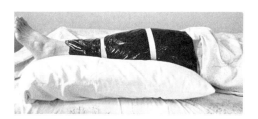

Figure 53.6

4. For the sterile soak, open the package containing the sterile basin and the sterile compress material (towels or gauze pads) without contaminating the contents. These may be opened onto a sterile towel. Pour the solution into the sterile basin. Don sterile gloves. Immerse the towel or gauze pad in the solution, wring it out, and wrap it around the site with the dominant hand. If additional compresses are needed, prepare them with the other hand, which is still sterile if it has not touched the client or any nonsterile surface.

The object of the sterile soak is to keep the sterile area from coming in contact with anything that is not sterile. Provide a sterile field, the towel, and open the sterile equipment onto it. After handling all of the nonsterile articles, the gloves may be donned and only sterile objects touched thereafter. If any nonsterile object is touched by the glove, it is no longer sterile and should not be reintroduced into the sterile field.

5. Place a conductive heating source, such as an aquamatic pad, over or next to the involved limb to maintain heat.

The moisture in the towel distributes heat around the limb. The heat source is *never* placed under the limb because this could cause excessive heat buildup, leading to burns.

ACTION	RATIONALE/AMPLIFICATION

Soaks

1. Fill a tub or basin with the desired soaking solution. (For the sitz or emollient bath, see Technique 28, Baths, Therapeutic.) Assist the client into a position of comfort for soaking the body part indicated.

Soaking of body parts may be done in a sink or a basin. If the client will be in a chair during the soak, place a water-resistant material under the basin to protect the rug or floor. Be sure that all dependent body parts are supported during the soak.

2. If the client cannot get out of bed, a soak may be done by saturation of a gauze bandage over the treatment area. Pad the bed and wrap gauze or towels around the area to be soaked. If the soak is sterile, use sterile towels and sterile technique to wrap the area. Pour the prescribed soaking solution onto the bandage until it is saturated. Keep a cover on the client to prevent chilling. After the soak, remove the saturated dressing and replace it with a dry one, if needed.

Padding the bed with plastic will prevent soaking the linens and the mattress. The object of the treatment is to soak a localized area.

Age-Specific Modifications

Great care must be exercised when applying heat and cold to the very young and the very old. Monitoring of the treatment area must be done at least every 5 minutes to ensure that trauma to the skin is prevented.

Clients who are particularly at risk during hot and cold treatments are those at the extremes of age and those with delicate or sensitive skin. Also, those persons with impaired circulation, those who are dependent on others for their physical care and protection, and those with paralysis are particularly susceptible to problems when being treated with hot and cold applications.

**Education/
Communication**

• Teach the client and family to

Perform the hot or cold application in the proper manner. Emphasize the difference between sterile and nonsterile applications. Be sure that the client and family understand why the therapy was ordered and the desired outcome.

Understand safety precautions involved in hot and cold applications. It is essential that safety precautions be emphasized because of the great potential for tissue injury involved in applying external heat and cold to the body. Emphasize that the maximum duration of any treatment should be 15 to 20 minutes. Stress the importance of checking the treatment area frequently during the treatment. Be sure that the family understands what signs and symptoms are indicative of tissue damage.

Perform sterile applications using proper sterile technique. Even if the applications are not sterile, they should understand what is clean and what is contaminated in order to prevent cross-contamination of themselves or others.

Keep the applications at the prescribed temperature for as long as possible. Ice packs must be replaced when the ice melts. Warm soaks for extremities may be kept warm by using an insulated styrofoam chest for the soak if it is not sterile. Compresses and packs may be kept warm by the application of an external heat source or cold by the application of an external source of cold, such as ice packs.

Referrals and Consultations

If the client and family cannot grasp the principles of sterile technique, a visiting nurse may be consulted to perform the sterile applications.

Evaluation of Health Promotion Activities

Quality Assurance/ Reassessment

- Observe the client and family performing the technique for the prescribed hot or cold application. Observe technique and adherence to safety precautions. If the technique is not adequate, demonstrate proper methods and answer questions.
- Inspect the client's skin in the treatment area for any signs of skin trauma that might indicate that the treatment is not being done properly.
- Reassess the treatment site periodically to determine the effectiveness of the treatment. Assess whether or not the client's condition is improving.

DOCUMENTATION

Charting for the Home Health Nurse
A progressive record of the appearance of the site and any problems stated by the client should be kept in order to assess the progress of the therapy.

Records Kept by the Client/Family
The family should keep a record of the duration and frequency of the hot or cold treatments. They may also make brief notes about the appearance of the site and any questions they might wish to ask the home health nurse during visits. This can be done in a small spiral notebook at the client's bedside.

Health Teaching Checklist

Name of Care Provider _____

Relationship to Client _____ Telephone #_____

Taught by _____ Date _____

	EXPLAINED	DEMONSTRATED
Importance of handwashing	_____	
Temperature measurement of client	_____	_____
Procedure for hot or cold application	_____	_____
Appearance of site	_____	
Possible side-effects		
Skin trauma	_____	
Pain	_____	
Anesthesia	_____	
Burns	_____	
Aquamatic pad		
Protective covering on pad	_____	_____
Control set on proper setting	_____	_____
Key to control kept in unit or at client's bedside	_____	_____
Pad placed in optimal position	_____	_____

Heat lamp

  Preparation of site   _____   _____

  60-watt bulb used   _____   _____

  Lamp 18 to 24 inches away from client   _____   _____

  Importance of checking client q 5 min   _____   _____

  Lamp left on client the prescribed time   _____   _____

  Safety precautions taken to see that the client or clothing do not come in contact with the bulb   _____   _____

Ice applications

  Preparation of ice appliance   _____   _____

  Cover for ice appliance   _____   _____

  Method of applying ice to the body   _____   _____

  Duration of treatment   _____

  Importance of checking client q 5 min   _____

Cool sponge bath

  Method of sponging the client   _____   _____

  Method of preventing chilling   _____   _____

  Ice packs applied to axillae, groin, and head areas   _____   _____

  Duration of sponge bath   _____   _____

  Desired outcome of sponge bath   _____

  Need for frequent temperature measurement   _____

Packs and compresses

  Sterile technique   _____   _____

  Sterile supplies, gloves, and equipment   _____   _____

  Correct size of compress or pack used   _____   _____

  Excess moisture squeezed from compress before application   _____   _____

  Client positioned in proper alignment with dependent parts supported   _____   _____

Body soaks

  Sterile technique   _____   _____

  Sterile equipment   _____   _____

  Affected part immersed slowly   _____   _____

  Dependent parts supported   _____   _____

  Client placed in a comfortable position   _____   _____

Product Availability

Aquamatic-K-Pad is available through hospital-supply houses. Instant ice packs are available at most pharmacies and drugstores.

54   Insulin Injection

Background

Since the major cause of diabetes is thought to be the lack of or inadequate use of insulin, diabetic therapy often includes the use of insulin in addition to dietary and exercise controls. If the diabetic has little or no insulin production capability in the pancreas, insulin is administered. Since insulin is a protein and is broken down in the stomach by gastrointestinal juices, it must be injected. The most common method is by the subcutaneous route. Whichever method of insulin administration is used, the client/family will be primarily responsible for performing the procedure on a daily basis. Emphasis must be placed on support and education of the client/family in insulin therapy.

Assessment of Self-Care Potential

Client/Family Assessment

- Assess the willingness and ability of the family to support the client in the treatment regimen required.
- Assess the family's financial situation to determine if purchasing of supplies and medications is feasible.

Physical Assessment

- Assess the client (and any assisting family member) for adequate fine motor coordination to manipulate the insulin injection equipment.
- Assess the visual acuity of the client (and any assisting family member) to determine if the markings on the insulin syringe can be read.
- Assess the body areas to be used for insulin injection to determine the presence of infections, inflammation, edema, tissue atrophy, or any other condition that could prohibit injections. Based on the assessment, develop a body log to indicate acceptable sites and rotations for injections.

Environmental Assessment

- Determine if the home contains a working refrigerator for storage of insulin.
- Assess the home to determine a space where the injections can be given without interruption. The area should have good lighting and should be clean. It should have provisions for safe storage of supplies needed during insulin administration. If the client has poor visual acuity, a magnifying glass can be used to provide necessary enlargement of markings on the syringes.

Planning Strategies

Potential Nursing Diagnoses

Skin integrity, impairment of

Knowledge deficit

Anticipatory anxiety

Expected Outcomes

Maintenance of skin integrity

Achievement of diabetic control through understanding of correct insulin administration

Reduction of anxiety related to self-injection

Health Promotion Goals

- The client and family will
  Adhere to aseptic technique in the process of insulin injections

Give the correct dosage of insulin at the prescribed times
Rotate sites according to the schedule developed
Correctly document the insulin administration
List and observe for complications arising from insulin injections and notify the nurse/physician of their occurrence

Equipment

Vials of prescribed insulin (Table 54-1)

Table 54-1. **SOME COMMERCIAL INSULIN PREPARATIONS**

MANUFACTURER	PRODUCT	AVAILABLE CONCEN-TRATION	SOURCE	ONSET (APPROX-IMATE)	PEAK (APPROX-IMATE)	DURATION (APPROX-IMATE)
Lilly	Regular	U-40 U-100	Beef* Pork* Beef-pork	15 min–1hr	2–4 hr	5–7 hr
Squibb	Regular	U-40 U-100	Pork	15 min–1 hr	2–4 hr	5–7 hr
	Regular	U-100	Pork†	15 min–1 hr	2–4 hr	5–7 hr
Nordisk	Velosulin	U-100	Pork†	15 min–1 hr	2–4 hr	5–7 hr
Novo	Actrapid	U-100	Pork†	30 min–1 hr	2½–5 hr	8 hr
Lilly	Semilente	U-40 U-100	Beef-pork	1–3 hr	2–8 hr	12–16 hr
Squibb	Semilente	U-100	Beef	1–3 hr	2–8 hr	12–16 hr
Novo	Semitard	U-100	Pork†	1½ hr	5–10 hr	16 hr
Novo	Protophane NPH	U-100	Pork†	1–1½ hr	4–12 hr	24 hr
Lilly	NPH	U-40 U-100	Beef* Pork* Beef-pork	1–3 hr	6–12 hr	24–28 hr
Squibb	NPH	U-40 U-100	Beef	1–3 hr	6–12 hr	24–28 hr
	NPH	U-100	Beef*	1–3 hr	6–12 hr	24–28 hr
Novo	Monotard	U-100	Pork†	2½ hr	7–15 hr	22 hr
Nordisk	Insulatard	U-100	Pork†	2–4 hr	4–12 hr	24–28 hr
Lilly	Lente	U-40 U-100	Beef* Pork* Beef-pork	1–3 hr	6–12 hr	24–28 hr
Squibb	Lente	U-40 U-100	Beef	1–3 hr	6–12 hr	24–28 hr
	Lente	U-100	Beef†	1–3 hr	6–12 hr	24–28 hr
Novo	Lentard	U-100	Beef-pork†	2½ hr	7–15 hr	24 hr
Lilly	PZI	U-40 U-100	Beef* Pork* Beef-pork	4–6 hr	14–24 hr	36+ hr
Squibb	PZI	U-100	Beef	4–6 hr	14–24 hr	36+ hr
Lilly	Ultralente	U-40 U-100	Beef-pork	4–6 hr	18–24 hr	36+ hr
Squibb	Ultralente	U-100	Beef	4–6 hr	18–24 hr	36+ hr
Novo	Ultratard	U-100	Beef†	4 hr	10–30 hr	36 hr
Nordisk	Mixtard (premixed) Regular—30% NPH—70%	U-100	Pork†	Like Regular and NPH when mixed		

* Iletin II (either purified pork or purified beef) available only in U-100
† Purified
N.B. Squibb and Novo recently merged to form Squibb Novo, Inc. The insulins Squibb and Novo have marketed will remain unchanged, but they will be packaged under this new company name.
(Published in *RN,* the full-service nursing journal. Copyright © 1982, Medical Economics Company Inc., Oradell, NJ. Reprinted by permission)

Alcohol swabs

Disposable insulin syringes with needles attached

Body log to guide injection-site rotation (obtained from American Diabetic Association)

Mechanism for safe disposal of syringes

A wall poster (obtained from the American Diabetic Association) detailing the steps of the injection procedure

Interventions/Health Promotion

ACTION	*RATIONALE/AMPLIFICATION*
1. Wash hands thoroughly.	Handwashing is an essential factor in preventing contamination.
2. Assemble equipment.	Having all equipment assembled prevents interruption of procedure with subsequent interruption of thought process and danger of break in technique.
3. Rotate insulin vial(s) in palms of hands.	Shaking insulin creates foaming; rotation mixes without foaming.
4. Cleanse the rubber top of the vials with an alcohol swab.	Cleansing is thought to remove some microorganisms from the top of the vial.
5. Pick up syringe, remove cap from the needle, and withdraw plunger to the approximate dosage prescribed. With vial standing upright, insert needle into top of vial, injecting the air from the syringe into the vial.	Caution must be used not to touch the needle or to let it touch anything else. Such contamination requires disposal of that syringe and the use of a new one.
6. With the needle remaining in the vial, turn the vial and syringe upside down and withdraw the required amount of insulin into the syringe by pulling the plunger 5 units past the dose. Then push the plunger back to the exact dose measurement.	Pulling the plunger beyond the required dosage and then pushing it back to the exact measurement removes any air bubbles that may be present. If any air bubbles remain, a flick of the finger on the syringe, with the syringe held needle up, will remove them.
7. Remove the syringe from the bottle and carefully replace the cap on the needle.	Replacing the cap will protect the needle from contamination until the injection site is prepared.
8. Select the injection site according to the log prepared (Fig. 54-1). Cleanse the site with an alcohol sponge in a circular motion, moving from the center outward (Fig. 54-2). Allow the alcohol to dry.	Cleansing the skin is thought to remove some microorganisms, thus assisting in the prevention of infection.

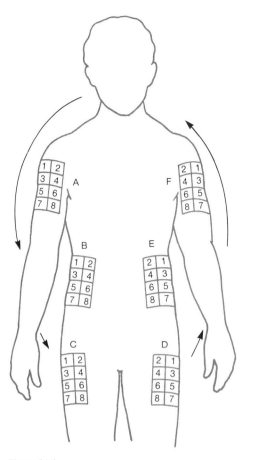

Figure 54.1
An example of a body log to guide injection site rotation. The client proceeds in a systematic fashion, counterclockwise, using all of the blocks marked 1, then all of those marked 2, and so forth. This ensures that the same site will not be used for injection too frequently. The log can be photocopied and the client can be instructed to "black out" the blocks as they are used.

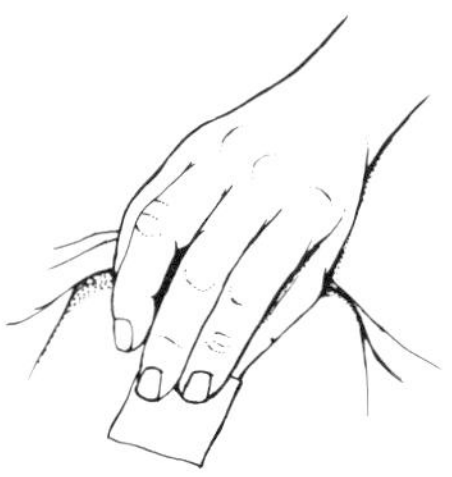

Figure 54.2
Cleansing the area of the selected site.

ACTION

9. Carefully remove the cap from the needle. Hold the syringe in the dominant hand. With the nondominant hand, pinch up a 2-inch fold of tissue.

10. With a smooth, quick motion, inject the needle into the subcutaneous tissue at an angle between 45 and 90 degrees (Fig. 54-3).

RATIONALE/AMPLIFICATION

Pinching separates the subcutaneous tissue from the underlying musculature. Pressure on the tissue also numbs the nerve endings, thus reducing pain.

Smooth, quick motions reduce discomfort.

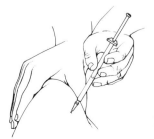

Figure 54.3
Inserting the needle at a 45-degree to 90-degree angle.

ACTION

11. Release the tissue. Pull back on the plunger to determine if the needle has entered a blood vessel (Fig. 54-4). If there is no blood return, inject the insulin (Fig. 54-5). If blood does return, do not inject the insulin. Withdraw the needle, select another site, and use a new syringe and needle for injection.

RATIONALE/AMPLIFICATION

Medications injected into the blood vessels are absorbed immediately. Insulin for diabetes control is intended to be absorbed during the longer period of time that occurs with the subcutaneous route.

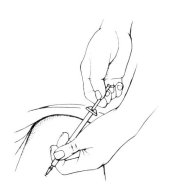

Figure 54.4
Withdrawing the plunger to determine whether the needle has entered a blood vessel. If blood returns, the needle has entered a blood vessel. Withdraw the needle and replace it with a new one. Using the new needle, begin the injection procedure again.

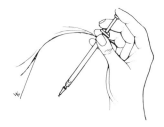

Figure 54.5
Injecting the insulin.

12. Replace the cap on the needle. Bend and break the needle. Dispose of the needle and syringe in a safe manner.

These measures are intended to prevent injury from the needle as well as misuse of the syringe and needle.

Filling the Syringe With a Combination of Long- and Short-Acting Insulin

1. Cleanse the vial tops with an alcohol sponge.

2. Inject air into long-acting insulin and withdraw the needle.

This creates a positive pressure for ease of withdrawing the solution later.

3. Inject air into the short-acting insulin and withdraw the prescribed number of units.

4. Insert the needle into the long-acting insulin vial and withdraw the prescribed number of units of insulin.

Related Care

1. Prepare a travel kit for all trips no matter how short.

The kit should contain all supplies needed for insulin injection. A small ice chest or insulated package with a chemical freeze pack can be used to keep the insulin cold.

ACTION	RATIONALE/AMPLIFICATION
2. Obtain and wear a Medic-Alert identification.	In the event of complications, the identification will alert others to take appropriate action.
3. Prepare a body log indicating the system to be used in rotating injection sites.	This poster can also be used as a method for recording injections. It should be posted in the area of the home being used to prepare injections.
4. Advise the client to carry hard candy at all times.	This is a precaution against hypoglycemic reactions following insulin injection.
5. Rotate sites on a systematic basis.	Rotation prevents lipodystrophy.

Education/ Communication

• Teach the client and family to
Select rotation sites according to a preset system
Keep the insulin properly refrigerated
Perform the injection appropriately and with aseptic technique
Assess injection sites for inflammation or other contraindications to their use
Observe for diabetic complications

Referrals and Consultations

• Consult the American Diabetic Association for assistance and information related to diabetes.
• Refer to a social worker if the client/family is unable to afford needed supplies.

Evaluation of Health Promotion Activities

Quality Assurance/ Reassessment

• Following the return demonstration of insulin injection, periodically visit the home at the time of injection to answer further questions and give surveillance.
• Reassess the injection sites for complications that might prohibit further use of the site.
• Assess the client for adherence to recommended exercise and dietary requirements and for diabetic complications.

DOCUMENTATION

Charting for the Home Health Nurse
• Note the condition of the injection sites.
• Document any verbalized concerns or anxieties.
• Note adherence to prescribed insulin regimen

Records Kept by the Client/Family
Sites of injection

Amount of insulin injected

Questions and concerns

Health Teaching Checklist

Name of Care Provider _____

Relationship to Client _____ Telephone #_____

Taught by _____ Date _____

	EXPLAINED	DEMONSTRATED
Handwashing prior to injection	_____	_____
Aseptic technique	_____	_____
Insulin withdrawal: proper dosage	_____	_____

	EXPLAINED	DEMONSTRATED
Insulin injection	_____	_____
Refrigeration of insulin	_____	
Rotation of injection sites	_____	

Product Availability

Insulin, syringes, alcohol sponges are available with prescription from any pharmacy. Medic-Alert bracelets are available through a pharmacy or through the American Diabetic Association. A travel kit can be improvised by the use of a shaving kit, a purse, or any other closing container. A body log for site rotation can be obtained from the American Diabetic Association or hand made. Free injection rotation guides are available from either Monoject, 1831 Olive Street, St. Louis, Missouri 63103, or Becton-Dixon Consumer Products, PO Box 500, Rochelle Park, New Jersey 07662.

Selected References

Up-to-date information is available from the American Diabetic Association, local affiliate.

55   Insulin Pumps

Background

The insulin pump is a small electromagnetic device that controls blood glucose levels by automatically infusing insulin in programmable doses at set intervals while permitting the client to manually infuse larger insulin dosages as needed, usually before mealtime. The insulin pump is not the treatment of choice for all diabetics. Usually the decision to use the insulin pump is based on highly structured criteria as well as counseling sessions and a determination of the client's history of adherence to prescribed insulin regimens. If the client is selected to use the insulin pump, careful attention to client and family education is required.

Assessment of Self-Care Potential

Client/Family Assessment

- Assess family motivation to assist the client in the successful use of the pump.
- Determine the client/family attitude toward diabetes and diabetes control.
- Assess client/family knowledge of the pathophysiological process of diabetes and diabetes control.
- Assess the visual acuity and fine motor coordination of the client and the family members who will be assisting in the operation of the pump. These should be adequate to administer glucagon in the event of an emergency as well as to operate the pump.

Physical Assessment

- Assess the site to be used for needle insertion for signs of irritation, inflammation, and infection.
- Assess the client's measured glucose levels periodically (client will also maintain close checks on these) to determine if a pattern of acceptable (above 60 mg) glucose levels is being maintained.
- Assess the client for symptoms of hypoglycemia:
  Sympathetic response caused by rapid drop in the blood glucose level: sweating, rapid heart rate, hunger
  Central nervous system response: confusion and loss of consciousness

Environmental Assessment

- Determine if there is a clean place in the home where the insulin can be added to the pump conveniently and without interruption.
- Determine a place in the home where the blood glucose level can be measured and recorded and where the supplies needed for the blood glucose level test prescribed can be stored.

Planning Strategies

Potential Nursing Diagnoses

Knowledge deficit: insulin pump, diabetes

Infection, potential for

Expected Outcomes

Maintenance of blood sugar balance by the use of the insulin pump

Prevention of infection

Health Promotion Goals

- The client and family will
  Maintain the insertion sites free of irritation, inflammation, and infection
  Maintain a pattern of blood glucose levels within 80 mg to 140 mg
  Wear the pump at all times except when playing contact sports, swimming, bathing, and, if desired, during sexual activity
  Change batteries as needed and maintain charged batteries
  Demonstrate the ability to fill the syringe with the prescribed amount and type of insulin
  Correctly insert the needle and secure it in place

Equipment

Recommended pump with charged batteries (Figs. 55-1 and 55-2)

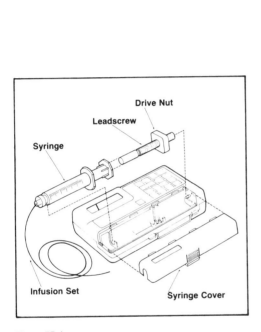

Figure 55.1
Illustration of insulin infusion pump. (Courtesy of Cardiac Pacemakers, Inc., St. Paul, Minnesota)

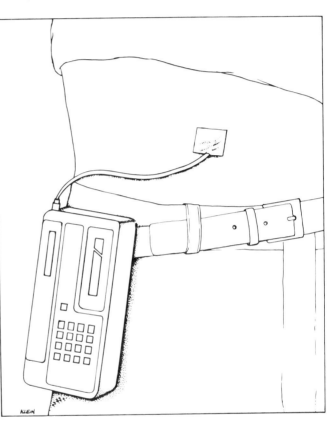

Figure 55.2
Insulin pump in place.

Prescribed type and amount of insulin

A syringe that fits the pump, fitted with a butterfly needle and polyurethane tubing (size 25 needle)

Dressing (1.5″ × 2″) of polyurethane or other see-through material to facilitate frequent monitoring of skin condition at the needle insertion site

Soap and water

Alcohol sponge or povidone-iodine sponge

Prescribed supplies for measuring blood glucose levels

Chart to document patterns of blood glucose determinations

Interventions/Health Promotion

ACTION	RATIONALE/AMPLIFICATION
1. Develop a familiarity with the pump.	Most pumps are equipped with alarm systems to warn of various problems such as run-down batteries, blocked needle or tubing, or uncontrollable delivery of insulin.
2. Develop a regular schedule of caring for the pump, to include charging and changing the batteries according to the manufacturer's specifications, and changing the syringe, tubing needle, and insertion site.	Developing a routine will set up a habit to assist in meticulous compliance with care recommendations. Frequent changing of the syringe, tubing, and insertion site is necessary to prevent skin breakdown and abscessing.
3. Fill the syringe each day with the prescribed amount of insulin to last one day.	The procedure for placing the syringe into the pump is dependent on the manufacturer's directions.

Changing the Needle, Tubing, and Insertion Site (Every 2 Days)

1. Prepare the site with soap and water, followed by applying povidone-iodine or alcohol.	The abdominal area is the site of choice because it has the best insulin-absorption capability. However, other subcutaneous sites can also be used, such as the back, hips, and arms.
2. Apply a skin barrier to the insertion site.	The skin barrier is similar to that used for ostomy clients to protect the skin from irritation caused by tape (Karaya products, for example).
3. Insert the needle at a 30- to 60-degree angle. Tape it in place by means of a see-through polyurethane patch. Adhere the tube with hypoallergenic tape or polyurethane.	Applying the polyurethane allows frequent visualization of the insertion site to observe for irritation, abscesses, or irritation from sensitivity to the needle.

Operation of the Pump

1. Wear the pump on the belt or in a pocket.	Sizes and weights vary. Many different pumps are on the market.
2. Attach a syringe with the prescribed amount of insulin (usually rapid-acting) daily.	Early models required insulin to be diluted with saline. Later models use undiluted insulin.
3. Inject a bolus of insulin prior to meals.	The increased injection provides greater flexibility of food ingestion at mealtime.

Related Care

1. Monitor the blood glucose closely to determine patterns of blood glucose levels.	Initially the blood glucose must be checked several times daily (1 to 2 hours before and after each meal) and once during the night. The monitoring will be done less frequently when patterns are well established.

ACTION	RATIONALE/AMPLIFICATION
2. Test the urine for ketone bodies if the blood sugar rises above 200 mg.	If ketone bodies are present, more insulin is administered and fluids taken. The blood glucose is tested every 1½ hours until it returns to normal and the urine is free of ketones.
3. Closely adhere to dietary and exercise prescriptions.	These affect the balance of glucose level.
4. Support the client/family in their adjustment to the pump.	Psychological adjustment is necessary for the successful use of the pump. Common complications are depression, boredom with the ongoing procedures, and frustration.

Age-Specific Modifications

The insulin pump is usually not prescribed for pediatric clients.

Education/ Communication

- Teach the client and family to
  - Care for the pump. This includes recharging and changing batteries as needed, filling and changing the syringe containing the insulin every day, and changing the tubing and needle every 2 days.
  - Insert the needle. This includes site selection, cleansing of the site, application of skin barrier, and application of a see-through bandage.
  - Program the appropriate level of insulin for continuous injection and injection of insulin bolus before meals
  - Understand alarm systems, take appropriate action, and turn off alarm
  - Perform blood glucose level testing and recording. In addition, the client and family should be taught to report blood glucose levels of over 200 mg and to maintain blood glucose between 80 mg and 120 mg.
  - Become involved in diabetes self-help group if available locally
  - Notify the physician or nurse if there are symptoms of hypoglycemia, resulting from increased activity or delayed food. These symptoms may change from those of a sympathetic nervous response (sweating, rapid heart rate, and hunger) to a central nervous system response (confusion and loss of consciousness).

Referrals and Consultations

- Refer to the American Diabetic Association, local affiliate, for continuous update on research and development of new equipment.
- Refer to a local diabetes self-help group, if available.
- Consult a social worker if the client is unable to finance the pump with existing insurance or Medicare.
- Consult a dietitian for difficulties with diet.

Evaluation of Health Promotion Activities

Quality Assurance/ Reassessment

- At every visit, assess the client's glucose level patterns.
- Inspect the needle insertion site to determine if it is free of irritation and/or infection.
- Assess the family's return to a normal lifestyle.
- Assess the family/client's progress in psychological adjustment to the pump.

DOCUMENTATION

Charting for the Home Health Nurse
- Note patterns of blood glucose levels.
- Document the condition of the needle insertion site.

- Note the functioning of the pump.
- Document family/client acceptance of the pump and adherence to the medical regimen.

Records Kept by the Client/Family

Results of blood glucose level monitoring

Dates of battery, needle, and tubing changes

Daily notation of skin condition at needle insertion site

Daily dosage of insulin added to the pump

Any symptoms of complications

Health Teaching Checklist

Name of Care Provider _____

Relationship to Client _____ Telephone #_____

Taught by _____ Date _____

	EXPLAINED	DEMONSTRATED
Care of insulin pump	_____	_____
Recognition of meaning of alarm systems	_____	_____
Addition of daily insulin	_____	_____
Changing of needle, tubing	_____	_____
Monitoring of blood glucose levels	_____	_____
Symptoms of complications	_____	

Product Availability

By prescription, the insulin pump is available through a hospital-supply firm or hospital pharmacy. The prescription will determine the type of pump to be used. Insulin can be purchased with a prescription at any pharmacy. Syringes, tubing, needles, skin barriers, and dressings can be purchased at any pharmacy.

Selected Reference

Brunner L, Suddarth D: Textbook of Medical-Surgical Nursing, 5th ed. Philadelphia, JB Lippincott, 1984

Background

Because of recent changes in the health-care industry encouraging early discharge from the hospital, increasing numbers of clients will require intravenous (IV) therapy at home. Home IV therapy can provide additional fluids and electrolytes, selected nutritional supplements, or a route for medications. Insertion of the IV cannula and initiation of the infusion will usually rest with the home health nurse. An exception to this might be a hemophiliac who administers clotting agents at home as required. The client or family members can be taught to monitor the infusion, add additional IV containers to the infusion, or to discontinue the infusion.

Types of IV Devices

Several styles of IV devices are available (Fig. 56-1). The catheter-over-the-needle device consists of a stainless-steel needle within a catheter. The vein is punctured with the needle, which serves as a stylet for the catheter, and the catheter is threaded into the vein over the needle. The needle is then removed, and the IV tubing is connected to the catheter hub.

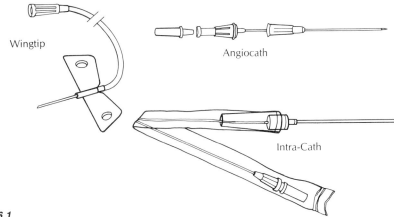

Wingtip

Angiocath

Intra-Cath

Figure 56.1

    The catheter-through-the-needle device consists of a stainless-steel needle through which the catheter is threaded into the vein. The catheter is protected by a plastic sleeve. Once the catheter is in place, the needle is withdrawn from the vein and the hub is engaged with the hub of the catheter. The plastic sleeve is removed, and the IV tubing is connected to the catheter hub. A protective clip is placed over the bevel of the needle to prevent damage to the catheter. This type of IV device is usually used for critically ill persons in the critical care unit. In special circumstances it may be used for home IV therapy.

    A butterfly device will be effective in a home IV program, particularly if long-term therapy is not indicated. Consider using a butterfly needle for children because it is easier to insert into smaller veins. The device consists of a short stainless-steel needle connected to plastic tubing. The IV tubing is connected directly to the hub of the plastic tubing.

    Intermittent infusion sets (IIS) or heparin locks are useful for the intermittent administration of medication. The client or family member can be taught to check the heparin lock for patency and to administer the medication. Heparin locks are similar in design to the butterfly device, but the hub is capped with a resealable injection cap. A catheter-over-the-needle device can be converted to an intermittent infusion device by disconnecting the IV tubing and applying a resealable injection cap to the hub of the catheter.

Heparin locks are kept patent by periodic flushing with a heparin flush solution. An infusion can be administered using a heparin lock by piggybacking the infusion using the resealable cap. Flush the device with a heparin flush when the infusion is complete. This technique is useful if medications must be diluted before administration. It is more comfortable for the client, decreasing the number of times entry into the vein is required.

Inline IV Filters

IV fluids may be administered through an inline filter, which removes particulate matter and bacteria, depending on the type of filter and the pore size of the membrane. Membrane filters will block the passage of air when wet. If a filter is used in home IV therapy, the 0.45-micron filter is most suitable. This filter will filter most bacteria and does not require an IV pump to maintain the rate. If an IV pump is used, a 0.22-micron filter can be used.

IV Drip Controller

As a safety factor in home IV therapy, a drip controller is desirable. The drip controller will monitor for air and will alert the client when the container is empty or if there are problems with the IV.

Assessment of Self-Care Potential

Client/Family Assessment

- Determine to what extent the client and family are willing and able to assume self-care activities related to home IV therapy. Assess whether the family will assume responsibility for adding IV fluids to the infusion, changing the dressing, or discontinuing the infusion. If a family member has a medical background, check that the person will be able to learn venipuncture. The feasibility of this will depend on the length of time the therapy will be necessary. Inserting a heparin lock allows the client or family to infuse fluids intermittently and does not limit mobility between infusions.
- Check that insurance counseling has been provided. Determine whether third-party payors will reimburse the client for home IV therapy.
- Assist the client to determine the most appropriate vendor to provide IV supplies and an IV pump. Determine whether rental of the IV pump is available. Check the availability of 24-hour service if problems develop or if the client is low on supplies.

Physical Assessment

- Determine the most appropriate mode of IV therapy for the client. This will depend on the reason for IV therapy (e.g., medication or fluid administration). Assess the gauge of IV device that will be required. Usually fluid and electrolyte administration for an adult requires an 18-gauge catheter. A 20-gauge catheter will be appropriate for children or if the drip rate is less than 75 ml per hour.
- Obtain a health history to determine if the client has a history of heart, respiratory, or renal problems. Take extra precautions, such as using a microdrip, to prevent fluid overload. Use the smallest container of IV fluid. Use a microdrip for pediatric clients to prevent fluid overload and allow slower drip rates.
- Check the client's intake and output to check for fluid retention. Check the ankles and sacrum for dependent edema.
- Assess the client for signs of congestive heart failure (i.e., rapid pulse rate, respiratory distress, moist cough, gallop rhythm).
- Assess the IV site for signs of infection (e.g., pain, inflammation, or swelling at the site, or increased temperature and pulse rate). Assess the IV for patency and infiltration.

Environmental Assessment

- Assess the basic sanitary practices used in the home. IV therapy is an aseptic procedure, and a home program cannot be implemented in unsanitary conditions.
- Determine a place in the home where IV supplies can be prepared. A clutter-free counter top in the kitchen or bathroom will be appropriate. Check that there is a place to hang the IV flask while priming the tubing. A door knob on a cabinet or a curtain rod will suffice. A coat hanger can be fashioned into a hook and suspended over a door also. A sink is required to drain IV fluid while priming the tubing.
- Determine the most comfortable place for the client during IV therapy. Unless the client is bedridden for other purposes, a reclining chair in a room where there is family activity will be appropriate. Check on the feasibility of using an IV pump with a battery pack so that the client can move with it. If the home has stairs or uneven surfaces, this may not be an option.
- Determine the best time for the IV infusion. If the client does not require constant infusion, running the IV at night might reduce necessary changes in activities of daily living (ADL). The IV pump will alert the client or family member if there are any problems. An adult will have to sleep close by if this is considered for a child.

Planning Strategies

Potential Nursing Diagnoses

Alteration in fluid volume

Alteration in nutrition, less than body requirements

Potential for injury: complications of IV therapy

Knowledge deficit: management of IV therapy at home

Expected Outcomes

Improvement of fluid balance

Improvement in nutritional status

Prevention of complications of IV therapy (phlebitis, systemic infection, fluid overload, air embolus, or hematoma)

Increased knowledge of home IV therapy program

Health Promotion Goals

- The client and family will
  Assume self-care activities in the home IV program according to their abilities
  Follow defined protocols to prevent complications of IV therapy

Equipment

IV solution/medications

IV tubing

Infusion device

Tourniquet

Razor or depilatory cream (if required)

Alcohol sponges

Sterile 4 × 4s

Iodophor ointment (optional)

Padded arm board

Freshly laundered bath towel to protect linen

IV drip controller

If using an intermittent infusion device (heparin lock)

Commercially prepared heparin flush or 10 ml of heparin flush solution in a syringe (1 unit heparin to 10 ml normal saline)

Interventions/Health Promotion

ACTION

RATIONALE/AMPLIFICATION

1. Wash your hands. Spike the IV fluid with the tubing. Prime the tubing and clamp it. Suspend the IV on an IV pole or substitute.

The drip chamber should be approximately 60 cm (24 inches) above the infusion site to prevent vein damage from higher pressures. Label IV tubing with date and time. This is important if more than one nurse may be visiting the client.

2. Thread the tubing through the IV drip controller.

Some drip controllers require special IV tubing.

3. Apply the tourniquet above the proposed puncture site (Fig. 56-2).

The tourniquet should impede venous flow but not arterial flow. The tourniquet is used to distend veins so that venipuncture is easier.

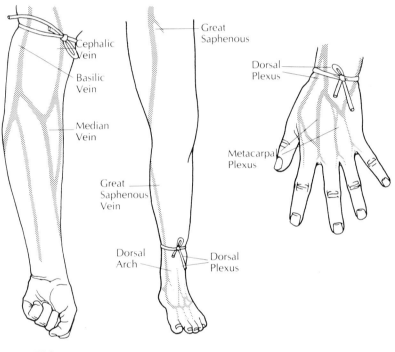

Cephalic Vein

Basilic Vein

Median Vein

Great Saphenous

Great Saphenous Vein

Dorsal Arch

Dorsal Plexus

Dorsal Plexus

Metacarpal Plexus

Figure 56.2

Select a puncture site. Release the tourniquet.

Prolonged application of the tourniquet may cause the vein to become tortuous. Sclerosed veins (in an elderly client) may be easier to puncture without a tourniquet.

4. Remove excess hair from the site if necessary, using a razor or depilatory cream.

Shaving is optional. Microabrasions caused by shaving are potential sites of infection.

5. Wash your hands thoroughly.

6. Prepare the insertion site with iodophor solution and allow it to dry. Reapply the tourniquet.

Remove a small amount of the iodophor with an alcohol sponge if the vein cannot be visualized.

ACTION

RATIONALE/AMPLIFICATION

7. Holding the needle bevel up and at a 45-degree angle, puncture the skin lateral to the vein (Fig. 56-3).

Support the extremity and anchor the vein, using the opposite hand.

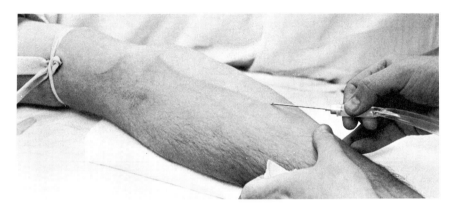

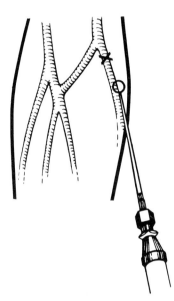

Figure 56.3

8. Reduce the angle of the needle to the skin, and gently insert the needle ½ cm (¼ inch) into the vein. Observe the flashback chamber or syringe for retrograde blood flow.

Blood in the flashback chamber indicates successful venipuncture.

9. Advance the device using the appropriate technique.
   For the catheter-through-the-needle device
   • Stabilize the needle with one hand. Advance the catheter through the needle with the opposite hand, until the full length has been inserted.

   A plastic sleeve protects the sterility of the catheter during advancement.

   • Engage the needle and catheter hub.

   If the catheter cannot be inserted the full length, withdraw the needle over the catheter to engage the catheter hub.

   • Withdraw the needle and catheter from the vein until about 4 cm (1½ inch) of the catheter is exposed. Remove the plastic sleeve. Withdraw the stylet.

   • Attach the primed IV tubing to the catheter hub and commence the infusion.

   Unclamp the tubing and follow the IV pump directions to start the infusion. This prevents damage to the catheter from the needle.

   • Apply the needle guard over the needle bevel.

ACTION   RATIONALE/AMPLIFICATION

For the catheter-over-the-needle
device
• Stabilize the needle hub with
  one hand. Advance the catheter over the needle and into
  the vein with the other hand
  (Fig. 56-4). Withdraw the needle from the catheter and connect the primed IV tubing.
  Commence the infusion.

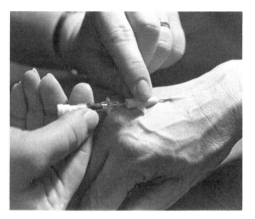

Figure 56.4

For the butterfly or heparin lock
• Gently advance the needle into   Care must be taken not to puncture
  the vein until the total length   the vein.
  has been inserted.
• For a butterfly device, remove
  the protective cap and connect
  the primed IV tubing. Commence the infusion.
• For a heparin lock, flush the
  tubing with a heparin flush by
  piercing the resealable cap
  (Fig. 56-5).

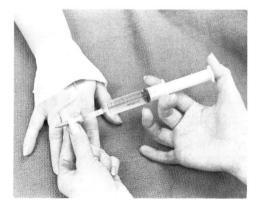

Figure 56.5

ACTION

10. Secure the infusion device with tape.

11. Apply iodophor ointment to the infusion site. (Optional:) Dress with a sterile 4 × 4 and an occlusive dressing (Fig. 56-6).

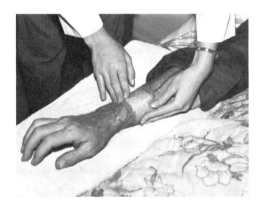

Figure 56.6

12. Write the date, time, type of device, and the person starting the IV on the tape. Adjust the infusion rate (Fig. 56-7).

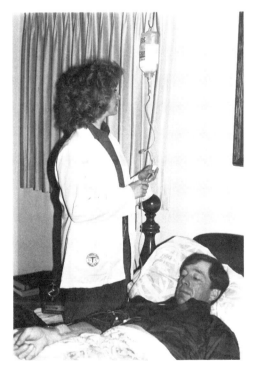

Figure 56.7

RATIONALE/AMPLIFICATION

Observe the infusion site after beginning the infusion. Swelling at the site indicates infiltration into the tissues. Remove the IV catheter and restart the IV at another site.

Use antibiotic ointment if sensitive to iodophor. A large adhesive bandage works well to dress the site.

ACTION	*RATIONALE/AMPLIFICATION*
Related Care	
1. Apply an arm board to immobilize the IV site if applicable.	An arm board can be made by covering a magazine, folded lengthwise, with a soft washcloth. Secure the washcloth with tape.
2. Change the IV tubing every 48 hours and the container every 24 hours. Palpate the site through the dressing for tenderness, and observe for signs of phlebitis every 8 hours. Attempt to rotate the site every 72 hours, if possible.	These are infection-control precautions. The rate of infection increases significantly after an IV device has been in place 72 hours.
3. Change the dressing if necessary, following the same procedure as when the IV was inserted.	
4. Keep the drip chamber at least half full of fluid to prevent air embolus.	
5. Give IV push medications using a heparin lock:	
• Prepare the medication.	The medication can be administered in a syringe or diluted in IV fluid. (50-ml containers of IV solution are available for this purpose). The mode of administration depends on the particular medication. Consult the package insert for instructions. If the medication is diluted in IV fluid, spike the container with IV tubing and prime the tubing.
• Swab the injection cap with an alcohol sponge.	Cleaning the injection cap prevents bacteria from being introduced into the bloodstream by the needle.
• Insert the medication needle into the injection cap. Check for patency of the heparin lock.	To check that the device is still in the vein, observe for a flashback of blood into the syringe when gentle back pressure is applied to the syringe. If using an IV piggyback, check for flashback by squeezing the rubber flash ball on the tubing and observing the tubing for a flashback of blood.
• If no flashback is observed, reposition the needle slightly by placing a folded 4 × 4 under the wings and retaping.	This can reposition a needle that is against the wall of a vessel. Do not push solution into the lock to try to clear a clotted needle. This releases clots into the circulation, causing emboli.
• Slowly inject the medication if using a syringe. Start the infusion if using a piggyback.	Inject or infuse the medication at a rate according to the package insert.
• Observe the client for side-effects of the medication.	
• Remove the needle when the medication has been administered.	Clamp the IV tubing before removing the needle.
• Flush the heparin lock using a heparin flush.	Heparinizing the lock prevents clotting of the needle.

ACTION	RATIONALE/AMPLIFICATION
6. Give intermittent IV fluids using a heparin lock, following the same procedure as above when administering medications diluted in IV fluid.	Using a heparin lock for intermittent fluid administration allows the client mobility between infusions.
7. Give IV medications by direct IV push using the venipuncture technique with a needle and syringe. Release the tourniquet before injecting the medication. Remove the syringe when the injection is complete. Apply pressure with a 4 × 4 or alcohol sponge until bleeding stops.	Medications are usually given diluted in IV fluid or normal saline to prevent damage to the vein or generalized reactions to rapidly administered medications. Consult the package insert before using this method.
8. Discontinue the IV when therapy is completed: • Clamp the tubing. Remove the dressing. Remove the cannula with one, smooth movement. Hold pressure on the site with a 4 × 4 until bleeding stops. Cover with an adhesive bandage. Dispose of equipment and cannula in the trash.	

Education/ Communication

• Teach the client and family to
Change the IV dressing if it is wet, soiled, or loose
Check the IV site for signs of infection. Monitor vital signs for elevated temperature or pulse rate indicating a possible infection.
Check IV fluids for the presence of particulate matter, cloudiness, or cracks. Do not infuse these solutions. Bring them to the attention of the home health nurse or vendor.
Maintain the integrity of the IV line. Remove air bubbles if they appear in the tubing. Keep the drip chamber at least half full to prevent air embolus.
Check the drip rate, and troubleshoot the IV line
Add new containers of IV fluid to the line when necessary
Monitor intake and output using household measuring devices and a flow sheet
Maintain and troubleshoot the IV drip controller
Discontinue the IV (if applicable). If the IV is accidentally discontinued, hold pressure on the site until bleeding stops. Cover with an adhesive bandage.
Cover the IV site with a resealable plastic bag or plastic wrap during bathing or showering. If showering is attempted, the extremity with the IV will have to be kept outside the shower. This is only feasible if a shower curtain is used. A wet dressing allows bacteria to penetrate and infect the IV site.
Wear clothing with a large sleeve opening so that the top can be removed while the infusion is in progress, if necessary. A robe is usually suitable, because the arm openings are larger. An oversized shirt is also appropriate.

Referrals and Consultations

• Refer the family to the home health nurse if problems develop with the IV therapy (e.g., signs of infection, mechanical problems with the IV or pump). Give a 24-hour number to the family.
• Refer the family to the vendor for problems or shortage of supplies.
• Refer the family to the physician or local emergency room for emergencies when the home health nurse cannot be reached.

Evaluation of Health Promotion Activities

Quality Assurance/
Reassessment

- Evaluate the client for complications of IV therapy.
- Check that the client and family can perform self-care activities following accepted protocols.

DOCUMENTATION

Charting for the Home Health Nurse

Intake and output flow sheet

Physical assessment findings

Condition of IV site

Ability of the family to manage IV therapy program

Records Kept by the Client/Family

Flow sheet: name of solution, amount of solution, number of bottle, date and time added, time of completion of bottle, tubing change (if appropriate), time IV discontinued (if appropriate)

Name of Care Provider _____

Relationship to Client _____ Telephone #_____

Taught by _____ Date _____

	EXPLAINED	DEMONSTRATED
Rationale for IV therapy	_____	
Intake and output flow sheet	_____	_____
Equivalents of household measures	_____	_____
Symptoms of IV therapy complications	_____	
Maintaining the drip rate	_____	
Adding IV fluids to the infusion	_____	_____
Discontinuing the IV	_____	_____
Changing the dressing	_____	_____
Maintaining and troubleshooting the pump	_____	_____
Troubleshooting the IV	_____	_____
Infection-control precautions	_____	_____
When to obtain assistance from health professional	_____	

Product Availability

IV therapy products are available from medical-supply companies listed in the yellow pages of the telephone book. Arrangements can be made with a local hospital pharmacy to supply IV fluids and additives. Medications are available by prescription from a pharmacy. IV therapy vendors supply a wide range of products and services.

Dressings are available from grocery stores and pharmacies.

Selected Reference

Metheny NM, Snively WD: Nurses' Handbook of Fluid Balance, 4th ed. Philadelphia, JB Lippincott, 1983

57 Oral Administration of Medications

Background

Oral administration of medications is the least expensive and the most convenient method for clients in the home. Physiologically, the oral route is also the safest one, since the skin and/or the vein do not have to be penetrated.

The major disadvantages of oral administration of medications relate to taste, effect on the gastric mucosa, irregular absorption from the gastrointestinal tract, and occasional effect on the teeth.

Closely related to the oral administration of medications is the administration of pharmaceuticals by the sublingual (under the tongue) and buccal (in the cheek) routes. Drugs given sublingually usually are intended to be absorbed into the blood vessels on the underside of the tongue. Those given bucally act locally on the mucous membrane or systemically in the saliva.

Assessment of Self-Care Potential

Client/Family Assessment

- Assess the client/family to determine their knowledge of the purposes for which each medication is intended; the distinguishing color, size, and identifying characteristics of each medication; and the prescribed time and schedule for taking medications.
- Assess the family/client's awareness of the danger of taking medications prescribed for other persons, as well as taking medications other than those prescribed.
- Determine if the client/family is aware of the need to keep medications in a place where children cannot get to them.

Physical Assessment

- Obtain information about medications currently being taken other than those prescribed: over-the-counter drugs; drugs prescribed by another physician; and illegal drugs or drugs prescribed for other family members.
- Assess the history of known or suspected drug allergies.
- Assess any indications of past dependency on drugs.
- Assess the client's history of taking antacids, alcohol, tobacco, coffee, tea, carbonated drinks.

Environmental Assessment

- If children are in the home or if children visit, assess the home to determine a safe place for medication storage. However, the storage place must not be so inconspicuous that the client forgets the location or forgets to take the medication.
- Assess the home to determine if other prescription drugs or over-the-counter drugs are present. Examine all bottles for expiration dates. Instruct the client to discard outdated ones and to consult the physician regarding the use of those drugs having interactive effects.
- If another person in the home has prescription drugs or is using over-the-counter drugs that might be harmful to the client, move those bottles of drugs to a separate location to avoid medication errors.

Planning Strategies

Potential Nursing Diagnoses

Knowledge deficit related to administration of medication

Expected Outcomes

Administration of the medication safely and accurately

Health Promotion Goals

- The client and family will
  Obtain prescribed medications
  Refrain from transferring medications from one container to another
  Refrain from using medications intended for another person, nonprescription drugs, or substances having an interactive effect with prescribed medications
  Consistently examine drugs for expiration dates and discard those outdated
  Notify the nurse if nausea or vomiting occurs following medication administration
  Document medications taken
  Take medications as ordered

Equipment

The prescribed medication with label indicating medication name, date of prescription, dosage, and route indicated

Glass of water, milk, crackers, or whatever substance desired

Safe storage place for medications

Sufficient lighting to prepare medications

Checklist for documentation

Memory jogger device if desired

MEMORY JOGGER DEVICES

If a client has several drugs to take at different times, or if the client tends to forget to take the medications as prescribed, recommend a device for remembering to take the medications. These can be purchased or made at home.

Purchased Memory Joggers

MedTymer. This device is built into the cap of a medication bottle. The electronic timer is set for the times the medications are to be given. The sound goes off at the specified time and continues to sound until the cap is removed. An added advantage is that its loud-tone sounds are in a lower frequency range that is easier heard by hearing-impaired elderly persons. In addition to the sound, a red light flashes for the hearing-impaired. It can be set for 1-, 2-, 3-, and 4-times a day schedules. It is available from HBK, Inc., 51 Brattle St. Suite 53, Cambridge, MA 02138; telephone (617) 492-7826.

One-day or one-week pill reminder. This plastic device has four small compartments marked "breakfast," "lunch," "supper," and "bedtime." In addition, the first letter of each word is marked in braille. These and similar devices can be obtained from pharmacies (Fig. 57-1).

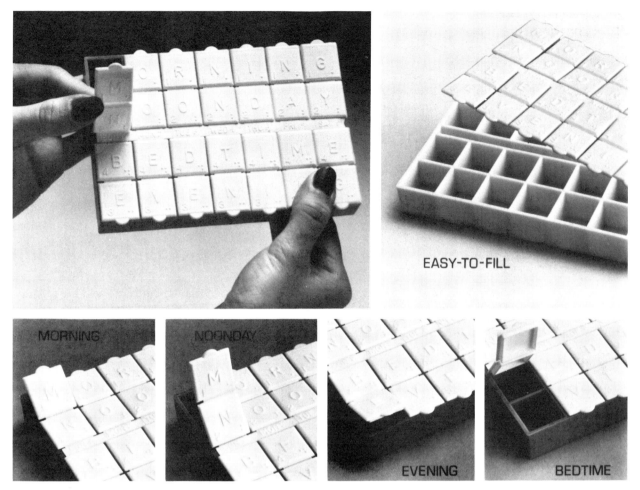

Figure 57.1
An example of a medication memory-jogging device found helpful by many clients. According to the manufacturer, it is easy to use and easy to fill. (Courtesy of Apex Medical Corporation, Bloomington, Minnesota)

Hand-Made Memory Joggers

A simple chart on the wall where the medications are stored will assist in sorting out confusing and different time schedules for medications. A simple one is as follows:

MEDICATION NAME	BREAKFAST	LUNCH	DINNER	BEDTIME

Another homemade but effective memory jogger can be assembled by using small matchboxes. The matchboxes are glued together and the boxes themselves are used as "drawers." Medications can be set up for one week or for several days. The number of matchboxes stacked upon each other relates to the number of times a day medications must be given. Add one row of boxes for each day of the week. Glue the box covers together. On the side of the stack, write clearly the time of day to be taken (breakfast, lunch, etc.); across the top, write the day of the week. If the client forgets whether the medication has been taken, a quick look in the "drawer" will answer the question.

Interventions/Health Promotion

ACTION	*RATIONALE/AMPLIFICATION*
1. Consult the checklist to recall medication to be taken, its route of administration, scheduled time of administration, and purpose.	Checking these essential elements prior to medication administration reduces the probability of error.
2. Wash hands.	Handwashing is the most effective means of preventing cross-contamination.
3. Select the medication container and compare label with directives on checklist.	This process of "double-checking" on route of administration, medication description, and time will reduce the probability of error.
4. Pour the medication: • If pill or capsule, pour indicated number into the bottle cap, then into the container from which it will be taken.	If medication is spilled or dropped on the floor, discard it.
• If liquid, pour with the label up to prevent soiling the label. Hold the container into which the liquid will be poured at eye level and if possible on a flat surface.	These measures will increase the accuracy of measurement.
5. Take the medication with the required or recommended substance.	Some substances (milk, crackers, food) prevent gastric upset.
6. Record the medication administration on the checksheet provided for that purpose.	Documentation of all medications is essential to determine the effect of the medication.
7. Replace medications. Record any side-effect.	Document time and date, and describe side-effect. Notify nurse or physician of side-effect.

Related Care

1. If the client has difficulty swallowing pills, suggest that the pill be placed on the back of the tongue prior to taking the water, juice, or milk.	Stimulation of the back of the tongue produces a swallowing reflex that often aids in swallowing pills.
2. If the prescribed medication has a potentially harmful effect on the teeth or the oral mucosa, suggest the use of a straw for ingesting the medication and follow the medication with water.	Use of the straw bypasses the teeth and mucous membrane.
3. If the client finds the taste of the medication objectionable, suggest that ice chips be held in the mouth prior to taking the medication.	This deadens the taste buds, thus reducing the distaste of the medication. Objectionable taste can also be masked by taking the medication with applesauce, flavored gelatin, custard, or bread.

ACTION

RATIONALE/AMPLIFICATION

4. Store the medications where children and pets cannot get to them. Childproof lids should be applied if children visit or live in the home.

If the client is unable to remove childproof lids from the bottles, undertake other safety measures: locking the medications in a cabinet or drawer, for instance.

Age-Specific Modifications

- For infants and toddlers, specially made medication spoons and droppers can be obtained from a drug store for accurate measurement and for ease of administration.
- Children around 4 to 6 years of age can usually swallow pills. Instruct the child to place the pill near the back of the tongue and drink the liquid.
- A child's head should be elevated during medication administration to prevent aspiration of the medication.

Education/ Communication

- Teach the client and family to
  Administer the correct medication, of the correct dose, and at the correct time
  Observe for side-effects and interactive effects
  Take measures to decrease medication errors
  Notify the nurse of medication errors, side-effects, or interactive effects

Referrals and Consultations

- Notify the pharmacist to determine if medication is safe to take if
  The medication changes in color
  There is sediment in liquid medication
  New medication looks different than old medication
- Consult a social worker if financial difficulties or transportation problems prevent the purchase of medications when needed.

Evaluation of Health Promotion Activities

Quality Assurance/ Reassessment

- Evaluate if the desired effect has been accomplished without medication overdose, error, allergic reaction, or omission of a dose.
- Follow return demonstration of medication administration with a home visit at the time of medication administration to evaluate procedural accuracy.

DOCUMENTATION

Charting for the Home Health Nurse
- Record the schedule of administration of the medication.
- Record the achieved effect of the medications, as well as side-effects or allergic reactions.

Records Kept by the Client/Family
A suggested format for recording of medication administration in the home is as follows (Table 57-1). Use one sheet for each medication. Each sheet should contain enough spaces for a 2-week documentation.

Table 57-1. **MEDICATION ADMINISTRATION CHECKLIST**

DRUG: DESCRIPTION/PURPOSE	MAJOR SIDE-EFFECTS TO WATCH FOR	DATE	NUMBER TO BE TAKEN	TIMES OF DAY TO BE TAKEN (CROSS OFF WHEN TAKEN)
Aspirin: White pill	Ringing of ears, itching	Dec 18	2 every 4 hr	8 AM/12 noon/4 PM/8 PM/ 12 midnight/4 AM
		Dec 19		8 AM/12 noon/4 PM/8 PM/ 12 midnight/4 AM

**Health Teaching
Checklist**

Name of Care Provider _____

Relationship to Client _____ Telephone #_____

Taught by _____ Date _____

	EXPLAINED	DEMONSTRATED
Specific medications	_____	

Purpose
  Description
  Dosage schedule		

Checking label twice	_____	_____
Correctly measuring medication	_____	_____
Taking medication	_____	
Environmental safety regarding medications	_____	

Product Availability

Over-the-counter drugs should be used cautiously and with approval of health-care provider. Prescription drugs are available only with a physician's prescription and then must be purchased from a pharmacy.

Selected Reference

Lewis L, Fundamental Skills in Patient Care, pp 460–468. Philadelphia, JB Lippincott, 1984

58 Parenteral Administration of Medications

Background

Administering medication parenterally can be done by the subcutaneous, intramuscular, or intravenous route. The injectable method is the route of choice for many medications. Medication given parenterally is absorbed more quickly and does not have the gastrointestinal side-effects of the oral route. However, once the medication is injected the effect is irreversible. In addition, if the family is to administer the injection, or if the injection is to be self-administered, the educational process is more extensive and must include sterile technique, mixing of medications, if necessary, and the process of injection. Exact performance of each of these must be done to avoid abscesses and irritations at the injection site.

Assessment of Self-Care Potential

Client/Family Assessment

- Assess the client/family to determine who will be taught to perform the injection. Even if the client will perform the injection personally, at least one family member should also be taught to perform the procedure in the event of client disability. If a family member is to perform the injection, another person should be taught the procedure to serve, likewise, as a backup in the event of an emergency.
- Assess with the client/family the ability to purchase needed medical equipment and supplies. Assess the client's health-care insurance and Medicare to determine if assistance is available.

Physical Assessment

- Assess the visual acuity of the person administering the injection to determine if that person can accurately see the markings on the syringe.
- Assess the fine motor movement of the person performing the injection to determine if that person is capable of withdrawing the medication and performing the injection.
- Examine the sites to be used for injections to determine if they are free of complications and can be used for injection.

Environmental Assessment

- If the medication is to be kept cold, a place should be reserved in the refrigerator for medications only, for example, a specially marked box.
- The site for storage of medication and injection equipment should be clean. The storage site should not be accessible to children or visitors in the home.
- A receptacle for disposing of syringes should be placed in the home. Syringes should not be disposed of with the normal household waste.
- Adequate lighting should be available in the area where the injection is to be prepared.
- Privacy and lack of interruption should be provided to the client or family member in the process of preparing the injection and administering it so as to allow for concentration and prevention of error.

Planning Strategies

Potential Nursing Diagnoses

Physical injury, potential for, related to medication error

Skin integrity, potential impairment of

Knowledge deficit regarding medications

Expected Outcomes

Administration of the proper medications as prescribed

Prevention of complications resulting from faulty injection procedure

Understanding of the reasons, expected actions, and side-effects of the drug

Health Promotion Goals

- The client and family will
  Obtain the prescribed medication and syringes
  Demonstrate appropriate aseptic technique for injection procedure
  Demonstrate proper injection procedure
  Store supplies in a clean place that is safe from children and visitors
  Dispose of needles and syringes in a safe manner
  Correctly rotate sites of injection
  List purpose of medication, dose to be given, expected side-effects, and inter-action effects, if any, with tea, coffee, alcohol, or other substances being used in daily living

Equipment

Syringes (individually packaged, disposable, presterilized, of appropriate size)

Needles (may be attached to syringe, or may come separate; should be disposable, presterilized, individually packaged, and of appropriate size)

The prescribed medication
  Ampule (An ampule contains a single dose of the medication. It is made of glass and has a constricted neck that is usually scored for ease of opening.)
  Vial (A vial is a small glass bottle of medication closed with a rubber stopper. A vial contains multiple doses.)

Alcohol sponges

A chart to indicate rotating injection sites

Interventions/Health Promotion

ACTION	*RATIONALE/AMPLIFICATION*
1. Wash hands thoroughly.	Handwashing is the most effective method of preventing contamination.
2. Select the ampule or vial with the prescribed medication. Read the label twice and compare with medication-recording chart.	Double-checking labels prior to withdrawing medication reduces the probability of error.
3. Select the sterile syringe and needle of appropriate size.	Generally a 2-ml syringe with a 25-gauge needle is used for subcutaneous injections; a 20- to 23-gauge needle, 1½ to 2 inches, for intramuscular gluteal injections; a 23- to 25-gauge needle, ⅝ to 1 inch, for deltoid intramuscular injections; and a 20- to 22-gauge needle for intravenous therapy.

ACTION	RATIONALE/AMPLIFICATION

ACTION

4. Prepare the medication:

Vial

- Mix solution, if necessary, by rolling the vial in the palms of the hands.
- Remove the metal cap protector and cleanse the rubber stopper by rubbing with alcohol sponge, using a circular motion.
- Remove the protective covering from the needle, pulling straight off.
- Holding the syringe, withdraw the plunger to fill the syringe with an amount of air equal to the amount of medication required.
- Inject the air into the vial. Inverting the vial and holding at eye level, withdraw the prescribed amount of medication (Figs. 58-1 and 58-2).

RATIONALE/AMPLIFICATION

Shaking causes foaming of solution.

Alcohol cleanses the stopper, thus preventing needle contamination during withdrawal of solution.

Removing without touching the needle prevents needle contamination.

This air will be injected into the vial to create positive pressure in the vial, allowing the solution to be withdrawn easily.
Solution must be measured at eye level to get correct measurement.

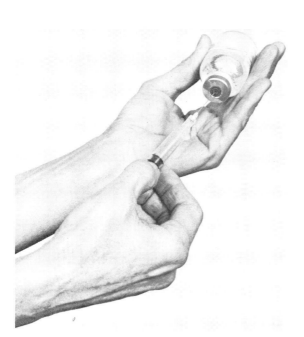

Figure 58.1
Invert the vial, insert the needle into the vial, and inject air into the vial.

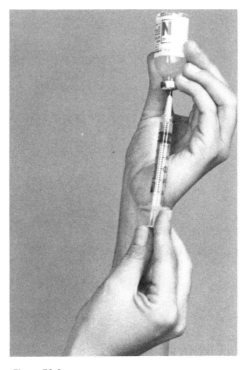

Figure 58.2
Withdraw the medication into the syringe, holding the syringe at eye level.

- Withdraw the syringe from the vial; replace cover on the needle.

Ampule

- Tap the upper end of the ampule several times with the finger.

Keeping needle covered until use maintains sterile condition of needle.

This causes the solution in the upper part of the ampule to move to the lower section for easier removal of solution.

ACTION	RATIONALE/AMPLIFICATION
• If the neck of the ampule is not color scored, file the neck of the ampule.	The filed line will assist in safely breaking the ampule.
• Place a piece of sterile gauze or other material around the ampule. Snap the top off, directing the break away from yourself (Fig. 58-3).	This prevents fingers from getting cut while breaking the ampule.

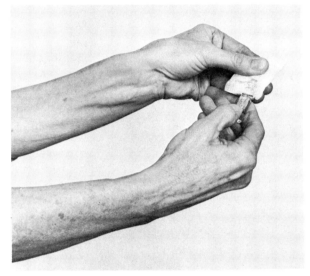

Figure 58.3
Use gauze to protect your fingers when breaking an ampule, and direct the break away from yourself.

• Remove the cap from the needle. Insert needle into solution and withdraw into syringe (Fig. 58-4).	Care must be taken to remove all solution from the ampule.

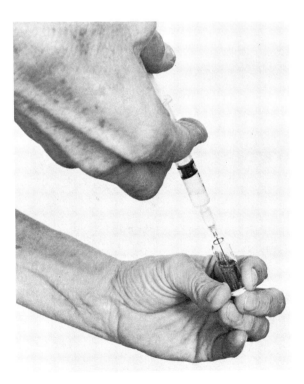

Figure 58.4
When withdrawing medication from an ampule, be cautious not to contaminate the needle by touching the rim.

ACTION	RATIONALE/AMPLIFICATION
Replace protective cover on needle	Replacing cover without touching needle maintains needle sterility.
5. Prepare the injection site:	
• Select the injection site.	The site should be free of tenderness, hardness, scarring, swelling, redness, itching, or pain. Sites should be rotated if a series of injections is to be given. A chart should be given to the client and kept where the medication is stored. If the chart is covered with acetate, a water-soluble pen can be used to mark where the last injection site was.
• Clean the selected site with the alcohol sponge. Cleanse the center of the site first, then proceed in a circular motion, widening the circle around the site.	Cleansing with an antiseptic agent reduces the number of microorganisms on the skin.
• Remove the protective cap from the needle while waiting for the antiseptic to dry.	Pull the protective cover straight off to avoid contaminating the needle.
• Invert the syringe and expel all but a drop of air from the syringe.	This drop of air will stay in the needle after the medication is injected, ensuring that all the medication has been injected.

Subcutaneous Injection

1. Select the site.

Any site with loose connective tissue is acceptable. Usual sites are the outer aspects of the thighs, backs of upper arms, and subcutaneous tissue of lower abdomen (Fig. 58-5).

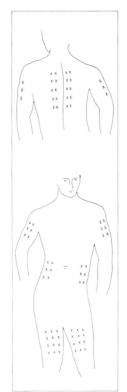

Figure 58.5
Appropriate sites for subcutaneous injections.

ACTION	RATIONALE/AMPLIFICATION

RATIONALE/AMPLIFICATION

If a series of subcutaneous injections is to be given, rotate sites according to a plan (Fig. 58-6).

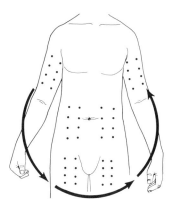

Figure 58.6
One method of systematically rotating injection sites.

ACTION

2. Grasp tissue with the nondominant hand, elevating it.

3. With the dominant hand, insert the needle smoothly and quickly at an angle from 30 to 90 degrees.

4. When the needle is inserted, release the tissue.

5. Pull back on the plunger to determine if the needle is in a blood vessel. If blood appears in the barrel, withdraw the needle and reinsert, again checking for entry into the bloodstream. If no blood returns, inject the medication slowly.

6. Withdraw the needle smoothly and quickly. Gently rub the site with the alcohol sponge to increase absorption and distribution.

7. Dispose of needles and syringes. Replace equipment.

8. Record injection and any side-effects.

Intramuscular Injection

1. Select the injection site (Figs. 58-7 to 58-10).

RATIONALE/AMPLIFICATION

Pinching the tissue is thought to desensitize it. Raising it separates it from the muscle tissue.

The angle of insert is determined by the amount of subcutaneous tissue present on the client.

Injecting solution into compressed tissue causes pain.

Medications injected into the bloodstream are absorbed immediately, with possible serious side-effects to the client. This possibility can be prevented by checking for entry into a blood vessel prior to injecting the medication.

Quick, smooth withdrawal prevents unnecessary pain.

Safe disposal prevents accidental puncturing by the needle and complications resulting from reuse.

Muscles with abrasions, bruises, or infections are not suitable for injection sites. No more than 2 ml should be given in the deltoid muscle; no more than 5 ml should be given in the gluteal muscle.

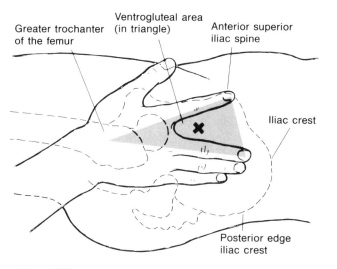

Figure 58.7
Ventrogluteal site for intramuscular injection.

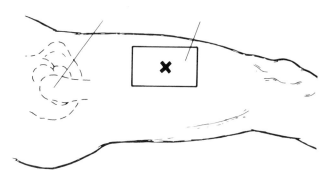

Figure 58.8
Vastus lateralis site for intramuscular injection.

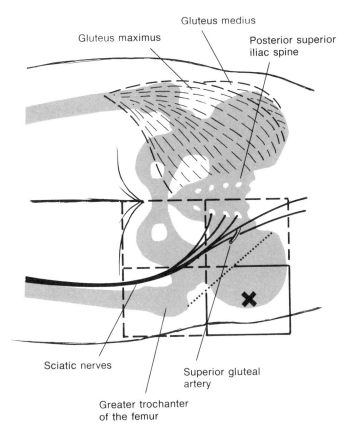

Figure 58.9
Gluteal site for intramuscular injection.

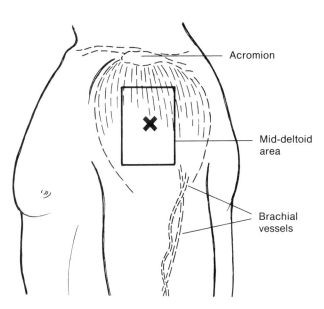

Figure 58.10
Deltoid site for intramuscular injection.

ACTION	**RATIONALE/AMPLIFICATION**
2. Cleanse the site with an alcohol sponge in a circular motion, starting at the center and rotating outward.	Cleansing the site reduces the presence of microorganisms.

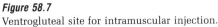

ACTION

RATIONALE/AMPLIFICATION

3. Remove the needle cover. Invert the syringe. Remove all but a drop of air from the syringe.

This amount of air will clear the needle of medication during the process of withdrawing the needle following the injection.

4. Using the nondominant hand, spread the skin at the site.

Spreading the skin makes it firmer. When the client is very thin, it may be necessary to hold the skin in a cushion-like fashion.

5. Insert the needle smoothly and quickly at a 90-degree angle.

A quick, smooth wrist motion lessens the pain of injection.

6. Pull back on the plunger to determine if the needle has entered a blood vessel. If blood appears in the syringe, remove the needle and select a new site, preparing a new syringe.

Accidental injection into the blood vessel results in immediate absorption via the circulatory system.

7. If no blood has returned, inject the solution slowly, holding the syringe steady.

This reduces discomfort to the client.

8. Withdraw the needle smoothly and quickly. Gently rub the site with an alcohol sponge.

Quick, smooth withdrawal prevents unneeded discomfort.

9. Dispose of needles and syringes. Replace equipment.

Safe disposal prevents accidental puncturing by the needle.

10. Record injection and any side-effects.

Intravenous Injection

1. For venipuncture, refer to Technique 56, Intravenous Therapy.

2. For an intravenous bolus
   • Draw medication into syringe.
   • Perform venipuncture.
   • Aspirate a small amount of blood into the syringe.
   • Release the tourniquet.
   • Inject the medication slowly.

This will ensure proper placement of the needle.

Check frequently by aspiration to ensure continued placement of the needle in the vein.

   • Observe the client carefully.

Observe for the indicated time for adverse reactions to the drug.

   • Place pressure over the injection site for at least 1 minute. Apply an adhesive bandage.

Pressure is indicated to stop bleeding at the venipuncture site after the needle is removed.

3. To add medication to intravenous solution
   • Add medication to solution prior to connecting it to the IV solution.

The drug is administered slowly and over a long period of time. One disadvantage to this method is that if the client does not receive all of the solution, the drug, too, is not all administered.

ACTION	RATIONALE/AMPLIFICATION
4. To add drugs to a volume-control meter (Fig. 58-11) • Clamp off the tubing of the intravenous fluid bottle.	This method is especially useful when the volume of fluid infused must be carefully controlled, as with elderly persons and infants. It allows drugs to be diluted in a very small amount of solution (*i.e.*, 50 ml to 100 ml).

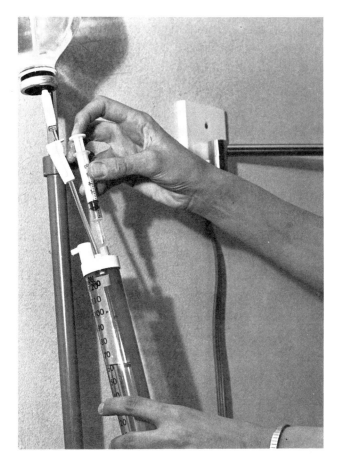

Figure 58.11
Adding drugs to a volume-control meter.

  • Inject medication into the volume-control chamber.
  • Allow all of the medication to be infused.
  • Open the intravenous fluid line.
5. The "piggyback" method (Fig. 58-12)

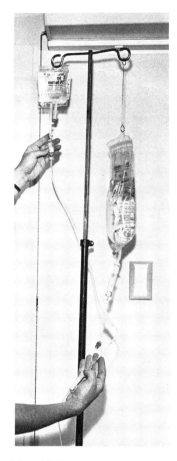

Figure 58.12
Giving intravenous medication, using the "piggyback" method. The medication in the small container will enter the venous system before the solution in the larger container.

ACTION	RATIONALE/AMPLIFICATION
• Dilute the medication in the amount of solution.	This tandem method allows the drug to enter the system more quickly than if mixed with the entire solution.
• Connect this solution to the IV tubing.	
• Close the clamp of the IV tubing until the "piggyback" has completed. Reopen the IV tubing.	
6. To introduce medication into the IV tubing (Fig. 58-13)	

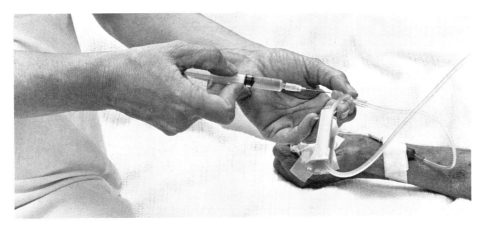

Figure 58.13
Introducing medication into the IV tubing.

ACTION	RATIONALE/AMPLIFICATION
• Prepare the prescribed drug.	The port for injecting medication is located near the distal end of the IV tubing.
• Cleanse the injection site on the tubing with an antiseptic swab. • Insert the needle into the injection site. • Clamp or pinch the IV tubing between the injection site and the IV solution. • Aspirate blood into the syringe to ensure that the solution will enter the client's vein. • Inject the drug slowly. • Open the IV tubing. • Remove the needle and syringe.	

7. Heparin lock (Fig. 58-14)

Insertion —
site

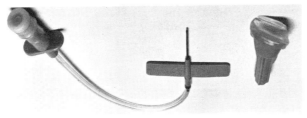

Figure 58.14
Equipment for a heparin lock.

• Clean the injection site with an antiseptic sponge.	Cleansing removes surface bacteria.
• Prepare 1 ml of heparinized saline in a syringe with a short needle. Aspirate to determine a blood return.	This ensures that the heparin lock is still in a vein.
• Inject a portion of the solution slowly. Remove the needle and cleanse the plug again with an antiseptic swab or sponge.	This determines that the needle is patent.

ACTION	RATIONALE/AMPLIFICATION
• Use a syringe or a piggyback with a short needle. Insert the needle into the insertion site and inject the prescribed medication slowly.	While the medication is slowly infusing, observe the client carefully for adverse effects of the medication.
• Remove the needle and again clean the insertion site with an antiseptic swab or sponge.	This prepares the site for the heparin to be injected.
• Inject 2 ml of heparinized saline into the plug.	This flushes the medication from the needle and ensures patency of the lock between injections by preventing the formation of blood clots in the tubing.
• Examine the injection site and plug every 8 hours and administer a small amount of heparinized saline if medication is not given at least that often (10 units is the usual amount given).	This ensures continued patency of the system.
• Change the heparin lock at least every 72 hours.	If the lock is clogged, it should be changed immediately.

Related Care

1. Never reuse syringes.

Reuse causes cross-contamination.

2. Prepare a travel kit for use by the client when away from home.

This kit should contain all supplies needed for medication injection while away from home. If medication must be refrigerated, a small ice chest with chemical cold pouches can be effectively used.

Age-Specific Modifications

1. In infants and children, the intramuscular injection can be given in the anterolateral thigh or deltoid muscle (Fig. 58-15).

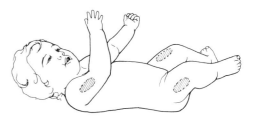

Figure 58.15
Intramuscular injection sites for infants and children.

2. If the buttock is used, determine the correct site by placing the thumb on the greater trochanter and the middle finger on the iliac crest. Select the site by letting the index finger drop in the middle between the middle finger and thumb.

Education/
Communication

- Teach the client and family to
  Keep syringes and medications stored safely from children and visitors
  Dispose of syringes and needles safely
  Wash hands prior to beginning the procedure. Observe sterile technique in
      the process of the technique.
  Select site for injection, and rotate sites if a series of subcutaneous or intra-
      muscular injections is to be given
  Observe injection sites for complications
  Withdraw the proper dosage of medication from an ampule or vial
  Document the procedure accurately
  Observe for effect of medication, side-effects, or interactive effects and notify
      the nurse/doctor if any occur

Evaluation of Health Promotion Activities

Quality Assurance/
Reassessment

- Document the accuracy of the procedure in relation to medication dosage,
  aseptic technique, and site selection.
- Evaluate the effect of the medication—the desired effect, any side-effects,
  allergies, or interactive effects.
- Inspect the condition of the injection sites for redness, warmth, edema.
- Observe the environmental safety features of the procedure—safe storage of
  the needles and syringes as well as safe disposal of the needles and syringes.

DOCUMENTATION

Charting for the Home Health Nurse

- Note the date of teaching and the person responsible for the injections or observation of the infusions.
- Note information from the medication documentation sheet being kept by the
  client (Table 58-1).
- Document any environmental safety factors related to the procedure such as
  whether the needles, syringes, and medications are being stored and disposed
  of safely.

Records Kept by the Client/Family

A suggested format for records in the home is as follows:

Use one sheet for each medication.

Each sheet should contain enough spaces for at least 1 week's documentation.

Table 58-1. MEDICATION DOCUMENTATION SHEET

DRUG NAME/DESCRIPTION	SIDE-EFFECTS	INJECTION SITE/DOSE	DATE AND TIME ADMINISTERED

Health Teaching
Checklist

Name of Care Provider _____

Relationship to Client _____ Telephone #_____

Taught by _____ Date _____

	EXPLAINED	DEMONSTRATED
Environmental safety features		
Storage	_____	_____
Disposal	_____	_____
Use of aseptic technique	_____	_____

	EXPLAINED	DEMONSTRATED
Drawing solution from ampule or vial	_____	_____
Site selection	_____	_____
Injection technique	_____	_____
Documentation of medication administration	_____	_____

Product Availability

Prescribed medications are available from a pharmacy. Syringes and needles can be purchased with prescription from a pharmacy as well. If the client is unable to purchase the medications and supplies, the insurance and/or Medicare should be examined carefully. If these do not offer assistance, consultation with a social worker should be sought for other possible sources of financial assistance.

Selected References

Lewis L: Fundamental Skills in Patient Care. Philadelphia, JB Lippincott, 1984

Wolff L, Weitzel MH, Zornow RA, Zsohar H: Fundamentals of Nursing, 7th ed. Philadelphia, JB Lippincott, 1983

59   Sterile Technique

Background

In the home setting, most care will be rendered in a clean environment. However, there are cases when sterile technique will be required. Sterile means free from microorganisms and their pathogenic by-products. The principles that apply to sterile technique include the following:

All objects used in a sterile procedure should be sterile, and their sterility should be maintained throughout the procedure.

Sterile objects become contaminated when they are touched by nonsterile objects, including the nonsterile hand.

Sterile items that are out of vision or below the waistline of the care provider are considered nonsterile.

Sterile objects may be contaminated by airborne microorganisms.

Fluids flowing in the direction of gravity may contaminate the sterile portion of equipment by fluid flowing from a contaminated area, such as where an instrument is held by the hand.

Moisture that penetrates through a sterile object draws microorganisms from unclean surfaces above or below the sterile surface.

The edges of a sterile field are considered contaminated along the 1-inch edge margin.

The skin cannot be sterilized and is considered contaminated.

When the sterility of an object is in doubt, the object is to be considered contaminated.

Assessment of Self-Care Potential

Client/Family Assessment

- Assess the understanding of the client and family regarding sterile technique. Determine their understanding of disease transmission by contact. Assess any previous experience they may have had with sterile technique in or out of the hospital.
- Assess the motivation of the client and family regarding the need to perform certain procedures using sterile technique. Assess their interest in learning how to do the procedure and their willingness to take the time and care necessary to maintain sterility.

Physical Assessment

- Assess the client's condition in regard to the need for sterile technique. Determine if sterile technique is needed or if clean technique would suffice.
- Assess the client and family regarding physical ability to maintain sterile technique. If the client or family have physical infirmities, such as palsy or paralysis, they may be physically unable to perform sterile procedures.

Environmental Assessment

- Assess the physical layout of the room in which the sterile procedure will be done. Determine if additional equipment or furniture will be needed to facilitate sterile technique. For instance, a table of some type is usually needed to set up the sterile field. A TV table or bedside cabinet may be used.

Planning Strategies

Potential Nursing Diagnoses

Knowledge deficit regarding performance of sterile procedures

Expected Outcomes

Maintenance of sterility during procedure

Prevention of cross-contamination

Health Promotion Goals

- The client and family will
  Learn to differentiate between sterile and nonsterile surfaces
  Understand how to perform procedures using sterile technique
  Know what to do if sterile technique is compromised
  Prevent cross-contamination of the client or themselves

Equipment

Sterile gloves

Sterile supplies pertinent to the procedure being done

Interventions/Health Promotion

ACTION

1. Thorough handwashing is essential before doing any sterile procedure. Even if sterile gloves are worn, the majority of the bacteria on the hands must be removed before the gloves are donned. This is accomplished by handwashing.

2. Produce a sterile field from which the procedure may be done. The sterile field must contain a surface onto which all sterile items may be placed. This is best accomplished by using the inside of the wrapper of a sterile package as the sterile field (Fig. 59-1). Once an item has been removed from this field and has touched a contaminated surface, it may not be reintroduced into the sterile field.

RATIONALE/AMPLIFICATION

Sterility depends on the absence or reduction of the number of microorganisms present. Handwashing is an effective way to remove most microorganisms.

Once a sterile item touches a nonsterile surface, it is contaminated.

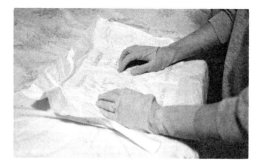

Figure 59.1

ACTION	RATIONALE/AMPLIFICATION
3. If equipment inside the sterile wrapper needs to be arranged, this can be done by means of sterile forceps or tweezers. Hold the forceps firmly and grasp the objects to be arranged. Do not replace the forceps into the sterile field when finished. Arrangement may also be done after the sterile gloves are donned.	Equipment is often packaged inside the sterile wrapper for safety and ease of storage. It must be rearranged before it can be used for the procedure. After touching the handles of the forceps, they are contaminated and may not be reintroduced into the sterile field.
4. If bottles of sterile liquid are needed for completion of the procedure, the container(s) may be set up with forceps and the liquid poured from bottles whose sides are not sterile. However, the liquid must be sterile or it will contaminate the sterile field. After the bottles are handled, the sterile gloves may be donned.	

Opening the Sterile Wrapped Package

1. Place the sterile wrapped package on a clean, dry surface. Place the package in the center of the surface so the edges will not hang over the side. If the package has been stored in a plastic container, tear where indicated and remove the sterile package before placing on the clean, dry surface.	If moisture penetrates the sterile wrapper, the package is no longer considered sterile.
2. Reach around the package and pinch the top flap on the outside of the wrapper between the thumb and forefinger. Pull the flap open, applying enough pressure to prevent the flap from returning to its original position.	Handling the outside of the wrapper protects the sterility of the inside of the wrapper.
3. Repeat with each flap, pulling it to the side toward which it opens. Open the left flap with the left hand and the right flap with the right hand.	During opening of the package, care should be taken to avoid reaching across the package because this may contaminate the contents.

ACTION	RATIONALE/AMPLIFICATION

Adding Items to the Sterile Field

1. Hold the item to be added in one hand by the outer wrapper with the upper flap away from the body. Using the other hand, open the package by grasping the outside of the flaps, pulling them away, and letting them fall to the sides (Fig. 59-2). Open the flap toward the arm last and lay the flap along the arm. With the free hand, gather the four corners of the wrap and hold them against the wrist.

The hands are contaminated and must not come into contact with the contents of the package or it is considered contaminated.

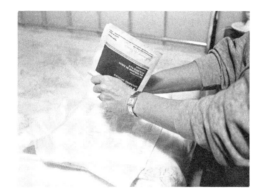

Figure 59.2

2. Drop the contents of the sterile package onto the sterile field (Fig. 59-3). Do not let any part of the flaps come in contact with the sterile field. Discard the wrapper.

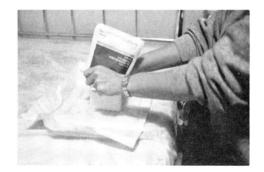

Figure 59.3

Glove Procedure

1. Place the package containing the sterile gloves on a flat surface. Open the outer package of the gloves. The outside of the package is now contaminated; however, the inside of the wrapper is still sterile. This opened wrapper may be used as the sterile field (Fig. 59-4).

The inside of the package in which the sterile gloves are wrapped will be sterile until it comes in contact with a contaminated object or becomes penetrated with a liquid.

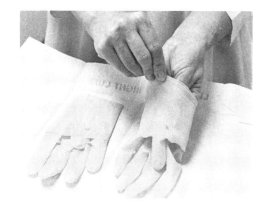

Figure 59.4

ACTION

2. The gloves should have a small (1-inch) cuff at the tops. With one hand, grasp the cuff of the opposite glove and slip the fingers of the opposite hand inside the glove. Pull the glove on by holding onto the cuff. Be careful not to contaminate the outside of the glove. Leave the cuff of the glove intact. Slip the gloved fingers under the cuff of the other glove and insert the ungloved fingers inside (Fig. 59-5). Pull the second glove on, leaving the cuff intact (Figs. 59-6 and 59-7). The areas inside the folded cuffs are considered sterile.

RATIONALE/AMPLIFICATION

Sterility is maintained as long as the bare hands touch only the inside of the gloves. The area under the cuff is sterile, so the gloved hand is not contaminated when it reaches under the cuff to pull on the second glove.

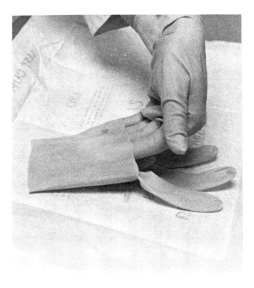

Figure 59.5

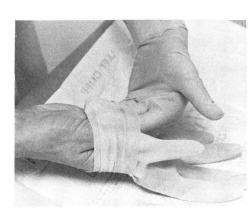

Figure 59.6

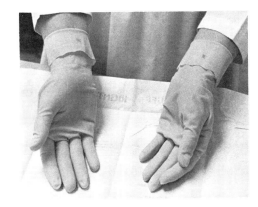

Figure 59.7

Education/ Communication

- Teach the client and family to
  Perform sterile procedures while maintaining sterile technique. Explain the procedure for opening packages and gloving.
  Understand the difference between a clean surface, a sterile surface, and a contaminated surface. Be sure that they understand the principles of sterile technique and can differentiate between what is sterile and what is not.
  Purchase supplies that meet the needs of the client. If clean supplies are adequate, they are generally less expensive than sterile supplies. However, some procedures require sterile technique. In these cases, it is dangerous to compromise in the purchase of supplies. Guide the family to avenues of financial assistance if they cannot afford the sterile supplies needed.

Evaluation of Health Promotion Activities

Quality Assurance/ Reassessment

- Observe the technique of the family and the client when sterile procedures are being done. Discuss the difference between sterile and contaminated surfaces to determine if the client and family have a good understanding of what is sterile and what is not.
- Absence of infection may be an indicator that sterile technique has been effective. The recurring wound infection or urinary infection in the catheterized client may lead to reassessment of the sterile technique involved.

Health Teaching Checklist

Name of Care Provider _____

Relationship to Client _____ Telephone #_____

Taught by _____ Date _____

	EXPLAINED	DEMONSTRATED
Handwashing	_____	_____
Sterile versus contaminated surfaces	_____	
Sterile field	_____	_____
Opening a sterile package	_____	_____
Arrangement of a sterile package	_____	_____
Sterile liquids	_____	_____
Introduction of sterile supplies into the sterile field	_____	_____
Donning of sterile gloves	_____	_____

Product Availability

Sterile gloves, packaged dressing change trays, catheter trays, and irrigation trays may be obtained at hospital-supply houses, pharmacies, and some drug stores.

60   Stump Care

Background

The term *stump* refers to that portion of an extremity remaining following an amputation procedure. While long-term care of the stump is essential for good fit of the prosthesis and for flexibility and use of the extremity, the client will, in addition, face many psychological and social adjustments such as body-image changes, experiences of phantom pain, and possibly employment change requirements. An essential element of care of the amputee, therefore, relates to psychological implications.

Assessment of Self-Care Potential

Client/Family Assessment

- Determine the willingness and ability of family members to assist the client during the initial phases of rehabilitation.
- Assess whether the client and family can meet the expenses of a prosthesis.
- Assess the client for body-image changes. Assess the family for acceptance of the altered body image.
- Determine the amount of support and teaching that will be necessary to teach and supervise the care of the stump.
- Assess the family/client to determine their commitment to total independence for the client.

Physical Assessment

- Assess the stump for irritation and/or drainage.
- Assess the stump for pain and determine if the client understands and has experienced phantom pain.
- Assess the range of motion and strength of the joint above the stump.
- Assess the client's current ability to use crutches, walker, cane, or prosthesis.

Environmental Assessment

- Note: as the client becomes skilled in using the prosthesis, necessary environmental alterations can usually be eliminated.
- Assess the home for hazards on the floors (throw rugs, etc.). In addition, assess the surfaces of the floors. If they are highly waxed they are slippery.
- Assess the areas of the home to be used by the client to determine if the furniture is arranged as simply as possible with regard to eliminating obstacles to the client.

Planning Strategies

Potential Nursing Diagnoses

Mobility, impaired physical

Body-image impairment

Joint contractures, potential

Self-care deficit

Expected Outcomes

Promotion of optimal mobility

Positive social adaptation to changes in body image

Prevention of contractures of the joint above the stump

Development of self-care abilities related to the care of the stump

Development of skill in use of the prosthesis

Total independence in daily living/job/school/lifestyle

Health Promotion Goals

- The client and family will
  Demonstrate stump dressing procedure accurately
  Observe for and report edema, redness, bleeding, and/or other drainage
  Perform recommended exercises regularly
  Verbalize feelings of anxiety, frustration, and anger as they arise
  Comply with recommendations for obtaining, fitting, and wearing the prosthesis

Equipment

One 4-inch elastic bandage

Gauze dressings (4 × 4s)

Cleansing solution: if no open sores or drainage, plain soap and water; if open sores or drainage are present, gloves and povidone-iodine solution

Receptacle for disposal of dressings

Interventions/Health Promotion

ACTION	*RATIONALE/AMPLIFICATION*
1. Wash hands and assemble equipment.	Handwashing is the most important factor in preventing cross-contamination.
2. Remove existing dressing and bandage.	The elastic bandage can be washed and reused if the elastic is still intact.
3. If open sores or drainage is present, put on gloves and cleanse area well with povidone-iodine solution.	Extreme care must be exercised to prevent spread of any existing infection to or from another household through self-contamination, or within the same household through lack of care in discarding soiled dressings or failure to wash hands.
4. If no drainage or open sores are present, wash with soap and water.	Cleanliness will assist in prevention of infection and/or irritation.
5. Rinse and dry well. Apply any prescribed medication. Apply nonadherent dressing if open sore.	It is essential to have the stump dry before applying dressings to prevent chafing.
6. Instruct the client to assume a sitting or semi-Fowler's position.	This position allows for ease in dressing the stump.
7. Apply gauze dressings to the stump loosely. Hold gauze dressings in place.	Gauze dressings provide padding between the end of the stump and the bandage.
8. Place the elastic bandage on the anterior portion of the extremity above the amputation.	If above-the-knee amputation, place Ace bandage on thigh, for example.

ACTION	*RATIONALE/AMPLIFICATION*
9. Bring bandage down diagonally to the end of the stump, around the stump, and back around the extremity above the stump, maintaining even pressure and forming a figure-8 (see Technique 45, Bandaging).	The figure-8 dressing maintains consistent pressure if properly applied and assists in preparing the stump for the proper fit of the prosthesis.
10. Bring the bandage around the extremity proximal to the joint above the stump. Continue the figure-8 until the stump is completely covered.	For an above-the-knee amputation, bring the bandage under the buttocks, front to the abdomen, and down diagonally again to the stump. For below-the-knee amputation, bring the elastic bandage from the stump to above the knee.
11. Secure the elastic bandage with clips, pins, or other securing devices.	As the stump heals, the gauze dressing may be eliminated.

Related Care

1. Keep appointments with the prosthetist and physical therapist.	The prosthetist should be actively involved in the client's rehabilitation planning.
2. Perform range-of-motion exercises of the joint adjacent to the stump on a regular basis.	These can be done actively or passively, and should incorporate the entire range of motion. Additional exercises may be recommended by the physical therapist or prosthetist.
3. Clear the environment of any articles that could serve as safety hazards to the client in the initial stages of use of the prosthesis.	Floors should not be highly waxed. Shoes should have non-skid soles and be low-heeled.
4. Assist the client and family to verbalize fears and concerns.	Altered body image creates psychological adjustment needs for both the client and family.

Age-Specific Modifications

For a child, home-bound schooling should be obtained if the rehabilitation phase is a lengthy one. However, independence in social activities should be encouraged as soon as possible.

Education/ Communication

- Teach the client and family to
  Discard soiled dressings appropriately. Elastic bandages do not have to be discarded each time. They can be laundered as long as the elastic is intact.
  Wash hands before beginning the procedure and after completing the procedure
  Wear gloves if drainage or open sores are present
  Document the condition of the end of the stump accurately
  Apply the elastic bandage with even pressure in a figure-8 configuration
  Perform the recommended exercises consistently
  Maintain level of use of the prosthesis as recommended

Focus on achieving independence as quickly as possible

Focus on the family and client's strengths rather than deficits

Referrals and Consultations

A prosthetist and physical therapist should be actively involved in the client's care from the beginning.

The state rehabilitation commission should be consulted for assistance in the purchase of the prosthesis and for employment retraining if that is necessary.

If home-bound, refer to Meals-on-Wheels and a senior citizens' group if it exists and is appropriate.

If a child, institutions such as a Shriners' hospital can assist with costs and/or services. For information, call the local Masons' Lodge or a social worker.

Evaluation of Health Promotion Activities

Quality Assurance/ Reassessment

- Visit the home initially on a daily basis to inspect the stump and to evaluate the progress of dressing, exercises, and use of the prosthesis. When the family has mastered these techniques, visits can occur on a less frequent basis.
- Note the progression toward independent functioning and acceptance of the altered body image.
- Note any experiences of phantom pain or other concerns.

DOCUMENTATION

Charting for the Home Health Nurse
- Document client/family demonstration of accurate performance of exercises and dressing changes.
- Note the quality of healing of the stump and client use of the prosthesis.
- Note attitudes toward independence and resumption of former lifestyle and social contacts.
- Document any verbalized problems related to body image, phantom pain, and other such concerns.

Records Kept by the Client/Family
Questions and concerns

Condition of the stump (e.g., presence of drainage, sores that develop, irritation)

Appointments to be kept

Health Teaching Checklist

Name of Care Provider _____

Relationship to Client _____ Telephone #_____

Taught by _____ Date _____

	EXPLAINED	DEMONSTRATED
Dressing change	_____	_____
Wrapping of stump	_____	_____
Exercises	_____	_____
Use of prosthesis	_____	

Product Availability

The prosthesis is custom fitted by a prosthetist, usually through the hospital where the amputation was performed. For replacement of prostheses, a prosthetist will again have to fit the prosthesis. Most insurances will assist with the cost of a prosthesis. If not, the vocational rehabilitation agency is consulted for direct assistance or for information as to other assistance agencies.

61 Traction

Background

Traction is applied for the purposes of immobilization and/or the application of force to a body part, usually an extremity. Traction is used to prevent movement of a body part, to decrease muscular spasm, to pull fractured or displaced bones into correct alignment, and to correct or prevent skeletal deformities.

Major types of traction are

Skin traction (Fig. 61-1): applied to the skin and soft tissue. Types are Buck's traction (using longitudinal traction with no suspension) and Russell's traction (using vectored or directional traction with balanced suspension).

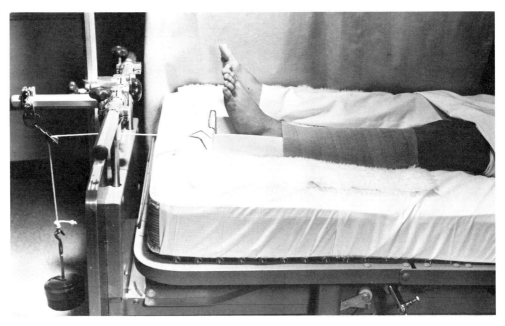

Figure 61.1
Skin traction. The client's left leg is in Buck's extension traction.

Skeletal traction (Fig. 61-2): applied by means of a pin directly to the bone or "skeletal" system. Common sites are the skull, arms, and legs. Skeletal traction is not ordinarily seen in the home.

According to body part, common types of traction are

Single leg traction: traction applied to one leg, either skeletal or skin type

Bilateral leg traction: both legs in traction, either skeletal or skin type

Pelvic: weights attached to the pelvic girdle, of skin type

Head or cervical traction: attached to the head, either skeletal or skin type

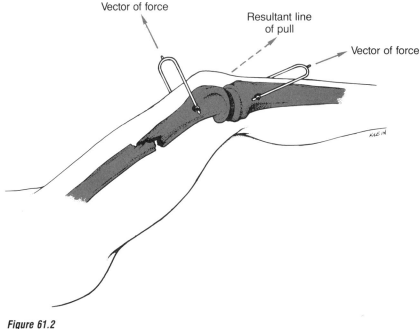

Figure 61.2
Skeletal traction. In this illustration, pins are applied to the right leg to achieve desired line of traction.

Assessment of Self-Care Potential

Client/Family Assessment

- Assess the willingness of the care provider to commit the time and energy necessary to provide the moderately extensive care required for a client in traction in the home.
- Assess the capability of the care provider to provide the care required.
- Assess the family adaptation to role change during this prolonged period, particularly if the client is the breadwinner, homemaker, or an active child who will miss school and other usual activities.
- Assess the family's financial status to determine their ability to rent needed equipment to care for the client properly.

Physical Assessment

- Assess the client's body alignment. Good alignment should be present when traction is applied.
- Assess the extremity in traction for warmth, swelling, color change, and sensation in comparison to the other extremity. Assess venous return to determine adequacy of circulation.
- Assess pressure areas of the extremity in traction for skin irritation and breakdown. Points of particular concern are the heel, the dorsalis pedis artery, the outer aspect of the calf just below the knee (the peroneal nerve lies close to the surface; compression can cause injury and foot paralysis), areas where adhesive is attached, and the sacral area of the back.
- Assess the dietary pattern of the client for fiber, protein, iron, calcium, and vitamins needed to prevent constipation.
- Daily, palpate the area over the traction tapes to detect pressure points.
- If leg traction, several times daily inspect the area over the Achilles tendon.
- If traction is of the arm, the area around the elbow where the ulnar nerve is located should not be wrapped tightly. Tension of the wrapping should be checked daily.
- Remove the wrappings three times a day and inspect the skin.
- Collect urine specimens periodically for laboratory analysis for impending renal calculi. Assess urinary output for changes in volume and character.

- Assess the traction apparatus:
  Bed position: determine if the foot is protected against footdrop. Assess if lateral support is provided to prevent external rotation of the extremity. Determine if support is provided to prevent inversion or eversion of the extremity.
  Traction device: determine if the adhesive strips are slipping at any point and if the pulleys are working freely. Inspect the ropes to determine if they are free from the bed or other obstruction. Determine if the footplate or spreaders are wide enough to prevent irritation but not so wide that the tapes tend to pull from the extremity. Note if the footplate contacts the end of the bed when the client slips down in bed. Check the knots to determine that they are securely tied. Determine if the rope is positioned to prevent it from digging into the mattress.

Environmental Assessment

- Observe the placement of the bed in the home. Since a client in traction will experience a moderately confining period of immobilization, the bed should be placed in a position conducive to psychological comfort and stimulation, such as near a window and in an area of the home where the client can participate in the daily activities of the family.
- Assess the availability of space to comfortably walk around the bed to provide work space for the care provider to bathe and/or otherwise conveniently care for the client. Adequate space must be present at the end of the bed to allow the traction device to hang freely and not encounter obstruction.
- Assess if there is adequate space near the bed to place chairs for visitors, to encourage sitting in chairs rather than on the bed (which will alter the tilt of the bed and thus the direction of pull applied to the extremity by the traction).

Planning Strategies

Potential Nursing Diagnoses

Mobility, impaired physical

Comfort, alteration in: pain

Skin integrity, potential impairment of

Alteration in bowel elimination: constipation

Expected Outcomes

Promotion of range of motion in unaffected limbs and joints

Prevention or control of pain and discomfort

Prevention of skin breakdown

Maintenance of adequate elimination patterns

Health Promotion Goals

- The client and family will
  Maintain proper functioning of the traction apparatus
  Prevent complications due to immobilization or inhibition of circulation caused by improper application or function of the traction
  Maintain physical well-being of the rest of the body by passive or active range-of-motion exercises
  Maintain usual activities of daily living within the physical limitations of the client

Equipment

If finances permit, rent or purchase a hospital bed for the period of traction application. A hospital bed will facilitate proper traction application and functioning, as well as provide various position-change capabilities.

If a hospital bed cannot be rented, a standing frame to hold weights can be rented from a home health rental agency.

Traction apparatus prescribed, to contain weights (either sandbags or waterbags, preweighted), pulleys, ropes, frames to hold the pulleys, weights, and ropes, and finally a method of securing the traction to the extremity. Skeletal traction is applied by a physician. Skin traction can be applied by a nurse or physical therapist on a physician's order.

Over-bed trapeze, hung from the frame of the bed to facilitate client movement

Interventions/Health Promotion

ACTION	RATIONALE/AMPLIFICATION
Applying Traction	
1. Inspect the skin for abrasions and/or circulatory disturbance. The extremity should be clean and dry.	The skin must be healthy to tolerate the traction.
2. Position the client in the bed in good alignment.	Good body alignment is essential for effective traction pull.
3. Pad the boney prominences with cast padding.	Padding will assist in preventing pressure sores and skin necrosis.
4. Apply foam-rubber padded straps with foam surface against the skin.	Begin at the proximal end of the extremity to be placed in traction; extend around heel (if a leg), leaving approximately 4 to 6 inches extended beyond the sole of the foot, and up the other side of the extremity.
5. Wrap an elastic bandage (Fig. 61-3) snugly and evenly around the extremity, beginning at the ankle (if a leg) and extending up to the tibial tubercle.	One person elevates and supports the leg while the other wraps it. The elastic bandage is used to secure the tape to the skin and prevent slipping.

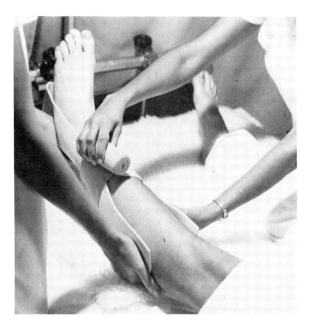
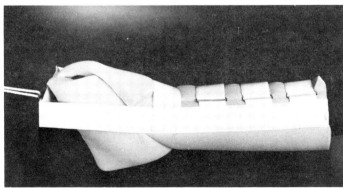

Figure 61.3
(*Left*) Applying elastic bandage over padded strips for Buck's extension skin traction. (*Right*) Another method of applying skin traction is to use the prepadded boot. (Photo of boot courtesy of All Orthopedic Appliances)

ACTION

6. Apply a spreader to the distal end of the tape.

7. Attach a rope to the spreader, pass it over a pulley at the foot of the bed (Fig. 61-4), and attach a weight to it (sand or water, either of which is premeasured). No more than 4.5 to 7 lb of traction can be used on a part with skin traction.

RATIONALE/AMPLIFICATION

This prevents pressure along the side of the foot.

Place a sheepskin under the extremity to reduce friction. Make sure the weight is secured by a knot.

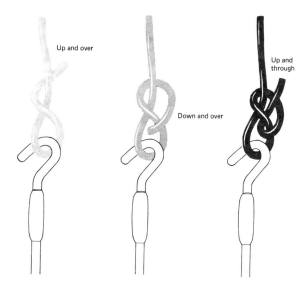

Figure 61.4
Tying traction knots correctly is essential to safe application of traction. The sequence of tying an effective knot can be remembered by memorizing "up and over, down and over, up and through." An added precaution is to secure all knots tightly with adhesive tape. (Courtesy of Zimmer Manufacturing Company)

Care of the Traction

Care relates to frequent assessments (see Physical Assessment and Environmental Assessment, earlier in this procedure).

Related Care

1. Instruct the client/family to notify the nurse if pain or related complications occur.

Common expressions of pain and the related complications are
Tingling sensation, numbness, coldness of affected part: compromise of the arterial blood supply
Numbness, tingling sensation, warmth of affected part; part is cyanotic, swollen: compromise of the venous blood return
Tingling, decreased sensitivity to heat, cold, touch; skin color and temperature are normal: local sensory nerve paralysis

ACTION	RATIONALE/AMPLIFICATION
2. Give a bed bath as frequently as desired.	Take care to keep the client's back clean and dry. The only precaution to be taken is not to allow the client's body alignment to be altered in the process of back care or bathing. This can be ensured by the use of an over-bed trapeze, instructing the client to use both hands to elevate the torso during the process of bedmaking or bathing.
3. Instruct the client/family in the use of active and passive exercises of all unaffected body parts on a frequent basis.	This enhances circulation and the prevention of emboli and produces a sense of comfort and well-being.
4. Encourage the engagement in any family activities that can include the client.	Encourage any interests or hobbies enjoyed by the client. Encourage visitors.
5. Assist the family to make temporary role changes within the family during the period of convalescence if necessary.	Efforts should be directed toward assisting with the role changes in a constructive manner, and also with the frequently occurring difficulty of role reversal following role change.
6. Increase fiber and bulk in the diet.	Constipation is a common problem. These alterations will assist in prevention.
7. Increase fluid intake to 1500 ml to 2000 ml daily.	Adequate fluid intake will help prevent renal calculi.
8. Do frequent range-of-motion exercises of all unaffected joints.	This will maintain movement and muscle tone of unaffected joints.

Age-Specific Modifications

If the child is of school age, acquire a substitute for absence from school, such as home-bound schooling.

Education/ Communication

• Teach the client and family to
  Understand the operation of the traction and the necessity to have the weights hanging freely; the ropes unincumbered by any obstacle; the knots tied securely; maintenance of the direction of traction; padding secured in all areas where skin pressure, friction, or traction might occur
  Observe for complications: expressions of pain, feelings of numbness, tingling, increased coldness or warmth of the extremity; absence of venous return to the affected extremity; diminished urinary output; constipation; irritation of back and other bony prominences
  Use the over-the-bed trapeze for assistance in lifting the torso
  Use/apply the bedpan and/or urinal if necessary
  Bathe the client in bed and give good back care

Referrals and Consultations

• Refer to a social worker if financial/employment assistance is necessary.
• Refer to the state rehabilitation commission if job retraining is needed.
• Consult with the Department of Human Services to determine availability and eligibility for participation in other local service agencies.

Evaluation of Health Promotion Activities

Quality Assurance/ Reassessment

- Make frequent home visits initially to determine the appropriate placement and pull of the traction.
- Observe the extremity for venous, arterial, or nerve interference.
- Inspect the back and sacral area to detect irritation or skin breakdown.
- Note if any difficulties are developing in the family relative to role-change or role-reversal requirements.
- Determine if financial difficulties are developing.
- Periodically bring a urine specimen to a laboratory for analysis.
- Assess the urinary and bowel elimination patterns.

DOCUMENTATION

Charting for the Home Health Nurse
- Note the presence of any complications.
- Document the status of the traction in relation to functioning of the apparatus as well as body alignment.
- Note any role change or employment problems being encountered.

Records Kept by the Client/Family
A checklist should be prepared for daily recording by the client/family. It should minimally contain the information shown in Table 61-1.

Table 61-1. TRACTION CHECKLIST

ITEM	SUN	MON	TUE	WED	THU	FRI	SAT
Bowel Movement							
Expressions of pain							
Numbness of limb							
Swelling of extremity							
Tingling of extremity							
Coldness or heat of limb							
Color changes of extremity							
Traction							
Weight hanging freely							
Ropes free							
Knots secure							
Trapeze secure							
Frame secure							
Padding in place							
Footplate in place							
Spreader in place							

Health Teaching Checklist

Name of Care Provider _____

Relationship to Client _____ Telephone #_____

Taught by _____ Date _____

	EXPLAINED	DEMONSTRATED
Collection of urine specimen	_____	
Dietary alterations	_____	
Use of trapeze	_____	_____
Active/passive exercises	_____	_____
Observation for complications	_____	
Observation of traction functioning	_____	_____
Documentation	_____	_____

Product Availability

All products needed can be rented from a hospital-supply rental agency.

Selected Reference

Brunner L, Suddarth D: Lippincott Manual of Nursing Practice, 3rd ed. Philadelphia, JB Lippincott, 1982

62   The Unna Boot

Background

The Unna boot is a gauze pressure bandage saturated with a gelatin and zinc oxide paste (some also have calamine lotion added). The purpose of the Unna boot is to promote healing of venous stasis ulcers while allowing ambulation. It in effect is a walking pressure boot.

Assessment of Self-Care Potential

Client/Family Assessment

- Assess the willingness of a family member to apply and remove the Unna boot.
- Assess the fine motor movement and coordination of the family member who will be applying and removing the Unna boot.
- Assess the availability of an alternate person to apply or remove the Unna boot if the primary assisting person cannot do so.

Physical Assessment

- Assess the stasis ulcer for depth and diameter prior to the first application of the Unna boot. Retain this information for use as baseline data.
- Assess the ulcer for inflammation, drainage, and bleeding.
- Each time the Unna boot is removed, assess the ulcer for depth, diameter, drainage, and bleeding, and compare this assessment to the baseline assessment.
- Assess the skin area under the boot for contraindications to use of the boot:
  Irritation of the skin
  Cellulitis
  Arterial ulcers
  Weeping eczema
  Foul-smelling drainage
  Cyanosis

Environmental Assessment

- Assess the home for general cleanliness. Dust or other irritants lodging in the ulcer can exacerbate the problem.

Planning Strategies

Potential Nursing Diagnoses

Health management deficit: assistance required to apply boot

Infection, potential for

Skin integrity, potential skin breakdown

Expected Outcomes

Proficiency in applying the Unna boot

Prevention of infection

Healing of the venous stasis ulcer

Health Promotion Goals

- The client and family will
  Correctly apply the Unna boot at scheduled times
  Ambulate with the Unna boot in place
  Frequently assess the affected leg for complications

Prevent complications

Cover the leg with a plastic bag while showering or bathing to prevent softening of the boot with the water

Maintain nutrition, social contacts, and independent functions of lifestyle

Equipment

Unna boot bandage (Many brands are available. The bandage must be stored at a temperature of not less than 30°F and not more than 86°F.)

A chair or stool that will allow the assistant to sit in front of the client while applying the boot

A bucket or other suitable container of warm water. It should be of sufficient size to allow the affected leg to be placed in it to soften the boot prior to removal.

Telfa or 4 × 4 gauze dressing as needed to cover the ulcerated area

A tube gauze roll or a 6-inch elastic bandage to cover the Unna boot to prevent soiling of clothing and furniture as well as to provide additional support to the leg

Interventions/Health Promotion

ACTION	RATIONALE/AMPLIFICATION
1. Apply the boot in the morning if possible. Change it every 2 to 3 days initially, then less frequently.	Applying the boot prior to ambulation is important because activity activates the boot.
2. Cleanse the leg thoroughly (shave if desired) with soap and water. Rinse the leg and dry thoroughly.	Sponging the leg with alcohol following drying provides additional dryness.
3. Instruct the client to assume a sitting position with the assisting person sitting on a stool or lower chair in front of the client. Flex the foot to a 30-degree angle.	Sitting so the client's foot can rest comfortably on the assistant's lap provides ease in the process of application.
4. Apply Telfa or a 4 × 4 gauze dressing to the ulcer if indicated.	A dressing should not be applied unless specifically ordered by the client's physician. The Unna boot is medicated with zinc oxide and sometimes calamine. The dressing will act as a barrier between the solution-impregnated boot and the ulcer.
5. Remove the Unna boot dressing from its package. Apply the boot, beginning wrapping on the inner aspect of the ankle and performing figure-8 turns (see Technique 45, Bandaging). Apply to the remainder of the leg, making overlapping turns as the bandage is moved up the leg.	Initial layers are wrapped snugly and cut or slashed frequently to aid in fit around the foot. Greatest pressure is applied at the ankle and lower third of leg. *Exercise caution not to apply it too tightly*. The bandage is not elastic and therefore has no "give."
6. Wrap the boot with tube gauze or a 6-inch elastic bandage around the leg covering the Unna boot dressing.	The covering provides additional support to the leg and protects clothing and furniture from soiling.

ACTION	**RATIONALE/AMPLIFICATION**
7. Allow the boot 30 minutes to dry prior to ambulation.	The client remains in bed or in a reclining chair with the leg elevated during the drying period. A fan or lamp can be directed on the boot to aid in drying.

Removing the Unna Boot

1. Instruct the client not to remove the boot alone.	Assistance is required for removal. If the boot is removed by the client, laceration of the skin with the scissors can easily occur.
2. Remove the elastic bandage or gauze wrap. Soak the bandaged leg in a container of warm water. After the boot has softened, unwrap it and discard.	The warm water softens the boot for ease of removal. An alternative method of removal is to cut the boot down the side of the leg with a bandage scissors. *Caution must be exercised not to damage the tender skin under the boot with the tip of the scissors.*
3. Assess the leg for complications, such as circulatory impairment and dermatologic complications, and the condition of the ulcer.	Notify the nurse or physician for guidance if any of these are noted.
4. Cleanse leg, dry thoroughly, and reapply the Unna boot.	

Related Care

1. Encourage ambulation.	Walking stimulates overall circulation. During ambulation, the boot acts as a rhythmic pump on the ankle, exerting even pressure on the leg veins.
2. Shower and/or bathe as desired.	Cover the leg snugly with a plastic bag to prevent softening of the boot with water.
3. Adhere to medication regimen as ordered.	The Unna boot is only a part of the treatment for venous stasis ulcers. Usually diuretics and antibiotics are also ordered.

Education/ Communication

- Teach the client and family to
  Remove the boot
  Assess the condition of the ulcer and remaining skin under the Unna boot.
    Comparing the measurement of the ulcer with previous measurements
      gives an indication of healing.
  Cleanse, dry, and reapply the Unna boot
  Ambulate freely
  Adhere closely to prescribed medication schedule

Evaluation of Health Promotion Activities

Quality Assurance/ Reassessment

Following return demonstration of the procedure and demonstration of ability to assess for complications, a home visit should be made the next day early in the morning to determine the accuracy of the application of the boot.

Comparisons of skin and ulcer quality and ulcer diameter to baseline data should be made frequently.

Positive reinforcement of accuracy of the procedure should be made.

DOCUMENTATION

Charting for the Home Health Nurse
- Note the presence or absence of complications.
- Document the condition of the ulcer: depth, diameter, inflammation, drainage.
- Note the adherence to prescribed medication.
- Note persistent or excessive pain.

Records Kept by the Client/Family
Questions and concerns

Condition of the ulcer: depth, diameter, inflammation, drainage

Condition of skin under the boot

Medications being taken

Health Teaching Checklist

Name of Care Provider _____

Relationship to Client _____ Telephone #_____

Taught by _____ Date _____

	EXPLAINED	DEMONSTRATED
Preparation of leg for boot application	_____	_____
Assessment of skin and ulcer condition	_____	_____
Documentation of assessment findings	_____	_____
Application of boot	_____	_____
Removal of boot	_____	_____

Product Availability

The elastic bandage can be purchased at any drug store or hospital-supply agency. The Unna boot is available from a pharmacy with a physician's prescription.

63   Wheelchair

Background

The wheelchair is the mobility aid of choice for the client who is unable to walk. It provides a means of independent mobility for a client who would otherwise be bedridden. Wheelchairs can be manually maneuvered or can be equipped with an electric motor for operation.

Assessment of Self-Care Potential

Client/Family Assessment

- Determine if the family is generally supportive of the client's mobility deficit needs and are willing and able to make necessary environmental adaptations.
- Assess the client/family's perceptions in relation to the deficit, that is, if they are oriented to achieving a high level of independence within the client's limitations or if they view the client as dependent and ill.
- Determine if a supportive family member is present and willing to assist the client during the initial learning phase of using the wheelchair.

Physical Assessment

- Determine if the client's arm and shoulder strength and coordination are sufficient to maneuver the wheelchair independently.
- Assess the client's visual acuity to determine if the client can foresee obstacles and judge depth and relative distances and widths.
- Assess the leg strength of the client to determine if it is sufficient to achieve transfer techniques in and out of the wheelchair.
- Assess the client's control of the torso to determine if props are required for good body posture while sitting in the wheelchair.
- Assess the client's desire and motivation to live as independently as possible.

Environmental Assessment

- Assess the doorways of rooms occupied and needed by the client to determine if the width is sufficient to allow passage of the wheelchair.
- If steps must be negotiated, assess the feasibility of covering them with ramps that will be relatively easy to negotiate.
- If the client must negotiate stairways inside the home, determine if it is feasible to install an elevator or other device.
- Assess the eating table, bathroom sink, and other areas needed by the client to determine if the wheelchair can approach closely enough to allow for use.
- Assess the bathroom to determine if the toilet seat is negotiable, either through transfer of the client to it or by use of a portable device applied to the toilet.
- Determine if the furniture in the home can be arranged along the walls and whether small items can be removed to allow for more convenient moving space.
- Assess the floor surfaces of the home to determine if they have either smooth surfaces that are not highly waxed or low-pile carpet.
- Determine if the telephone, stove controls, and refrigerator handle are within accessible range to the client.
- Assess the shower for accessibility. A stool with suction tips applied to the legs will assist in safety during showering. A hand-held showering device increases control of the water flow during the shower.

- Assess the floors of the home to determine if throw rugs are present and if they can be removed.
- Assess the bed to determine the possibility of installing an over-bed trapeze to aid in transfer techniques in and out of the bed.
- If strength in the legs is insufficient to accomplish transfer maneuvers, assess the bed area, bathroom, and other areas frequented by the client to determine if there is sufficient space to accommodate a mechanical lift to assist in transfer procedures.

Planning Strategies

Potential Nursing Diagnoses

Mobility, impaired physical

Body-image disturbance

Family processes, alterations in

Expected Outcomes

Resumption of independent activities of daily living

Environmental adaptation to provide optimal mobility opportunity

Promotion of an acceptable body image

Maintenance of supportive family relations

Health Promotion Goals

- The client and family will
  Develop adequate strength and coordination in upper body and arms to negotiate wheelchair and transfer procedures safely
  Master the technique of independent wheelchair mobility
  Demonstrate safe transfer techniques
  Make necessary environmental adaptations within the financial constraints of the family
  Contact medical-equipment rental agencies for assistance with equipment
  Contact social service agencies if needed for assistance with transportation, meals, finances, and job retraining and rehabilitation devices
  Maintain good nutrition, regular bowel habits, and normal urinary functioning

Equipment

Wheelchair with brakes and removable armrests and legrests if the client is unable to stand during the process of transfer procedures

Mechanical lift if general body weakness or disability is present

Pillows to prop the client if proper body positioning or comfort cannot be maintained without pillows

Transfer board to assist with transfer procedures if the client is unable to transfer independently or if a mechanical lift or assistant is unavailable

Interventions/Health Promotion

ACTION	RATIONALE/AMPLIFICATION
Demonstrate the appropriate transfer technique if the client is unable to transfer independently.	Transferring in and out of the wheelchair can be done safely by a lift method or a pivot method.
Lifting Technique	
	This technique is *not* used if the client is able to assist or move independently.

ACTION

1. Position the wheelchair parallel to the bed, brakes locked, armrest near the bed removed. If the bed is a hospital one, elevate it above the level of the chair and raise the head of the bed.

2. Cross the client's hands over the chest. One assistant stands behind the client, sliding hands beneath the client's axillae and grasping the client's wrists. The other assistant stands to the side of the client in front of the wheelchair and lifts under the client's knees and thighs.

3. At a signal given by one of the assistants, lift the client over the wheelchair and lower slowly into a sitting position.

4. Replace the armrest. Position the client to ensure good body alignment, comfort, and safety. Place a cover over the legs if the client desires. Support the dependent parts. Apply a waist restraint if the client is unable to support the body weight with good alignment.

Pivot Technique

1. Position wheelchair parallel to bed, facing the head of the bed, and, if possible, on the client's stronger side. Remove legrests and apply brake.

2. Bring client to a sitting position on the side of the bed, as close as possible to the front of the wheelchair.

3. Stand in front of the client. Put arms around the client under the axillae and clasp hands behind the client's back. Instruct the client to use the legs (or strong leg) to assist in rising to a standing position.

RATIONALE/AMPLIFICATION

Apply the brakes for safety. Removing the armrests and elevating the bed reduce the energy required to perform the transfer.

This allows full support of dependent parts as well as a feeling of security.

The two assistants must move in unison so that the weight of the client is evenly distributed and the client feels secure.

Proper body alignment, comfort, and safety prevent complications due to immobilization, undue pressure, and poor body alignment.

This technique is used when there is only one assistant available. It can be used to transfer a client from wheelchair to toilet, wheelchair to car, wheelchair to bed, wheelchair to shower, and return to wheelchair.

Proper positioning minimizes the distance of the move and ensures safety.

Ask the client to assist as much as possible to increase independent functioning and reduce muscular strain to the assistant.

ACTION	RATIONALE/AMPLIFICATION
4. Allow a few seconds for the client to gain equilibrium. The assistant and client then pivot together so the client's back is turned to the chair. Instruct the client to grasp the armrests to assist in lowering the body into the wheelchair (Fig. 63-1).	A short pause is often necessary to ensure balance following a major position change.

Maneuvering Techniques

ACTION	RATIONALE/AMPLIFICATION
1. For going down a ramp, if the ramp is not steep, maneuver the wheelchair down the ramp in a normal manner. If the ramp is steep, turn the wheelchair around and descend the ramp backward.	Descending a steep ramp facing the normal way may create a hazard, such as the client falling out of the wheelchair or the feeling of falling out.
2. Climbing and descending a curb or one step. *Ascending:* maneuver the wheelchair to the edge of the curb or step. With hands on the handles and one foot on the foot brace at the back of the wheelchair, tip the wheelchair back to a height to raise the front wheels over the curb or step. Then ease the large wheels up on the curb or step. *Descending:* turn the wheelchair around so the back of the wheelchair is facing the curb. Ease the large wheels down, followed by the small wheels.	Turning the wheelchair around prevents accidentally falling from the wheelchair. Perform each of these maneuvers gently to prevent a "jerky" and insecure feeling for the client.

Related Care

ACTION	RATIONALE/AMPLIFICATION
1. Use caution going through narrow spaces and approach them slowly.	Since the hands are on the outside of the wheel, it is easy to skin them on narrow doorways or other passageways. If this persists as a problem, the client may wish to wear gloves until maneuvering mastery is achieved.
2. Take measures to prevent constipation caused by limitation of exercise.	Adequate bulk and fiber in the diet, active and passive exercises, and adequate fluid intake assist in achieving regular bowel elimination.
3. Administer skin care on a regular basis.	Pressure areas can occur from sitting in one position for long periods of time as well as from improper positioning.
4. Encourage desired diversionary activities (visitors, senior citizens center, social activities, etc.).	Use these as a means to discourage isolation and dependence.
5. Adapt the environment to encourage independent functioning.	See Environmental Assessment, earlier in this technique.

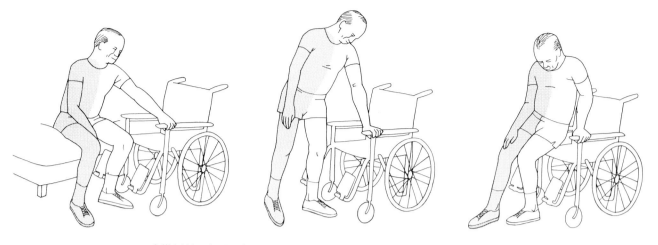

A. Weight-bearing transfer from bed to chair. The patient stands up, pivots until his back is opposite the new seat, and sits down.

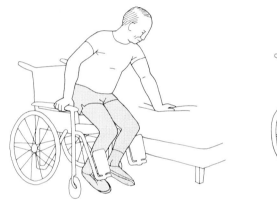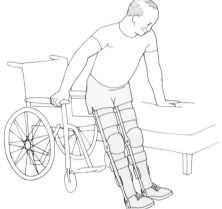

B. (*Left*) Non-weight-bearing transfer from chair to bed. (*Right*) With legs braced.

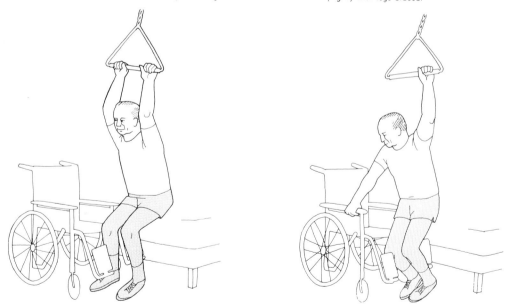

C. (*Left*) Non-weight-bearing transfer, pull-up method (*Right*). Non-weight-bearing transfer, combined method.

Figure 63.1
Independent transfer from bed to wheelchair. The wheelchair is in a locked position. (Redrawn from Hirschberg GG, Lewis L, Vaughan P: Rehabilitation, Philadelphia, JB Lippincott)

ACTION	*RATIONALE/AMPLIFICATION*

Age-Specific Modifications

1. For a child, rent or purchase a pediatric-size wheelchair.

2. For a child or teenager, contact the school district for assistance with home-bound schooling or school attendance.

Education/ Communication

- Teach the client and family to
  Make environmental adaptations as finances permit:
  Bathroom: create access to toilet, shower, wash basin; apply suction tips to a stool to create stability in the shower; apply a hand-held shower device; remove throw rugs or other obstacles from the floor.
  Dining area: create access to dining table; move furniture to provide maneuverability of wheelchair.
  Steps and stairways: provide ramps or elevating device.
  Bedroom: rearrange furniture for maneuverability of wheelchair.
  Floors: remove obstacles and throw-rugs; if purchasing floor covering, obtain smooth covering such as linoleum or low-pile carpet.
  Teach transfer techniques (from bed to wheelchair and other transfers needed to accomplish independent functioning). Encourage as much independence as possible. Rent or purchase a mechanical lift if the client is unable to transfer alone and assistants are not easily available.
  Provide active and/or passive exercises. See Technique 1 for active/passive exercises.

Referrals and Consultations

- Refer to the state rehabilitation commission if the mobility deficit is a lengthy one and job retraining or employment alterations are necessary.

Evaluation of Health Promotion Activities

Quality Assurance/ Reassessment

- Visit the home periodically to assess safe use of the wheelchair.
- Assess pressure areas for skin irritation and/or breakdown.
- Assess bowel and urinary functions. Note if active/passive exercises and dietary alterations need to be made.
- Assess the independent functioning of the client in regard to daily home activities as well as school and/or work responsibilities.

DOCUMENTATION

Charting for the Home Health Nurse
- Note client success in mastering wheelchair maneuverability and transfer techniques.
- Note any difficulties related to activities of daily living and job performance. Document provisions made for assistance in those areas and whether they have been accomplished.
- Note results of surveillance of skin care, urinary and bowel status, and dietary and exercise recommendations.

Records Kept by the Client/Family
Any questions or concerns related to care, wheelchair use, transfers, or referrals

Any indication of bowel, urinary, or skin complications

Health Teaching Checklist

Name of Care Provider _____

Relationship to Client _____ Telephone # _____

Taught by _____ Date _____

	EXPLAINED	DEMONSTRATED
Maneuvering of wheelchair	_____	_____
Transfer procedures	_____	_____
Climbing and descending curbs or one step	_____	_____
Environmental adaptations	_____	_____
Skin care	_____	_____
Active/passive exercises	_____	_____

Product Availability

Wheelchairs, over-the-bed trapezes, mechanical lifts, toilet adaptation devices, and waist restraints are available for purchase or rent through any medical-supply rental/purchase firm.

Selected Reference

Nursing Photobook: Providing Early Mobility. Springhouse, PA, Springhouse Corporation, 1984

64　Walker

Background

A walker is an ambulation assistive device. Walkers are available with or without wheels, are adjustable in height, and are available in collapsible types for ease in travel. Most walkers are made of light-weight aluminum.

Assessment of Self-Care Potential

Client/Family Assessment

- Assess the willingness and ability of the care provider to provide support and assistance to the client during the early use of the walker until the client feels competent in its independent use.
- Assess the willingness and ability of the family to make necessary environmental alterations to assist in the safe and convenient use of the walker by the client.

Physical Assessment

- Assess the client's arm strength and hand grip. Some strength in the arms and ability to grip will be necessary to manipulate the walker and lift it with each step.
- Assess the balance and coordination of the client.
- Assess the leg strength of the client.
- Determine the height of the client for use in adjusting the height of the walker.

Environmental Assessment

- Assess the living and social environment of the client to determine if steps must be climbed. One step can be easily mastered. Climbing more than one step requires personal assistance or the installation of a ramp.
- Assess the environment for the presence of a strong, sturdy, comfortable chair with strong armrests and a broad base, to provide assistance to the client while rising and sitting.
- Assess the doorways, hallways, and bathroom area to determine if adequate space is available for easy manipulation of the walker by the client.
- Determine if the vehicle in which the client will ride can accommodate the walker and if the client can get in and out of the vehicle comfortably. The seat on which the client sits should be next to a door. The height of the vehicle should be low and manageable.

Planning Strategies

Potential Nursing Diagnoses

Mobility, impaired physical

Body image disturbance

Expected Outcomes

Independent and safe use of the walker

Resumption of former daily activities with little alteration

Family adjustment to necessary adjustment in lifestyle

Promotion of an acceptable body image

Equipment

Appropriate walker

Shoes with non-skid soles and a broad heel base

Secure, comfortable chair with strong armrests

Interventions/Health Promotion

ACTION

1. Select the appropriate walker:

   The stationary walker (Fig. 64-1).

RATIONALE/AMPLIFICATION

Consult a physical therapist if desired.

This walker is light-weight and inexpensive. It has handgrips and no movable parts. It is available in a collapsible form for ease of storage and travel. The client must have *good balance and arm strength* to use this walker. A *three-point-and-one gait* is used with this walker.

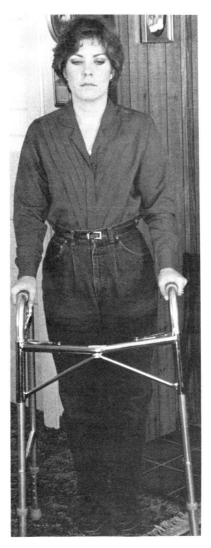

Figure 64.1
Client using a walker of appropriate height.

ACTION	RATIONALE/AMPLIFICATION
The reciprocal walker	This walker is light-weight and has handgrips, four legs, and a *hinge mechanism allowing one side to be advanced ahead of the other.* It is more stable than the stationary walker and therefore can be used with clients having *decreased arm strength and balance.* Clients using the reciprocal walker use a *two-point or four-point gait.* It is adjustable in height.
The rolling walker	This walker has four wheels and is larger, heavier, and more expensive than the stationary or reciprocal walkers. It can be equipped with a seat and a flexible backrest. It is adjustable in height. It is recommended with caution, since it is *hazardous for clients lacking coordination and balance.* The seat must also be adjusted to height, with the knees and hips flexing at 90 degrees in the sitting position.
2. Adjust the height of the walker.	The height of the walker is determined by having the client stand behind the rear legs of the walker, holding the hand grips. The walker should come to the client's hip joint with elbows flexed approximately 30 degrees.
3. Advise the client to wear non-skid shoes with a broad-based heel.	Supportive shoes assist in preventing falls.
4. Until the client is walking independently, apply a strong belt around the client's waist during walking practice.	This allows the assistant to stand at the client's side, holding the belt to offer assistance.
5. Instruct the client to look straight ahead while walking rather than at the feet.	This improves posture while walking.
6. Teach the appropriate gait (one of the following).	The gait may have been prescribed by a physical therapist.

The Two-Point Gait (Fig. 64-2)

The client begins by standing with weight evenly distributed between legs and the walker. One side of the walker is simultaneously advanced with the opposite foot. The client continues in the same manner, alternating sides.	This gait is used with a reciprocal walker.

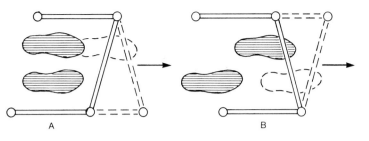

Figure 64.2
Two-point gait.

ACTION	RATIONALE/AMPLIFICATION

The Four-Point Gait (Fig. 64-3)

This gait is done in four steps. Begin with weight evenly distributed between walker and legs:

1. Move left side of walker forward.
2. Move right foot forward.
3. Move right side of walker forward.
4. Move left foot forward.

Continue in same manner.

This gait is used with a reciprocal walker.

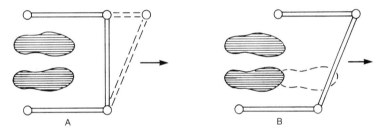

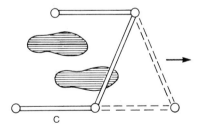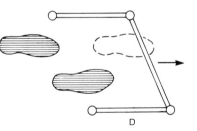

Figure 64.3
Four-point gait.

ACTION	RATIONALE/AMPLIFICATION

The Three-Point Gait (Non-weight-Bearing) (Fig. 64-4)

Begin with weight distributed evenly between the unaffected leg and the walker.

This gait is used with a stationary walker.

1. Shift weight to unaffected leg.
2. Lift and advance walker.
3. Using arms, bear all weight on the walker. Swing the unaffected leg forward.

Repeat in same manner.

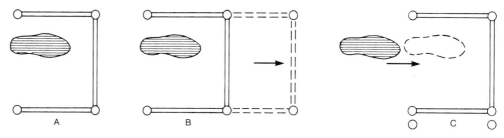

Figure 64.4
Three-point gait.

The Three-Point-and-One Gait (Partial Weight-Bearing) (Fig. 64-5)

Begin with weight distributed mostly on the strong leg and the walker (some weight will be borne on the affected leg).

Used with a stationary walker.

1. Shift all weight to the unaffected leg.
2. Move the walker and the affected leg simultaneously.
3. Shift weight to unaffected leg and walker.
4. Move unaffected leg forward.

Continue in same manner.

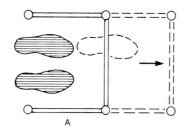 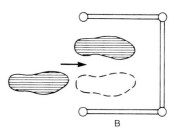

Figure 64.5
Three-point-and-one gait.

ACTION	*RATIONALE/AMPLIFICATION*

Sitting and Rising From the Sitting Position

1. Instruct the client to stand in front of the chair so the backs of the legs touch the seat of the chair. The weight is shifted primarily to the stronger leg. Place the weaker leg behind the other. Grasp the armrests with the hands. Bearing weight on the armrests and the legs, lower the body into the chair. Place the walker beside the chair.

Bearing weight on the armrest assists with balance as the body is lowered into the chair.

Establishing a habit of moving the walker to the side of the chair is for convenience of the client and safety of others walking near the client's chair.

2. For rising from the sitting position, position the walker in front of the client. Place the right leg under the chair with the left leg forward. Slide the body forward in the chair. Distribute the body weight between the arms and legs, raising the body up to a standing position. Support the body with the left hand and right foot, and grasp the walker with the right hand. The client is then ready to ambulate with the walker.

Using the strength of both arms and legs increases the balance and coordination until a standing position is assumed.

Related Care

1. Apply a device with armrests to the toilet.

The armrests will assist in rising and sitting.

2. Install a stool with rubber suction cups on the legs in the shower.

The suction tips prevent slipping while showering.

3. Mount a container such as a basket or other container to the front crossbar of the walker.

These will allow items to be carried while using the walker.

4. If desired, purchase a set of long tongs with magnetic tips.

This device can be used for picking up small items such as needles and pins.

Education/ Communication

- Teach the client and family to
  Function as independently as possible. The normal routine of living should be resumed as closely as possible. Travel in a car and social engagements should be encouraged.
  Use the appropriate gait with the walker
  Rise and sit safely
  Make environmental alterations as necessary: remove obstructing items from the areas used by the client; install a ramp in areas where there are more than two steps.

Referrals and Consultations

- Refer to the state rehabilitation commission if assistance in job retraining is needed and for the latest developments in assistive devices and rehabilitation technology.
- Refer to a physical therapist for assistance with walker selection and gait.

Evaluation of Health Promotion Activities

Quality Assurance/ Reassessment

- Periodically visit the home to assess the safe and effective use of the walker.
- Reassess the home to determine if recommended environmental alterations have been made and if additional ones should be made.
- Determine if the client and family are resuming their usual social contacts and former lifestyles as much as possible.

DOCUMENTATION

Charting for the Home Health Nurse

Progress of the client in achieving the gait recommended, and sitting and rising procedures

Questions and concerns verbalized by the client/family

Progress in making environmental alterations

Records Kept by the Client/Family

Questions and concerns

Occurrences of any accidents (falls, slipping, etc.)

Health Teaching Checklist

Name of Care Provider _____

Relationship to Client _____ Telephone #_____

Taught by _____ Date _____

	EXPLAINED	DEMONSTRATED
Appropriate gait technique	_____	_____
Sitting and rising from sitting	_____	_____
Safety factors	_____	_____

Product Availability

The walker can be rented or purchased from a hospital-supply firm. A basket to attach to the walker to contain items being carried can also be obtained from a hospital-supply firm.

Selected Reference

Nursing Photobook: Providing Early Mobility. Springhouse, PA, Springhouse Corporation, 1984

65   Wound Care

Background

A wound is a break in the integrity of the body tissue. It may be internal (closed) or external (open). A wound is clean when it does not contain any pathogenic organisms. Wounds may also be contaminated or infected. Wounds cannot be considered sterile since normal flora that inhabits the skin is present in the wound. The normal response of the body to wounds is inflammation, a condition characterized by swelling, redness, heat, pain, and impaired function of the involved part. Inflammation is a natural attempt of the body to destroy or dilute the invading agent, repair damage, and prevent the spread of the condition. The goal of wound care is to prevent infection and hasten healing.

Assessment of Self-Care Potential

Client/Family Assessment

- Assess the familiarity of the client and family with wound care. Determine if any of them have had previous experience with surgical procedures.
- Assess the ability of the family and client to tend to the wound. Some persons are very squeamish about the sight of wounds and blood.

Physical Assessment

- Assess the extent of wound healing and any potential or present problems. Determine the cause of the wound and the stage of healing.
- Assess the extent of the wound or incision in relation to the client's level of activity to determine which type of dressing will achieve the desired purpose.
- Assess the skin around the wound to determine if the dressing itself is causing any problems. Determine if the dressing may be too tight or if the client may be exhibiting an allergy to the tape used.

Environmental Assessment

- Assess the area where the procedure will be done to determine if lighting is adequate. Determine if there is a table or cabinet on which the sterile supplies may be placed with reasonable security.

Planning Strategies

Potential Nursing Diagnoses

Actual impairment of skin integrity

Activity intolerance

Alteration in comfort due to pain (acute)

Expected Outcomes

Prevention of infection

Satisfactory healing of wound

Return of client to previous level of activity

Control of pain

Health Promotion Goals

- The client and family will
  Change the dressing in such a manner as to prevent complications and promote healing

Understand the principles of sterile technique in changing the dressing
Feel comfortable about activity expectations and care of the wound
Understand the importance of exercise and nutrition in proper wound healing

Equipment

Sterile dressing tray (available commercially) or
Sterile forceps, hemostats, or tweezers
Waxed or plastic bag or disposal of the contaminated dressing
Sterile saline (if the dressing tends to adhere to the wound)
Sterile towel
Antiseptic cleanser
Gauze pads or cotton balls
Sterile gloves
Dressings
Tape
Additional equipment needed for T-tube wound care
Soap
Povidone-iodine solution and ointment
Swabs
Alcohol and hydrogen peroxide
Velcro belt
Sterile, disposable paper cloth
Sterile 4 × 4 gauze pads (5)
Additional equipment needed for suture or skin staple removal
Sterile scissors or skin staple remover
Sterile skin strips

Interventions/Health Promotion

ACTION	*RATIONALE/AMPLIFICATION*
1. Explain to the client what will happen during the dressing change. It may be necessary to remind the client not to move suddenly or to touch the wound area each time the dressing is changed.	If the client moves during the dressing change or touches the wound area, contamination of the incision site may occur.
2. Prevent cross-contamination by careful handwashing before and after the dressing change. Loosen the tape and remove the outer dressing by touching the surface only. Place the outer dressing in a waxed or plastic bag and set it in an accessible place out of the dressing change area. Be careful not to dislodge drains when removing dressings (Fig. 65-1).	Handwashing has proven to be one of the best methods of controlling the spread of infection. The inner aspect of the dressing is contaminated and should not be touched. The bag should not be permeable so that drainage from the dressing will be contained.

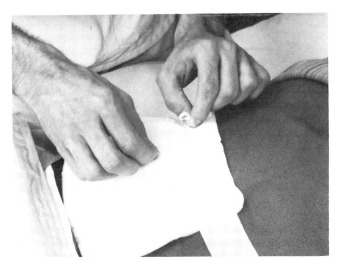

Figure 65.1

ACTION

3. Open the sterile hemostats, forceps, or tweezers and use the instrument to remove the inner dressing from the wound. These forceps are now contaminated and should not be placed near the sterile area. Place the dressing in the waxed or plastic bag (Figs. 65-2 and 65-3).

RATIONALE/AMPLIFICATION

The wound is considered contaminated and anything that comes in contact with it is contaminated. If the dressing adheres to the wound, a small amount of sterile saline may be poured over the area to facilitate removal.

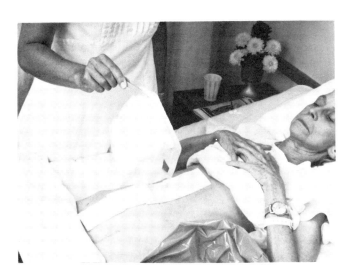

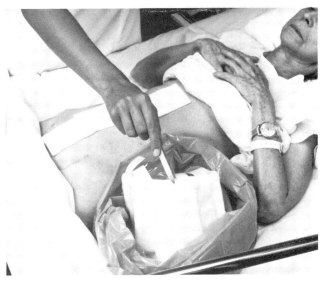

Figure 65.2   *Figure 65.3*

ACTION

RATIONALE/AMPLIFICATION

4. Open the sterile towel on the bedside table or on the corner of the bed where it is within reach but not in danger of being contaminated. Open the sterile gauze pads or cotton balls onto the sterile towel. Pour some of the antiseptic onto the pads. Don sterile gloves and use the gauze pads or cotton balls to clean the wound area. Clean from the wound outward for an area of 2 inches. Use a new sterile pad for each stroke. A sterile applicator may be used to clean the wound (Fig. 65-4). Sterile forceps may be used to perform this cleansing procedure if a second pair is present; however, do not reintroduce the original pair into the sterile field because they are contaminated once they touch the contaminated dressing.

The sterile towel provides a sterile field on which new items may be introduced without contaminating them. The cotton balls should not be saturated heavily or the antiseptic will soak through the sterile towel. Once a sterile cloth has been saturated with liquid, it is no longer considered sterile. The wound is cleaned with an outward movement to prevent bringing contamination into the wound site.

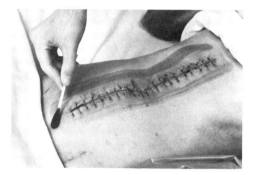

Figure 65.4

5. Cover the wound with a dry, sterile dressing (Fig. 65-5). A nonpenetrable or nonstick substance, such as a Telfa pad, may be used next to the skin to reduce the chance of the dressing sticking to the wound. The next layer of the dressing should be thick enough to absorb drainage (Fig. 65-6). However, large bulky dressings should be avoided. Change the dressing more frequently, if necessary, using a moderate dressing each time. Extra padding may be needed over drains.

A dry, sterile dressing inhibits the growth of microorganisms. If the wound can be prevented from sticking to the dressing, there will be less trauma when the dressing is removed. Large, bulky dressings inhibit movement, are uncomfortable, and encourage the growth of microorganisms since they tend to be changed less frequently. To decrease the chance of cross-contamination, dress the suture line before dressing the drain site.

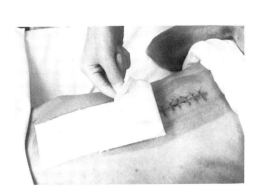

Figure 65.5

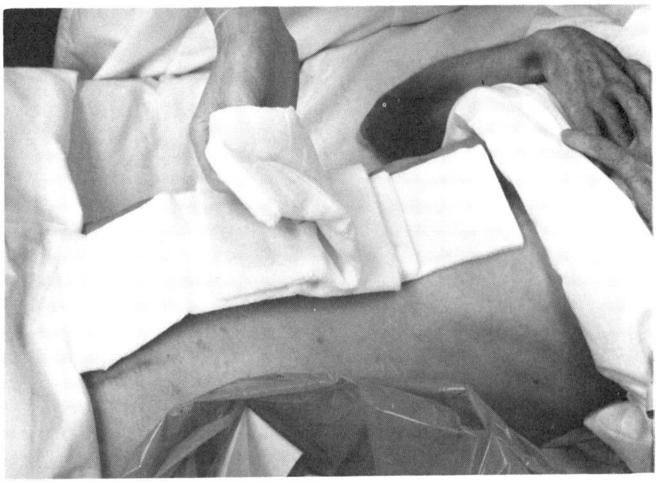

Figure 65.6

ACTION

6. Secure the dressing with some type of tape. Silk and paper tape cause less skin reaction and are easier to remove. If frequent dressing changes are necessary, Montgomery strips may be applied. Place the strips on both sides of the wound with the holes facing the wound (Fig. 65-7). Lace gauze strings through the holes and tie them in the center to the dressing over the wound (Fig. 65-8). To remove the dressing, untie the gauze, change the dressing, and retie. These strips are commercially available or may be made from 1-inch or 2-inch tape.

RATIONALE/AMPLIFICATION

The dressing must remain in place to prevent contamination of the wound site. Montgomery strips can prevent trauma to the surrounding tissue, which can occur when tape is applied and removed frequently.

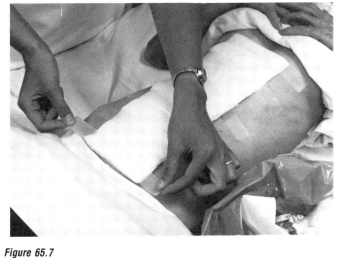

Figure 65.7

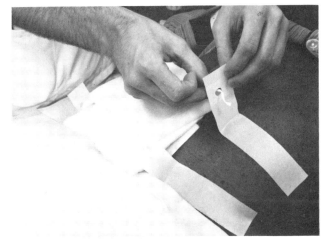

Figure 65.8

ACTION	*RATIONALE/AMPLIFICATION*
7. Remove the waxed or plastic bag containing the soiled dressing. Tape the top shut and dispose of this bag in the trash. Wash hands when the dressing change is finished.	The soiled dressing may contain organisms that are pathogenic if introduced into the environment of the home. Handwashing will decrease the chance of cross-contamination.

Related Care

Dehiscence or Evisceration

If the integrity of the wound is interrupted and the suture line breaks open, cover the area with sterile towels soaked in sterile saline. Notify the surgeon at once.	Dehiscence is the sudden breaking open of the suture line. Evisceration is the protrusion of the viscera through an abdominal incision. Both of these are emergencies requiring prompt surgical intervention.

Suture or Staple Removal

1. Remove the dressing and cleanse the incision. Inspect incision area to ensure that there is no break in the integrity of the suture line before removing sutures or staples.	Removal of sutures and staples depends on the development of enough tension for the wound to remain closed without the support of the sutures or staples. Silk sutures should be removed in 6 to 8 days to prevent scars.
2. With a sterile forceps or hemostat, grasp the suture and elevate it so that the portion of suture below the knot is clearly visible. With sterile scissors, cut the suture below the knot (Fig. 65-9). Avoid cutting the knot. Succeeding interrupted sutures are removed by repeating the cutting process for each suture. Succeeding continuous sutures are removed in the same manner, except that each portion to be cut is grasped by the suture itself since there is no knot for each stitch.	Direct visualization allows cutting at the proper position. Cutting the suture near the point of insertion into the skin prevents drawing the contaminated exposed portion of the suture through the tissues.

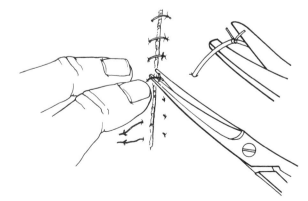

Figure 65.9

ACTION	*RATIONALE/AMPLIFICATION*
3. Remove the suture in a smooth continuous motion. Remove every other suture from one end of the incision to the other. Check to see if the tension on the wound causes any problems. If the suture line seems stable, remove the remainder of the sutures. Reinforce the suture line with the application of small adhesive strips applied directly to the skin over the suture line.	If the wound begins to separate after the removal of part of the supporting suture line, there is a good chance that it will be even more compromised with the removal of additional sutures since tension on the suture line will be increased. Sutures may be replaced with small wound closure strips, which provide the needed support until healing is sufficient.
4. Remove skin staples with a staple remover in one motion. Place the staple remover between the staple and the skin and gently pull the staple from the skin. Remove every other staple to check for incision line integrity.	If the incision begins to open after the removal of several of the staples, leave the remainder in place and notify the physician. Complete removal may cause dehiscence.

T-Tube Care

1. Wash hands. Remove the soiled dressing and place in the sack.	Prevent the chance of cross-contamination.
2. Prepare a sterile field with a sterile towel or sterile paper. Open the 4 × 4 pads onto the sterile surface. Open the bottles of cleansers (the alcohol, sterile saline, and the hydrogen peroxide) and place the lids with their tops down. Pour a small amount of the solutions on three different 4 × 4 pads.	The sterile towel or paper will offer a location in which sterile equipment may be kept in readiness for use during the procedure. This prevents delays.
3. Don sterile gloves. With the saline pad, wash around the wound site with a motion moving outward from the point of insertion of the T tube in a circular fashion to a point about 3 inches (7.5 cm) from the wound. Repeat the procedure using the hydrogen peroxide pad.	Once a gloved hand comes in contact with the skin, wound, or drainage, it is no longer sterile and should not be reintroduced into the sterile field. The skin is cleaned from the wound outward to reduce the risk of bringing pathogenic microorganisms from the skin into the wound area.
4. With the alcohol pad, wipe the tubing itself from the point of insertion away from the body for about 6 inches (15 cm).	Alcohol is an effective antiseptic when cleaning equipment. Cleaning proceeds away from the incision site to reduce the chance of cross-contamination.
5. Wipe the wound with the povidone-iodine swabs, cleaning outward from the wound. Apply the povidone-iodine ointment to the wound by squeezing the packet and letting the ointment drop onto the wound. Spread the ointment over the wound area with a dry 4 × 4.	Medicated ointments will help prevent infection during healing.

ACTION	RATIONALE/AMPLIFICATION
6. Open the remaining 4 × 4 and completely encircle the T tube at the wound site. Tape this dressing to the abdomen. Also, tape a section of the tubing itself to the abdomen.	The gauze dressing will absorb any drainage from the incision. If the T tube is taped to the abdomen, pressure on the insertion site is reduced and the chance of inadvertent removal is reduced.

Age-Specific Modifications

1. Infants and small children may require restraint in order to keep the dressing intact and in place. Avoid large, bulky dressings.	Infants do not understand the need for dressings to remain in place. Restraint of the hands with some room for mobility may solve the problem.
2. Place a cylindrical piece of stockinette or an old stocking or nylon hose with the end cut off over the infant's hand. Tape the material securely in place, being careful not to compromise circulation. Fold the material back over itself, pulling it over the infant's hand. Tie the long end of the stocking or stockinette to the bed frame or pin it to the sheet (Fig. 65-10). Allow the infant as much freedom of movement as possible without jeopardizing the dressing.	The infant's hands and fingers are enclosed within the cylinder of the stocking or stockinette so that fingers cannot handle and pull tubes and dressings. This method may also be used on confused adults.

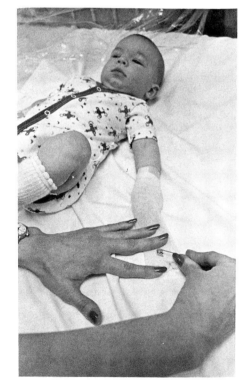

Figure 65.10

Education/ Communication	• Teach the client and family to Feel comfortable with the fact that the suture line will hold during activity. Fear of the suture line breaking may create tension and anxiety and may cause the client to become immobile. Since the immobility itself may cause complications after surgery, it is imperative to convince the client and family that sufficient tension has been applied to the wound by the sutures to prevent breaking when the client turns, coughs, hyperventilates, and moves about the area. Wear loose-fitting clothing over the dressing so that the wound site will not be irritated nor will drains be occluded. If the client has a T tube, good clothing should not be worn while it is draining because the bile stains clothing. Explain that these stains may be removed by soaking the garment in a combination of detergent, baking soda, and bleach. Maintain proper hygiene during the time the dressing is worn just as at other times. A shower is generally preferable to a tub bath to reduce the risk of bacteria entering the wound area. Recommend that the period immediately after the shower is a good time to do wound care. Avoid heavy lifting and strenuous activities that might strain the incision or drain site. Teach incisional splinting (holding a pillow against the incision area) to be used when the client needs to cough or sneeze. Understand postoperative care of the wound regarding significant signs and symptoms that should be reported. If bright red blood is noted on the dressing, particularly during the first 48 hours after surgery, hemorrhage may be occurring. The surgeon should be notified. Painful swelling, low-grade fever, and purulent drainage may signify infection and should be reported. Care for the T-tube drainage bag. Advise that the drainage bag be emptied at the same time each day. Show the client how to drain the bag by releasing the spout at the bottom of the bag. Caution against releasing the T tube from the connecting tube since this can be an avenue of infection. Demonstrate how the client may coil up the connecting tubing. A Velcro belt may be used to secure the tubing and the drainage bag to the abdomen. Emphasize the importance of securing the drainage bag at a level below the incision site so that gravity will drain the bile through the T tube into the bag and not from the bag back into the T tube, which may cause infection.

Evaluation of Health Promotion Activities

Quality Assurance/ Reassessment	• Prevention of infection is a good indicator of the success of the dressing change procedure. • Observe the client and family changing the dressing. Determine if they understand the principles of sterile technique. Ask them to point out what is sterile and what is contaminated. Observe if they reintroduce contaminated objects into the sterile field. • A progressive record of the condition of the wound and the amount and appearance of the drainage will offer insight into the effectiveness of the healing process.
DOCUMENTATION	*Charting for the Home Health Nurse* • Chart the condition of the wound and the amount and appearance of drainage at each visit. • Note any undesirable side-effects along with the name of the person to whom they were reported. • Note the date of suture removal and the condition of the wound thereafter.

Records Kept by the Client/Family

The client should keep a record of how many times the dressing is changed every day. The approximate amount of drainage should be noted in relation to the previous day. In most cases, drainage should gradually diminish until it disappears. Recording should especially note if there is a sudden increase in drainage. If the client has any type of drain bag that is emptied regularly, the amount and characteristics of drainage should be recorded.

Health Teaching Checklist

Name of Care Provider _____

Relationship to Client _____ Telephone # _____

Taught by _____ Date _____

	EXPLAINED	DEMONSTRATED
Sterile technique	_____	_____
Dressing change		
Removal of outer dressing	_____	_____
Removal of inner dressing	_____	_____
Cleansing of incision	_____	_____
Application of dressing	_____	_____
Securing of dressing	_____	_____
Dehiscence and evisceration	_____	
Suture removal technique	_____	_____
Skin staple removal technique	_____	_____
T-tube care		
Cleansing of skin around tube	_____	_____
Cleansing of tubing	_____	_____
Safety precautions	_____	_____
Removal of drainage from drain bag	_____	_____
Infant restraint for dressings	_____	_____
Signs and symptoms to watch for at home	_____	

Product Availability

Steri-strips, Montgomery strips, and dressing change kits can be obtained at most pharmacies and drug stores.

Selected References

Flynn M, Rovee D: Wound healing mechanisms. Am J Nurs 82(10):1544–1558, October, 1982

Neuberger G, Reckling J: A new look at wound care. Nursing '85 15(2):34–41, 1985

Quinless F: Teaching tips for T tube care at home. Nursing '84 14(5):63–65, 1984

Teaching/Learning

66   Bedmaking

Background

There are two ways to make the bed: with the client out of the bed and with the client in the bed. When a person must spend extended periods in the bed, such as during illness, it is essential to make the bed as comfortable as possible. A tightly spread sheet and clean environment not only contribute to the client's comfort and well-being, but are also important in preventing skin breakdown.

Assessment of Self-Care Potential

Client/Family Assessment

- Assess the frequency with which linens are changed on the beds in the family home.
- Assess the understanding and acceptance of the client and family regarding the need for the client to remain in bed for extended periods or continually.

Physical Assessment

- Assess the physical limitations of the client that might preclude getting out of bed while bedmaking is being done. Determine if the client is weak or dizzy.
- Assess the ease with which the client can turn from side to side in the bed. Assess the need for siderails on the bed, which the client can use to assist in turning from side to side.

Environmental Assessment

- Assess the situation in the client's bedroom. Note the height of the bed and whether or not it abuts a wall or large furniture.
- Assess the amount of linen in the home. Determine how many changes of sheets can be dedicated to the client's use when helping to determine the linen-changing schedule.
- Assess the presence of laundry facilities in the home to determine the frequency with which linens could reasonably be expected to be laundered. If there are no laundry facilities in the home, determine who does the laundry and where it is done.

Planning Strategies

Potential Nursing Diagnoses

Alteration in comfort: pain

Potential impairment of skin integrity

Activity intolerance

Expected Outcomes

Provision of a clean, comfortable environment for the duration of the illness

Prevention of skin breakdown and infection

Prevention of muscle strain

Health Promotion Goals

- The client and family will
  Understand how to make the bed with the client in it with minimal exertion of the client and utilization of proper body mechanics
  Demonstrate an understanding of how to make the bed so that it is a place of comfort and safety
  Be able to recognize signs of skin breakdown or pressure and know what actions to take to prevent further trauma

Equipment

Contour sheets and flat sheet (or two flat sheets)
Pillowcase(s)
Turning sheet or pad
Spread or blanket

Interventions/Health Promotion

ACTION

RATIONALE/AMPLIFICATION

Unoccupied Bed

1. With the client in a secure place, strip the linens from the bed. Place the soiled linens in a hamper or pillowcase, not on the floor.

2. If the bed is adjustable, raise it to its highest position for linen change. Place the bottom sheet on one side of the bed and secure at the upper and lower corners. Push the bulk of the remaining linen to the center of the bed. If the bottom sheet is flat, secure it with mitered corners. Align the lower edge of the sheet with the foot of the mattress. Place the upper edge of the sheet under the top of the mattress. Raise the side edge of the sheet onto the bed. Tuck the remaining portion under the mattress. Fold the entire side section over the side of the mattress and secure it under the edge of the mattress (Fig. 66-1, 66-2, and 66-3).

The floor area provides a mechanism for spreading infectious agents when it comes in contact with such items as linen.

Raising the bed eliminates the need to stoop during bedmaking, which may cause back strain. Contour sheets fit neatly over the corners of the mattress. Flat sheets must be secured to keep the surface smooth. Generally only the upper edge is secured with mitered corners since the mitered corner of the top sheet at the foot of the bed will help secure the lower edges of the bottom sheet.

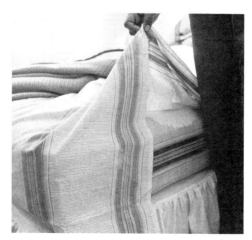

Figure 66.1

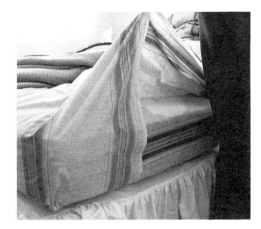

Figure 66.2

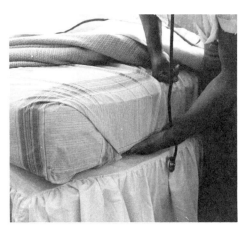

Figure 66.3

ACTION

3. If a turning sheet is used, place it on the bed next. Place the center fold of the turning sheet in the center of the bed and pull one side over to secure it under the edge of the mattress.

4. Place the center fold of the top sheet in the center of the bed and align it with the upper edge of the bed at the desired height. Tuck the top sheet under the lower edge of the mattress and secure with a mitered corner. To miter the foot section of the upper sheet, the raised side edge is lowered to the side of the bed rather than being tucked under the side of the mattress. Apply the spread in the same manner as the top sheet.

5. Move to the other side of the bed and repeat the process. When securing the bottom and turning sheets, tighten them and secure with no wrinkles on the bed surface. Tighten by using the body weight applied through the large muscles of the legs and buttocks, keeping the back straight.

RATIONALE/AMPLIFICATION

The turning sheet is used to assist in turning the client from side to side. It is tucked securely under the mattress when the client is in bed. The appropriate side is loosened when the client is being turned. It is then pulled taut and tucked again under the edge of the mattress. Materials appropriate for a turning sheet may be a regular flat sheet folded in half so that it can be tucked under both sides of the mattress, or a twin bed sheet. Sheepskin or soft pads may be placed under the client for protection of skin integrity and comfort.

The mitered corner at the foot of the bed helps secure the top sheet and prevents it from being pulled out during the course of the client's stay in bed. The spread and top sheet may be folded into a mitered corner at the same time.

A taut, wrinkle-free foundation lessens the discomfort and pressure on the client's skin. Using one's weight as a counterbalance against the sheets and keeping the vertebral column straight prevent strain on the smaller, weaker muscles of the back.

ACTION	RATIONALE/AMPLIFICATION
6. Loosen the top linens at the foot of the bed to form a pleat (Fig. 66-4).	A pleat at the foot of the bed allows room for the feet without confining, restrictive pressure from tight covers.

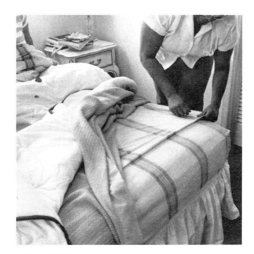

Figure 66.4

Occupied Bed

1. The client is rolled from one side of the bed to the other so that one side of the bed is made while the client lies on the other (Fig. 66-5). Raise the siderail on the side to which the client will turn. If no siderails are present, ask a family member to stand at the opposite side of the bed so the client will not fall from the bed.	Some means of securing the client's safety must be used to prevent falls. If siderails are not present and no one is available to assist, place a straight-back chair in a secure manner against the side of the bed to which the client will turn. Turn the client toward the chair but do not allow the client's full weight to press on the chair to prevent falls. If the client cannot offer any assistance, use a turning sheet to facilitate turning.

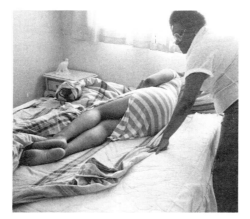

Figure 66.5

ACTION	**RATIONALE/AMPLIFICATION**
2. With the client rolled to the opposite side of the bed, loosen the linens on the vacated side and tuck them under the client (Fig. 66-6). Place the clean linens on this near side of the bed and secure them in place. Fold this clean linen over the top of the soiled linen and push as far as possible under the client.	If the linens that are to be removed are soiled with body fluids or excreta, place a towel or protective covering over them before the clean linens are placed on top and tucked under the client. This will prevent soiling the clean linens.

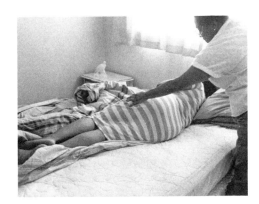

Figure 66.6

3. Tell the client to expect a large lump in the bed during turning (Fig. 66-7). In one smooth movement, roll the client over the soiled and clean linens toward the clean side of the bed. Have the siderail up or assistance on the clean side to which the client will now be turning. After the client has turned, move to the other side and finish changing the linen. Remove the soiled linen and place it in a container or bag. Pull the clean linens from under the client and secure them. If a turning sheet is used, pull it taut using the stronger muscles of the legs and buttocks. Place the top linen over the top of the client and secure it at the foot of the bed.	Rolling the client is much easier and causes less strain than lifting. The siderail can be used as a turning assistance device as well as a support for the client in the side-lying position. Pulling the linen tight with the leg and gluteal muscles will provide a desirable environment for the client without undue strain on the care provider's lower back muscles.

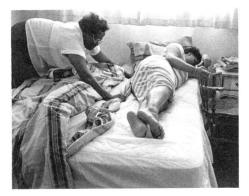

Figure 66.7

ACTION	*RATIONALE/AMPLIFICATION*
4. Place the client's accessories in a convenient place. They should be within reach but out of the way so they are not dropped or broken. If siderails are present, they should be left raised.	Accessories, such as liquid refreshments, telephone, tissues, and diversional materials, may be kept at the bedside on a small table. Siderails can prevent falls by the confused or weak client.

Education/ Communication

- Teach the client and family to

  Make the bed with the client in the bed. Explain the method of turning the client only once during the process in order to conserve strength.

  Make the bed in an efficient manner with the client out of the bed. The desirable effect is a smooth, wrinkle-free surface. Remind the family to watch the client closely when out of bed to determine stamina and physical capabilities. If tiring becomes evident, return the client to bed at once and proceed with making an occupied bed.

  Recognize when the bed should be made. The frequency of linen changes will depend on the needs and desires of the client as well as the availability of replacement linens and laundering facilities. If the client has a draining wound or is incontinent, a pad should be placed in the area most likely to receive the drainage to protect the linen. When the linen becomes soiled, it should be changed. For the bedridden client, the linens should be pulled taut to remove wrinkles several times a day. The object is to keep the client comfortable. Advise the family to use common sense and to be sensitive to the wishes of the client regarding frequency of linen changes and bedmaking.

  Adapt linen to the bed. If contour sheets are not available, they may be made by sewing small pieces of elastic to the corners of flat sheets, which will fit over the corners of the mattress and hold the linen in place. This method will also work if the sheets are too small to tuck securely beneath the edges of the mattress.

  Empathize with the bedridden client. Emphasize to the family members that although they do not notice wrinkles in their bed linen during the course of an 8-hour night, the client who must remain in the bed for extended periods becomes very sensitive to the condition of the linens. Also, if the client must take meals in bed, crumbs and debris may become very annoying during the course of the day.

Evaluation of Health Promotion Activities

Quality Assurance/ Reassessment

- Check the condition of the bed when visiting the client. Note the condition of cleanliness of the linens and determine the amount of wrinkling.
- Inspect the skin on the client's back, buttocks, legs, and arms. Large red creases in the skin may indicate that the client has been lying on wrinkled bedding.
- Allow the care provider to demonstrate making the bed. Note proficiency at such unfamiliar methods as mitering a corner and making one side of the bed at a time. Demonstrate any areas in which deficiencies are noted.

Health Teaching Checklist

Name of Care Provider _____

Relationship to Client _____ Telephone # _____

Taught by _____ Date _____

	EXPLAINED	DEMONSTRATED
Method of making an unoccupied bed	_____	_____
Mitering the corners	_____	_____
Making one side of the bed at a time	_____	_____
Safety precautions for the client while out of bed	_____	_____
Methods of making an occupied bed	_____	_____
Mitering the corners	_____	_____
Turning the client safely	_____	_____
Removing the linen	_____	_____
Frequency of bedmaking	_____	
Frequency of linen changes	_____	

Product Availability

Hospital beds may be rented or purchased from hospital-supply houses. Usually siderails are available for an additional charge. Generally, twin-size contour sheets will fit these beds.

67 Breast Self-Examination

Background

In the United States, one out of every 11 women develops breast cancer. Most breast cancers are discovered by the woman herself. Monthly breast self-examination (BSE) allows for early detection of breast cancer. There is an excellent chance for cure if breast cancer is found early and treated promptly.

Mammography

Mammography is an x-ray of the breast that can locate lesions too small to be palpated during BSE or by the physician. Mammography has been particularly beneficial in women over the age of 50 and who have no symptoms of breast cancer. The American Cancer Society recommends the following guidelines for early detection of breast cancer: Women between the ages of 20 and 40 years should perform BSE every month and be examined by a physician every 3 years. A baseline mammogram between the ages of 35 and 40 can be used for later comparison if needed. Those over age 40 should do BSE monthly and have a physical examination every year. The American Cancer Society recommends a mammogram every year routinely after the age of 50. Women aged between 40 and 49 years should be guided by their physicians regarding mammography.

Assessment of Self-Care Potential

Client/Family Assessment

- Determine whether the client is willing to learn and practice BSE.
- Assess whether the spouse or sexual partner can offer encouragement to the client to examine her own breasts.

Physical Assessment

- Assess the client for risk factors for breast cancer, that is, advancing age, previous history of breast cancer or a history of breast cancer in the immediate family, never having children or having the first child after age 30, onset of menstruation before age 12 or menopause after age 55, obesity, or chronic cystic mastitis.
- Determine the normal menstrual cycle. The breasts are best examined about 1 week after a menstrual period when they are not tender or swollen.
- Check whether the client is postmenopausal. The breasts should be checked on the first day of each month.
- Determine whether the client has had a hysterectomy. If on hormone therapy posthysterectomy, the client should consult the physician regarding the best time of the month to perform BSE.

Planning Strategies

Potential Nursing Diagnoses

Knowledge deficit, breast self-examination procedure

Expected Outcomes

Early detection of breast lumps

Increased knowledge of self-care activities

Health Promotion Goals

- The client will
  Examine her breasts monthly
  Be examined by a physician and obtain a mammogram according to American Cancer Society guidelines

Interventions/Health Promotion

ACTION

1. Examine the breasts during a bath or shower. With the fingers flat, move the hand gently over every part of each breast. Use the right hand to examine the left breast, left hand to examine the right breast. Note any lump, hard knot, or thickening.

2. Stand before a mirror with arms by your sides. Raise arms high overhead. Look for any changes in the contour of each breast.

3. Rest the palms of the hands on hips and press down firmly to flex the chest muscles. Look for changes in the contour of each breast.

4. Lie down and place a pillow or folded towel under the right shoulder. Place the right hand behind the head (Fig. 67-1).

RATIONALE/AMPLIFICATION

Hands glide easily over wet skin, making examination easier.

Changes could include swelling, dimpling of the skin, or changes in the nipple. A breast lesion can change the breast contour.

The left and right breast will not exactly match. One breast is larger in most women.

Placing the hand behind the head distributes the breast tissue evenly.

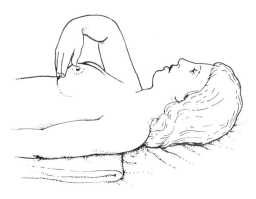

Figure 67.1

5. With the left hand, fingers flat, palpate the right breast gently using a small circular motion, around an imaginary clockface (Fig. 67-2). Begin at 12 o'clock and move to 1 o'clock, and so forth, back to 12 o'clock. Move 1 inch (2 cm) toward the nipple and repeat. Examine every part of the breast in this way, including the nipple.

Examining every part of the breast requires at least 4 circles. A ridge of firm tissue in the lower curve of each breast is normal.

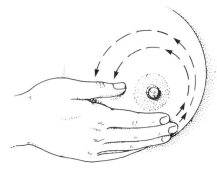

Figure 67.2

ACTION	*RATIONALE/AMPLIFICATION*
6. Repeat the technique for the left breast using the right hand to palpate. Place the pillow or rolled towel under the left shoulder.	
7. Finally, gently squeeze the nipple of each breast between the thumb and index finger.	Report any discharge to the physician immediately.

Education/ Communication

- Teach the client to
  Perform BSE monthly:
  About 1 week after a period when the breasts are not tender or swollen
  On the 1st day of each month if postmenopausal
  Depending on hormone therapy if posthysterectomy (check with the physician)
  Examine her breasts initially in the shower
  Use a circular motion to palpate breast tissue
  Distinguish normal breast tissue from abnormal lesions. Not all lesions are malignant. Only the physician can make that diagnosis.

Referrals and Consultations

- Refer the client to the American Cancer Society (ACS) for literature and step-by-step instructions on BSE. ACS also has a film on BSE and breast models that can be used for teaching. Using the models allows the client to practice finding lesions in the breast.
- Refer the client to a physician if any abnormalities are noted during BSE, such as thickening of breast tissue, swelling, dimpling, or discharge. Refer the client to a physician or nurse practitioner for regular breast examinations according to ACS guidelines.

Evaluation of Health Promotion Activities

Quality Assurance/ Reassessment

- Observe a return demonstration of BSE to check the client's technique.

DOCUMENTATION

Charting for the Home Health Nurse
Effectiveness of client's technique for BSE

Assessment findings

Health Teaching Checklist

Name of Care Provider _____

Relationship to Client _____ Telephone #_____

Taught by _____ Date _____

	EXPLAINED	DEMONSTRATED
Breast self-examination	_____	_____
Schedule for BSE	_____	
Findings to report	_____	

Selected Reference

Bates B: A Guide to Physical Examination, 3rd ed. Philadelphia, JB Lippincott, 1983

Ventilation

68

Breathing Exercises and Chest Physiotherapy

Background

Breathing exercises are used to assist in the removal of pulmonary secretions. They may also be prescribed in preparation for surgery and to build up stamina for the respiratory impaired. Breathing exercises are often used in conjunction with postural drainage, which involves the utilization of gravity to enhance removal of secretions from the respiratory tract. Air enters the lungs through the respiratory tract. In the smallest portions of the respiratory tract, the alveoli, the oxygen in the inspired air is exchanged for carbon dioxide. In order for an adequate amount of oxygen to reach the alveoli, the respiratory tract must be open and operational. When the amount or quality of inspired air is compromised, alveolar exchange is inadequate and the body does not have the oxygen required for life. Breathing exercises help to clear the respiratory tract so that air may be inspired at the needed rate.

Assessment of Self-Care Potential

Client/Family Assessment

- Assess any family history of respiratory disease. Note particularly whether or not anyone has ever suffered asthma, chronic bronchitis, hay fever, or emphysema.
- Assess the family members regarding the use of tobacco. Note who uses tobacco and the type and the amount of smoke to which the client is subjected daily.

Physical Assessment

- Assess the respiratory patterns of the client. Determine if there is any cyanosis. It is also important to know the respiratory rate in order to compare the rate during and after the exercises. Assess whether respiratory difficulty occurs on inspiration or expiration.
- Assess the client's breath sounds. Auscultate the chest to determine the presence of rales, grunting, or other unusual sounds. Assess the presence of sternal retraction or the use of accessory muscles during breathing.
- Assess skin color as well as the color of the nail beds.
- Assess the client's history of respiratory problems. Determine previous occurrences of pneumonia, asthma and allergies, shortness of breath, tuberculosis, and any other difficulties with breathing.
- Assess the client's history of tobacco use. Determine the type of tobacco used and the duration and frequency of use.
- Assess the general physical condition of the client in relation to being able to perform breathing exercises. If the client is very weak, exercises may have to be spaced between other periods of exercise and activity.

Environmental Assessment

- Assess the ventilation of the home. Determine if the client has access to clean, fresh air. Determine if the home has air conditioning and how the client tolerates its presence or absence.

- Assess the room in which the breathing exercises will occur. Assess the ability of the client to achieve the required positioning. If the client is a child, determine the type of furniture in the home and select a chair which will support the care provider and the child safely and comfortably.
- Assess the environment for smog. Determine if smog is a possibility, if it is heavier at times, and how the client tolerates the usual environment.

Planning Strategies

Potential Nursing Diagnoses

Ineffective airway clearance due to chronic respiratory problems

Ineffective breathing pattern due to chronic respiratory problems

Impaired gas exchange resulting from inadequate aeration

Sleep pattern disturbance due to inability to breathe adequately

Expected Outcomes

Removal of secretions from the airway and bronchial tree with resulting clearing of airway and improvement in respiratory rate

Expulsion of air and fluid from the pleural space

Adequate aeration of the tissues

Improvement of sleeping patterns; adequate rest

Health Promotion Goals

- The client and family will
  Learn to do the breathing exercises as needed or prescribed in order to produce optimal aeration of the lungs
  Understand safety precautions involved in breathing exercises

Equipment

Inspiratory or expiratory incentive device (such as a balloon or a commercial device) or incentive spirometer

Vibrator

Emesis basin, towel, and tissues

Pillows

Bed elevators (for postural drainage)

Stethoscope

Interventions/Health Promotion

ACTION	*RATIONALE/AMPLIFICATION*
Breathing Exercises	
1. Wash hands before assisting with breathing exercises.	Handwashing helps eliminate the chance of cross-contamination.
2. Breathing enhancement may be encouraged by offering the client a small, hand-held respiratory incentive device (Fig. 68-1). Some resistance is offered by the device to either inspiration or expiration.	After surgery, deep breathing is an important part of the prevention of complications. Commercial devices are available to offer inspiratory resistance. A balloon will offer expiratory resistance.

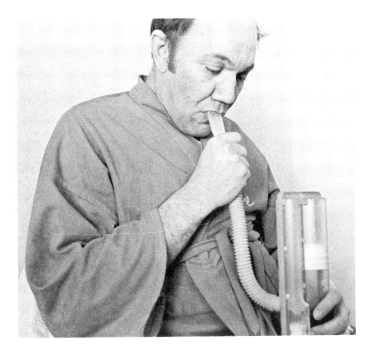

Figure 68.1

ACTION

3. Positive-pressure-breathing treatments can help inflate the client's lungs. Medication can also be administered by this route. A special machine is used to force pressurized air into the client's lungs. A humidification source and oxygenation source are needed in addition to the machine. Because of the hazards involved, positive-pressure apparatus should be used only by those who have specialized knowledge and training in the use and care of these machines. The principles may be taught to the client and family, but frequent monitoring is essential. (See Technique 74, Pressure Breathing Treatments.)

4. For exercising the diaphragm, place the fingers on the client's anterior lower ribs. During *inhalation,* ask the client to push the chest out forcefully against the light pressure of the fingers. During *exhalation,* ask the client to contract the abdominal muscles.

5. For exercising the apex of the lungs, apply light pressure just below the clavicle when the client *inhales.* When the client *exhales,* apply pressure to the sternum with the heel of the hand.

RATIONALE/AMPLIFICATION

Positive-pressure machines usually deliver the gases to the lungs at a pressure of 10 to 20 lb/inch. The prescription of amount of pressure, frequency of treatments, and medications should be carefully regulated by a respiratory-care specialist.

The diaphragm lines the lower thorax area. Expanding and contracting this muscle will help to strengthen it.

Counterpressure forces the client to bear down, thus strengthening the breathing muscles and aerating larger lung areas.

ACTION

RATIONALE/AMPLIFICATION

6. For exercising the posterior portions of the lungs, position the client on the side or prone. Place both hands over the lower portion of the client's thorax posteriorly. Apply pressure when the client *exhales.* Relax the pressure during *inhalation.*

Gravity is used as a counterpressure along with the manual force of the hands.

7. For exercising the lateral lower rib area, encourage the client to *exhale* completely. Place both hands lightly on the lateral aspect of the client's lower ribs. Instruct the client to expand the ribs against the pressure of the hands during *inhalation.* During *exhalation,* ask the client to tighten the abdomen and pull the ribs as pressure is placed over the lower rib cage area.

Tensing and relaxing strengthens those muscles used in breathing. Complete exhalation encourages maximum expansion of the rib cage.

Postural Drainage

1. Position the client according to the portion of the lung that is involved. Use pillows or a reclining chair to prop the client into the desired position (Fig. 68-2). Encourage the client to cough up the secretions. Do not do postural drainage immediately before or after meals.

Gravity is used to assist in the evacuation of secretions from the lungs. The area of congestion should be uppermost, above the area of entry of the bronchi into the lungs, because this is the vehicle for expelling the secretions from the lungs. Postural drainage may require a great deal of exertion; therefore, the client should be allowed to rest before and after eating to reduce the chance of vomiting.

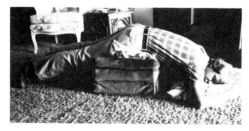

Figure 68.2

2. Active postural drainage occurs when the client assumes a position in which the affected area of the lung can be drained. Place the area to be drained uppermost. Position the client across pillows or on a slanting board with the head below the rest of the body and the affected lung uppermost. Place an emesis basin nearby into which the client can expectorate secretions. Encourage the client to cough vigorously for 2 or 3

The client actively attempts to expectorate secretions by coughing while in the desired posture. Gravity and thumping of the chest wall help loosen and drain secretions.

ACTION	RATIONALE/AMPLIFICATION

minutes. Percussion or vibration may be used in conjunction with posturing (Fig. 68-3).

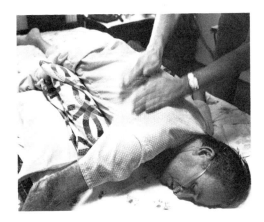

Figure 68.3

3. Drainage may be enhanced by percussion and vibration. To percuss the client, cup the hand and strike the chest wall in the involved area. A hand-held vibrator may be placed against the chest wall in the involved area during the *exhalation* phase (Fig. 68-4). Percuss or vibrate for 5 exhalations in succession and allow the client to rest.

The objective of percussion is to loosen the secretions by the resonating thumping or vibration on the chest wall. Cover the skin with a towel if percussion directly onto the skin is uncomfortable.

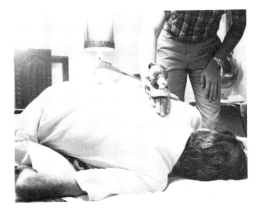

Figure 68.4

ACTION

RATIONALE/AMPLIFICATION

4. Passive postural drainage occurs when the client is too weak or confused to participate actively in the treatment. It is accomplished by positioning. Place the client supine in the bed. Elevate the foot of the bed approximately 20 inches above the level of the bed plane. Place the emesis basin nearby to catch secretions as they are expectorated. Leave the client in this position for approximately 15 minutes. Encourage coughing during the last few minutes if the client is able.

For the weak or physically debilitated, active postural drainage may be too taxing on the physical condition to be therapeutically effective. Gravity will cause the secretions to drain and pool. Short sessions of coughing will then be effective for partial or total removal of the secretions. The foot of the bed may be elevated on blocks or the foot of the mattress may be propped upward with pillows.

5. Posturing to facilitate breathing or for relief of congestion may be done by placing pillows under the client's mattress if a hospital bed is not available. The mattress may be propped at the foot or the head.

If the client has difficulty sleeping at night, elevation of the head may relieve congestion enough to allow rest.

Age-Specific Modifications

1. Postural drainage and breathing exercises may be done with the infant or small child held on the lap. The proper position may be gained by keeping the area to be drained uppermost. Hold the child securely to prevent falls.

It is difficult to gain cooperation from the infant or small child regarding remaining in the desired position for the desired time period. Therefore, holding the child seems to be more effective in postural drainage of small children.

Education/ Communication

- Teach the client and family to
  Recognize when breathing exercises or postural drainage are indicated by the respiratory status of the client. They should be taught how to relieve breathing problems effectively by exercises or drainage or by a combination of both.
  Perform breathing exercises or postural drainage safely. Emphasize the anatomical landmarks around the rib cage area and show them where to place their hands when placing resistance against which the client will breathe.
  Recognize desirable and undesirable breath sounds so that they will know when treatments should be done. They should also be able to assess the effectiveness of the treatments by auscultation.
  Recognize the differences between adults and small children regarding needs when breathing exercises and postural drainage are done. In the infant, the chest wall is thin with little musculature and the rib cage is very soft and pliant. The amount of counterpressure required for infants and small children is much less than that required for adults.
  Learn about the client's physical condition and limitations. Encourage physical activities that will increase the respiratory efficiency, such as swimming and walking, unless these are contradicted by the client's physical condition.

Referrals and Consultations

Consultation with a respiratory-care specialist may be needed if sophisticated ventilatory assistance is to be used in the home.

Evaluation of Health Promotion Activities

Quality Assurance/ Reassessment

- Assess the effectiveness of the breathing exercises and postural drainage activities by the change in respiratory rate and effort after the treatment. The client will be tired immediately after the treatment. However, after resting for a short time, the respiratory status of the client should be improved. The amount of expectoration may also indicate the effectiveness of the treatment.
- Observe the family doing percussion or vibration of the client to determine if the technique is satisfactory and effective.
- Allow the family member to listen to the client's breath sounds and evaluate where percussion or auscultation is needed. Then auscultate and determine how effectively the family member assessed the situation.

DOCUMENTATION

Charting for the Home Health Nurse
- Note breath sounds and the appearance and amount of expectoration during each visit. These indices will help determine if the client's condition is progressing satisfactorily.

Records Kept by the Client/Family
- Ask the client and family to keep a record of the frequency, duration, and results of the breathing exercises and postural drainage. This record may be used to determine the optimal time of day and length of treatment. It may also be used to determine if the client's condition is getting progressively better or worse.

Health Teaching Checklist

Name of Care Provider _____

Relationship to Client _____ Telephone #_____

Taught by _____ Date _____

	EXPLAINED	DEMONSTRATED
Signs and symptoms that indicate the need for chest physiotherapy or breathing exercises	_____	
Method of using breathing-enhancement device (balloon or incentive spirometer)	_____	_____
Breathing exercises	_____	_____
Postural drainage	_____	_____
Safety precautions for infants and small children	_____	_____
Auscultation of breath sounds	_____	_____
Propping of mattress to facilitate breathing	_____	_____

Product Availability

VOLDYNE, a volumetric exerciser for incentive deep breathing to maintain and improve inspiratory volume and respiratory fitness, may be obtained from Chesebrough-Ponds, Inc., Greenwich, CT 06830.

Hand-held vibrators may be obtained at most pharmacies and drug stores.

69 Chest Tube

Background

Loss of integrity of the pleural space because of surgery, trauma, or spontaneous rupture of a lung bleb requires the insertion of a chest tube connected to a drainage system to restore normal respiratory function. Air entering the pleural space interferes with normal intrathoracic pressure and prevents expansion of the lung (Fig. 69-1). Should air continue to enter the pleural space after the lung is totally collapsed, enough pressure can develop to push the mediastinal structures toward the unaffected side, causing a tension pneumothorax (Fig. 69-2). This is an emergency condition that requires immediate insertion of a chest tube to restore normal breathing.

In the hospital, the chest tube is connected to an underwater-seal drainage system that prevents air from reentering the pleural space but allows air and fluid to drain. This drainage system is cumbersome and difficult to manage at home. When the person is ready for discharge, the chest tube can be connected to a Heimlich valve, which is much easier to manage. A Heimlich valve allows fluid and air to drain from the pleural space through a tube that resembles a collapsed Penrose drain. Air is unable to enter the pleural space because of the "one-way" effect of the valve (Fig. 69-3). The tube is secured in place by a suture, so there is no danger of it falling out.

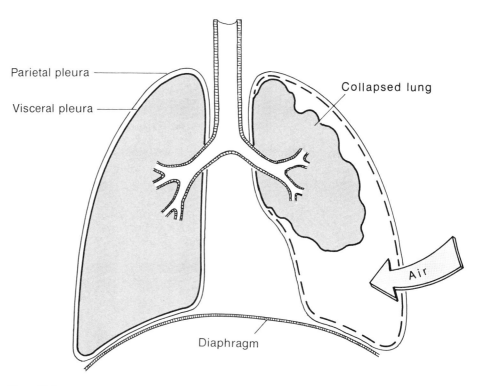

Figure 69.1
Loss of integrity of the pleural space caused by interruption of the pleural lining.

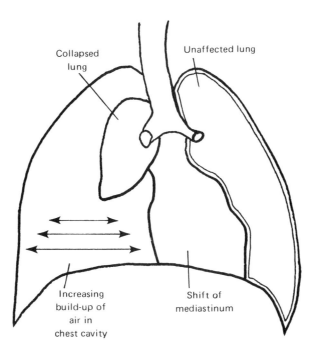

Figure 69.2
Tension pneumothorax.

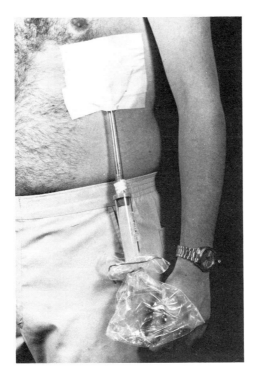

Figure 69.3
Heimlich-valve chest-drainage system using a
resealable plastic bag for drainage. (Photograph
by Ernie Farino, Former Chief, Medical Media,
Veterans Administration Medical Center,
Amarillo, Texas)

Terminology

Hemothorax: Collection of blood in the pleural space. Occurs as a result of trauma or surgery.

Pneumothorax: Air in the pleural space. Occurs as a result of penetrating chest trauma, surgery, or spontaneous rupture of a lung bleb, which can occur in persons with chronic obstructive pulmonary disease.

Hemopneumothorax: Blood and air in the pleural space.

Assessment of Self-Care Potential

Client/Family Assessment

• Determine the willingness and the ability of the client and family members to care for the chest tube.
• Assess their understanding of the importance of keeping the drainage system intact so that air will not enter the pleural space.

Physical Assessment

• Assess the client's respiratory system and oxygenation. Palpate the chest wall for crepitus, a crackling sensation that can be palpated if air is escaping into the subcutaneous tissues. Crepitus occurs in the presence of a pneumothorax, when air cannot escape from the pleural space. Observe for respiratory distress, which could also indicate that the drainage system is not patent.
• Check the integrity and patency of the drainage system.
• Assess the color, character, and amount of fluid draining from the chest tube.
• Check the stab wound (chest tube insertion site) and suture line (if postoperative) for inflammation indicating infection.
• Check vital signs for indications of infection (elevated temperature and pulse).

Environmental Assessment

• Check the home for cleanliness. Wound care cannot be managed if basic sanitation practices are not used in the home.

Planning Strategies

Potential Nursing Diagnoses

Breathing pattern, ineffective: tension pneumothorax due to nonpatent drainage system

Knowledge deficit: management of chest drainage system

Injury, potential for, pneumothorax: accidental removal of chest drainage tube or disconnection of Heimlich valve

Infection, potential for: inability to follow infection-control practices

Expected Outcomes

Reexpansion of the affected lung

Increased knowledge of chest drainage system

Prevention of accidental premature removal of chest tube

Implementation of emergency procedures in the event of accidental tube removal

Prevention of infection

Health Promotion Goals

• The client and family will
Maintain the chest drainage system intact and patent
Use infection-control precautions to prevent infection
Give emergency care in case of the accidental removal of the tube or interruption of the drainage system

Equipment

Resealable plastic sandwich bags *or*
Urinary drainage bags
4 × 4s
Combine dressing (if necessary)
Tape
Iodophor solution and cotton-tipped swabs *or*
Iodophor swab sticks
Paper bag for disposal of dressings

Interventions/Health Promotion

ACTION	*RATIONALE/AMPLIFICATION*
1. Place the client in a comfortable position. Wash hands thoroughly. Assemble the equipment conveniently on a nightstand or table.	Be sure there is adequate light to be able to check the site adequately.
2. If a dressing is in place around the tube, remove it and place it in the paper bag. Check the insertion site for drainage or inflammation indicating infection.	
3. Clean around the tube insertion site and a small portion of the tube using iodophor swab sticks. Begin close to the tube and work outward using a circular motion. Do not return to the insertion site with the used swab. Repeat the procedure until all blood or crusty secretions are removed.	Cleaning outward from the insertion site prevents contaminating the area already cleaned.
4. Cut a slit in a 4 × 4 and place it around the tube. Cover the 4 × 4 with tape.	
5. Disconnect the plastic resealable bag from the Heimlich valve and replace it with a clean bag. Record the character and amount of drainage. Discard the bag in the paper bag.	A plastic resealable bag is suitable if the drainage is small. For larger amounts of drainage use a urinary drainage bag. Empty the drainage bag into a container, taking care not to contaminate the system. Change the bag every 48 hours. Discard the drainage into the commode to prevent spreading infection.
6. Wash hands.	

Related Care

1. Wash urinary drainage bag and container used for emptying contents in hot soapy water. Rinse in clear water. Hang the drainage bag over the bathtub to drain. When it is dry, place it in a plastic bag until ready for use.

ACTION	*RATIONALE/AMPLIFICATION*
2. Remove the chest tube when requested by the physician:	The chest tube can be removed when the accumulation of air and fluid has ceased.
• Prepare an occlusive dressing of sterile petroleum jelly on a 4 × 4 or use a commercially prepared occlusive dressing.	An occlusive dressing prevents the recurrence of a pneumothorax by forming a seal over the opening created by the chest tube.
• Cut the skin suture holding the chest tube in place, using a sterile scalpel blade or small scissors.	
• Place a linen protector on the client's bed. Clamp the tube between the fingers and remove steadily with one motion. Place the tube on the linen protector.	
• Have the client perform a Valsalva maneuver by bearing down as the tube is removed.	This increases the intrathoracic pressure and serves to force remaining fluid or air from the pleural space, while preventing air from reentering the pleural space.
• Quickly cover the chest tube insertion site with the sterile occlusive dressing before the client inhales. Tape the dressing in place. Discard the tube.	This prevents entry of air back into the chest. The dressing should remain in place 48 to 72 hours.

Education/ Communication

• Teach the client and family to
Redress the tube daily. Empty drainage daily or more often if required.
Maintain the integrity of the drainage system at all times. If the Heimlich valve is disconnected, air can enter the pleural space. If the valve is accidentally disconnected, reconnect it to the chest tube. Having the client cough several times will force the air that has entered the pleural space out through the chest tube.
Provide emergency care should the chest tube accidentally be removed. Cover the site with a combine dressing or clean folded washcloth while the person inhales. Remove the pad during exhalation. This prevents air from entering the chest during inhalation and allows air to be forced from the chest during exhalation. Contact the physician or take the client to the nearest emergency room.
Use good handwashing when manipulating the tube or dressing

Referrals and Consultations

The client or family should contact the home health nurse if the person experiences respiratory distress. This could indicate that the drainage system is not patent.

The client should also report signs of infection (purulent drainage, elevated temperature or pulse rate, redness at the site).

The family should contact the physician if the tube is accidentally removed, after taking emergency measures.

Evaluation of Health Promotion Activities

**Quality Assurance/
Reassessment**

DOCUMENTATION

Charting for the Home Health Nurse
Ability of the family to care for the chest tube

Condition of the site

Patency of the drainage system

Amount and quality of the drainage

Respiratory assessment

Vital signs

Records Kept by the Client/Family
Amount and quality of the drainage

**Health Teaching
Checklist**

Name of Care Provider _____

Relationship to Client _____ Telephone #_____

Taught by _____ Date _____

	EXPLAINED	DEMONSTRATED
Daily chest tube care	_____	_____
Emergency measures for accidental tube removal or disconnection of Heimlich valve	_____	_____
Signs of infection	_____	
Care of drainage bags	_____	_____
Infection control precautions	_____	_____

Product Availability

Resealable plastic sandwich bags are available in grocery stores. Urinary drainage bags are available through medical-supply companies. Combine dressings, 4 × 4s, iodophor solution, and cotton-tipped applicators are available at drug stores.

70   Heimlich Technique

Background

Many deaths each year are attributed to obstruction of the airway by a foreign body. Airway obstruction most often occurs during eating, particularly in persons who have ingested alcohol, who chew food poorly, or who have dentures. Often the airway obstruction is mistaken for a heart attack. This is why the phenomenon has been called the *cafe coronary*. Many restaurants have special forceps for removing a foreign body. The use of these should be reserved for a person who has been trained in their use.

The universal sign for choking is grasping the throat with both hands (Fig. 70-1). Immediate attention is necessary to remove the obstruction and restore normal respiration. The Heimlich maneuver can be used on a conscious or unconscious victim. If the obstruction cannot be removed in an unconscious victim, rescue breathing may force enough air around the obstruction and into the lungs to sustain life until the person can be transported to a medical facility.

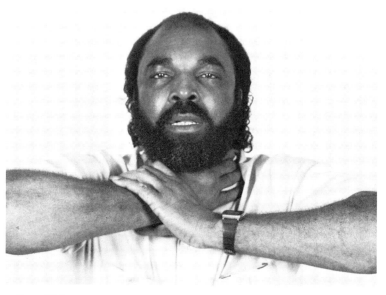

Figure 70.1
Universal choking sign.

Assessment of Self-Care Potential

Client/Family Assessment

- Determine whether family members are willing to learn the Heimlich technique. Assess whether family members have any physical limitations to prevent performing the technique (e.g., adaptations will have to be made for a child to perform the technique on an adult).

Physical Assessment

- Note whether the distressed person uses the universal choking sign to signify an airway obstruction.
- Assess the person to determine whether there is a partial or complete airway obstruction. With a complete airway obstruction, the person will be unable to speak.

- Determine if the client has an effective cough. Encourage coughing attempts. Often this is sufficient to dislodge the foreign body.
- Assess the person for crowing respirations or cyanosis, indicating poor air exchange.
- Determine whether the victim has lost consciousness. (See Technique 5, Basic Life Support, for Heimlich maneuver on an unconscious person.)

Environmental Assessment

- Check whether special forceps are available for removing a foreign body from the throat.

Planning Strategies

Potential Nursing Diagnoses

Breathing pattern, ineffective: due to airway obstruction

Airway clearance, ineffective: due to airway obstruction

Injury, potential for respiratory arrest: due to airway obstruction

Expected Outcomes

Restoration of normal breathing pattern

Removal of airway obstruction

Prevention of cardiorespiratory arrest

Health Promotion Goals

- The client and family will
  Assess a person in respiratory distress for obstruction of the airway
  Perform the Heimlich maneuver on a choking victim

Interventions/Health Promotion

ACTION	RATIONALE/AMPLIFICATION
1. Identify complete airway obstruction by determining if the victim is able to speak.	If there is a complete obstruction, the person will be unable to speak because air will not pass through the vocal chords.
2. If the back blows do not dislodge the foreign body, stand behind the victim and wrap your arms around the victim's waist. Grasp one fist with the other hand, with the thumb side of the fist against the person's abdomen in the midline between the waist and the ribs.	For pregnant or obese clients, wrap arms around the lower rib cage above the abdomen.

ACTION

3. Give 4 quick thrusts with an inward and upward motion (Fig. 70-2).

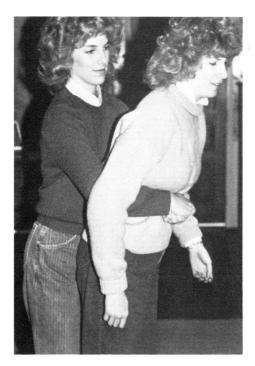

Figure 70.2
Heimlich maneuver to relieve airway obstruction in an unconscious person.

4. If the maneuver is not effective, repeat the sequence as necessary.

5. If the victim loses consciousness, proceed with basic life support and the Heimlich maneuver for an unconscious person (see Technique 5, Basic Life Support).

Age-Specific Modifications (Pediatric)

A child can perform the technique on an adult, using the astride position with the adult supine.

RATIONALE/AMPLIFICATION

Considerable effort is required to dislodge a foreign body. The Heimlich maneuver works on the "popping the cork from the bottle" principle by using air remaining in the lungs. Aim for the maximum effect the first time. Each attempt may force a small amount of air from the lungs, decreasing the chance of success.

Education/ Communication

- Teach the client and family to
  Perform the Heimlich maneuver if assistance is not available by falling across a chair. The force against the abdominal area has a similar effect as the Heimlich maneuver.
  Use the universal choking sign
  Prevent choking by cutting food into small pieces and chewing well, avoiding laughing and talking while chewing and swallowing, taking particular care if wearing dentures, avoiding excessive alcohol intake before or during meals, restricting children from running or playing with food or foreign objects in their mouths, and keeping small foreign objects away from children and infants

Referrals and Consultations

- Refer clients to the American Heart Association or the American Red Cross for training programs in basic life support, including the Heimlich maneuver.

Evaluation of Health Promotion Activities

Quality Assurance/ Reassessment

- Check clients' knowledge of the Heimlich maneuver with return demonstrations.

DOCUMENTATION

Charting for the Home Health Nurse
Competency of clients in performing the technique

Health Teaching Checklist

Name of Care Provider _____

Relationship to Client _____ Telephone # _____

Taught by _____ Date _____

	EXPLAINED	DEMONSTRATED
Universal choking sign	_____	_____
Heimlich maneuver	_____	_____
Adaptations for pregnancy, obesity	_____	_____
Prevention of choking	_____	
Availability of basic life support classes	_____	

Product Availability

Training equipment, including manikins, cut-away models, films, and literature, is available through the American Heart Association and the American Red Cross.

Selected Reference

Herrin TJ, Montgomery WH: Instructors Manual for Basic Life Support. Dallas, American Heart Association, 1985

Laryngectomy Care

Background

Laryngectomy is the complete or partial removal of the larynx. Total removal of the larynx results in immediate and total loss of the voice (Fig. 71-1). If one of the two vocal cords can be preserved, "normal" speech is maintained. Laryngectomees are total or partial neck breathers. It is important to note that, even with the total removal of the larynx, the person is not necessarily a total neck breather. Surgical reconstruction of a new communication between the trachea and hypopharynx for sound production converts the total laryngectomee into virtually a partial neck breather (Fig. 71-2). Additionally, most laryngectomees are recovering from cancer, although in some cases, injury, burns, or infection may necessitate a laryngectomy.

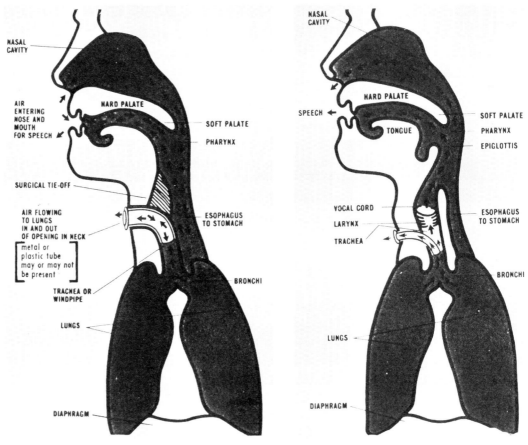

Figure 71.1
Physiology of the head and neck after total laryngectomy. (Reprinted with permission of the American Cancer Society)

Figure 71.2
Partial neck breather. (Reprinted with permission of the American Cancer Society)

To keep the stoma patent, a laryngectomy tube (metal or plastic) may be worn. Immediately postoperatively, the laryngectomy tube worn by the person resembles a tracheostomy tube, except that it is somewhat larger in diameter and shorter in length (Fig. 71-3). A laryngectomy tube consists of an outer cannula, inner cannula, and obturator. The obturator is used to occlude the outer cannula during insertion of the tube and is replaced by the inner cannula when the tube is in place.

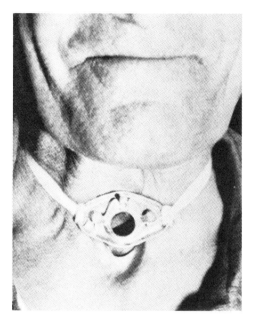

Figure 71.3
Laryngectomy tube. (Lauder E: Self-Help for the Laryngectomee, 1983–84 edition. San Antonio, Lauder Publisher, 1979)

Assessment of Self-Care Potential

Client/Family Assessment

- Determine whether the client will be able to return to former occupation. Check whether vocational counseling is available if a change of occupation will be necessary. Determine whether the state employment office can be of assistance. If the client will be unable to return to work, assist the person to apply for Social Security benefits (if applicable).
- Check whether a third-party payor will reimburse the client for home health visits.
- Determine whether the client and family will be able to care for the laryngectomy. Determine the input that will be required from the home health nurse.
- Assess the client's motivation to learn to communicate. The average laryngectomee learns to speak in 1 to 4 months. Determine whether esophageal speech or a speech aid will be desirable for the client (Fig. 71-4). Check whether a speech pathologist or laryngectomee trained in esophageal speech is available to the client.

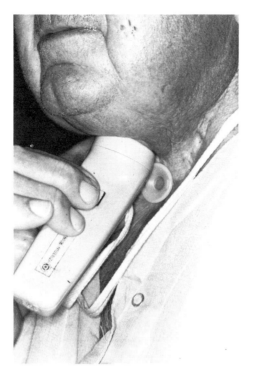

Figure 71.4
Artificial larynx. (Photograph by Keith Mitchell,
Veterans Administration Medical Center,
Amarillo, Texas)

- Assess whether the successfully rehabilitated client is a candidate to visit new laryngectomees or to become involved in teaching alaryngeal speech. Training programs are provided through the International Association of Laryngectomees. Assess whether this would give the client new purpose in life.

Physical Assessment
- Determine whether the client will prefer to wear a laryngectomy tube all of the time or only at night. Immediately postoperatively, the client will probably be instructed by the physician to wear it at all times until the stoma heals. Determine whether the client prefers to wear a plastic button that helps keep the stoma open (Fig. 71-5). A physician's prescription is required to order buttons for the first time. The physician should insert the button initially.
- Assess respiratory status.
- Assess the amount, color, and character of mucus. Determine whether the client is able to clear mucus from the respiratory tract by coughing or whether suctioning is required.

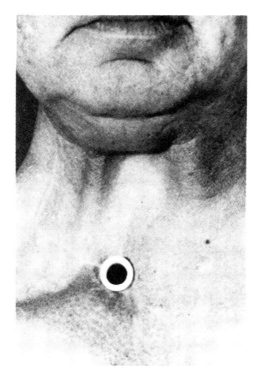

Figure 71.5
A plastic button helps keep the stoma open.
(Reprinted with permission from Lauder E:
Self-Help for the Laryngectomee, 1983–84
edition. San Antonio, Lauder Publisher, 1979)

Environmental Assessment	• See Technique 76, Tracheostomy Care.

Planning Strategies

Potential Nursing Diagnoses	Airway clearance, ineffective: loss of normal clearance mechanisms due to laryngectomy
	Infection, potential for: loss of normal respiratory defense mechanisms
	Home maintenance management, impaired: changes in activities of daily living due to laryngectomy
	Self-concept, disturbance in: body image, laryngectomee
	Powerlessness: inability to communicate verbally
Expected Outcomes	Maintenance of a patent airway
	Prevention of infection
	Healing of laryngectomy stoma
	Incorporation of laryngectomy care into activities of daily living
	Acceptance of body-image changes
	Mastery of alaryngeal speech or communication aid
Health Promotion Goals	• The client and family will Assume total responsibility for care of the laryngectomy Protect the respiratory tract from dust and respiratory irritants Make appropriate adaptations in the client's activities of daily living Accept body-image changes Enroll the client in a speech therapy program

Equipment

Disposable paper cups or reusable containers (2)

4 × 4s

Scissors

Small brush or pipe cleaners

Twill ties

Suction equipment

Small makeup mirror

Cotton swabs (long)

Pickups

Hydrogen peroxide

Saline or distilled water

A & D Ointment

Stomahesive (optional)

Interventions/Health Promotion

ACTION	*RATIONALE/AMPLIFICATION*
1. Assemble supplies needed to clean the inner cannula. Wash hands thoroughly. Pour hydrogen peroxide and saline or distilled water into containers.	See Technique 74, Pressure Breathing Treatments, for saline recipe.
2. Position a small makeup mirror so that the stoma can be visualized, or use the bathroom mirror.	See Technique 76, Tracheostomy Care.
3. Suction the stoma.	See Technique 75, Suctioning. Manipulation of the tube will induce coughing.
4. Remove the inner cannula and place it in the peroxide. Use pipe cleaners or a brush to remove mucus. Rinse the cannula in saline or distilled water. Replace the cannula, taking care to secure it in position.	Hydrogen peroxide is very effective in removing organic material from the tube.
Replace the ties with fresh ties. If a family member is unavailable to hold the tube in place while this is done, attach new ties to the tube before removing the old ties. If secretion management is a problem, cut a slit in a 4 × 4 and place it around the tube. Apply A & D ointment to the skin around the tube to prevent excoriation. Cut Stomahesive and apply to the skin to allow healing of excoriated skin if necessary.	The ties hold the tube in place. Continual secretions can cause irritation of the skin. See Technique 76, Tracheostomy Care.

ACTION	*RATIONALE/AMPLIFICATION*
5. When instructed by the physician, remove the entire tube for a specified period each day: • Cut the ties securing the tube. • Remove the entire tube. • Clean the tube ready for replacement. To reinsert the tube • Remove the inner cannula from the outer cannula. • Insert the obturator into the outer cannula. • Reinsert the tube carefully into the stoma. • Remove the obturator and reinsert the inner cannula and lock it in place. Replace the ties.	The tube will be removed for increasing lengths of time to promote healing of the stoma, and so that eventually the tube can be left out entirely. The obturator forms a rounded tip to facilitate inserting the tube.
6. When it is no longer necessary for the client to wear the laryngectomy tube, swab the inside and the circumference of the stoma each morning and evening with a cotton-tipped applicator dipped in saline or warm tap water.	To prevent the possibility of dropping the applicator into the stoma, use the long wooden stick applicators rather than the short applicators sold for baby care.
7. If a plug of dried mucus has formed and cannot be removed with the applicator, remove it with a pair of pickups or forceps.	Do not use eyebrow tweezers because there is a danger of dropping them into the stoma, and forceps will be easier to use. Manipulation of the stoma will cause coughing.

Related Care

1. Insert stoma button if indicated.	A stoma button may be used by clients to keep the stoma tract open. It is inserted in place of the laryngectomy tube.
2. Maintain an adequate fluid intake.	Fluids liquefy mucus, enabling the client to clear the airway effectively.

Education/Communication

• Teach the client and family to

Suction the stoma as necessary to keep it patent (Fig. 71-6). Provide a small makeup mirror so the client can suction the stoma unassisted. Expect increased mucus production if the client catches a cold.

Place an open container of water near the home heat source during the winter to increase the humidity. Use a humidifier or vaporizer in the home, and especially at night. Low humidity, air conditioning, and heating cause problems for laryngectomees who benefit from high humidity because air enters the trachea directly.

Maintain an adequate fluid intake to liquefy mucus

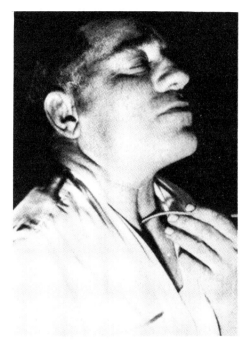

Figure 71.6
Suctioning a laryngectomee. Note that the person is not wearing a laryngectomy tube. (Reprinted with permission of the American Cancer Society)

• Teach the client to

Wear a laryngectomy collar or bib to prevent foreign material from entering the trachea (Fig. 71-7). Soft cotton bibs or plastic collars with replaceable filters are available. If living or working in dusty, dry surroundings, wear two bibs and dampen the outer one with water to help catch the dust.

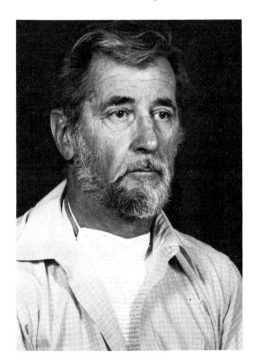

Figure 71.7
Home-made laryngectomee collar. (Photograph by Keith Mitchell, Veterans Administration Medical Center, Amarillo, Texas)

Carry a medical emergency card at all times (Fig. 71-8)

Cover the collar with an ascot tie or clip-on ready-made tie (men), or scarf or high-necked clothing (women)

Wear dentures (if applicable) except at bedtime. Properly fitting dentures aid the person's ability to compress air and produce more understandable speech. Improperly fitted "clicking" dentures can also interfere with phonation and intelligibility of speech.

Bathe carefully to avoid getting water in the stoma. Expect a bout of severe coughing when even the smallest amount of water gets into the stoma. Wear a shower collar if showers are preferred.

Not plan to participate in water sports. Fishing or boating from larger boats or from the shore does not create a problem. Avoid situations where falling in the water is a possibility. Laryngectomees can drown much more easily than other people.

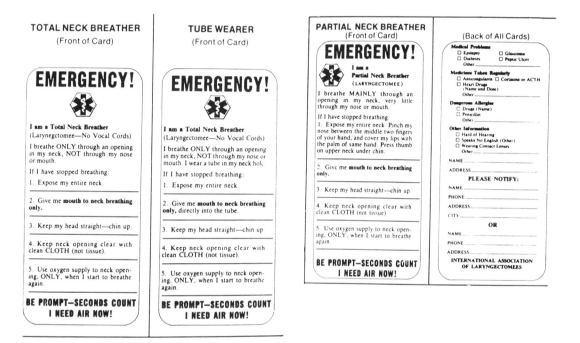

Figure 71.8
Medical emergency cards to be carried in the shirt pocket or outside pocket of a woman's handbag.

- Teach the family to
  Perform cardiopulmonary resuscitation (CPR) on a "neck breather." Use a manikin for practice. Show the film "Three Critical Minutes" to assist with instruction.

Referrals and Consultations

- Refer the client to a speech pathologist trained in teaching laryngectomees or a lay laryngectomee instructor. Consult the International Association of Laryngectomees (IAL) Directory of Instructors of Alaryngeal Speech (the address is given below. The directory is free to laryngectomees.)
- Refer the client and family to the International Association of Laryngectomees for information on local Lost Chord clubs, referrals, and educational literature.

- Refer the client and family to the following audiovisuals (or arrange for them to view them):

  "To Speak Again"
  Produced by Washington Hospital Center
  Washington, DC
  Sound, color, 20 minutes
  16-mm format, 8 mm and super 8 mm for Fairchild projector
  (Code # 4526)
  Suitable for new laryngectomees

  "A Second Voice"
  International Association of Laryngectomees
  Sound, color, 15 minutes
  16-mm format, 8 mm and super 8 mm for Fairchild projector
  (Code # 4525—English)
  (Code # 4536—Spanish)
  Describes complete rehabilitation of the laryngectomee

  "Three Critical Minutes"
  Color, sound, 17 minutes
  16-mm format
  Produced by International Association of Laryngectomees and Wisconsin Division of the American Cancer Society
  (Code # 4539)
  Suitable for instructing the general public in first aid methods for laryngectomees

Evaluation of Health Promotion Activities

Quality Assurance/ Reassessment

- Periodically observe the client's technique in caring for the laryngectomy. Check for adherence to infection-control precautions.
- Assess the family's acceptance of the body-image changes caused by the laryngectomy.
- Assess the status of the respiratory system.

DOCUMENTATION

Charting for the Home Health Nurse
Respiratory assessment

Acceptance of body-image changes by the client and family

Condition of the stoma and surrounding skin

Color, amount, and character of mucus

Ability of the client to perform self-care

Health Teaching Checklist

Name of Care Provider _____

Relationship to Client _____ Telephone #_____

Taught by _____ Date _____

	EXPLAINED	DEMONSTRATED
Laryngectomy care	_____	_____
Airway clearance measures	_____	_____
ADL changes (clothing, activities)	_____	
Importance of speech therapy	_____	
Resuscitation of a "neck breather"	_____	_____
Infection control precautions	_____	_____

Product Availability

Pickups or forceps can be purchased in drug stores or obtained from medical-supply companies listed in the yellow pages of the telephone book.

Stoma buttons are available from

Stoma Button Company
PO Box 984
Baker, Oregon 97814-0984

Laryngectomee collars (100% cotton) are available from

Romet
PO Box 132
Westerly, Rhode Island 02891
(404) 322-0454

Plastic stoma covers with replaceable filters are available from

Cardinal Manufacturing Co.
1055 E 52nd Street
PO Box 55223
Indianapolis, Indiana 46205

Instructions for crocheting laryngectomee bibs can be obtained from the American Cancer Society, listed in the telephone book (see Fig. 71-7).

Shower collars are available from

Mr. CL Sheldon
PO Box 128
Watertown, Massachusetts 02172
$8.25 each, mailed postpaid in the United States and Canada

Vaporizers and humidifiers are available in drug and grocery stores.

Distilled water, hydrogen peroxide, and saline are available in drug and grocery stores.

Medic-Alert bracelets inscribed with the words "Neck Breather" are available from

Medic Alert Foundation Inc.
Turlock, California 95380
Bracelets cost approximately $10.

International Association of Laryngectomees
219 E 42nd St
New York, New York 10017
(212) 867-3700

A & D Ointment is available without a prescription from drug and grocery stores. Stomahesive or a similar product is available from drug stores or medical-supply companies that sell ostomy supplies.

An artificial larynx is available from AT&T. Check with the local telephone company.

The Communicaid voice amplifier is available from

Communicaid
1560 West William Street
Decatur, Illinois 62522

The aid is designed to increase the voice volume of laryngectomees and others with weak voices.

Selected References

International Association of Laryngectomees: First Aid for (Neck Breathers) Laryngectomees. New York, International Association of Laryngectomees

Veterans Administration, Department of Medicine and Surgery: Laryngectomy: Orientation for Patient and Family. Washington, US Government Printing Office, 1986

Lauder E: Self-Help for the Laryngectomee, 1984, 11115 Whisper Hollow, San Antonio, Texas 78230

72　Mechanical Ventilation

Background

Advances in respiratory support over the past two decades have resulted in increased survival rates for victims of trauma and persons with neuromuscular diseases. Many of these people who cannot be weaned from the ventilator have been in intensive care units or long-term-care beds for extended periods of time. This practice consumes acute-care resources and provides an institutional existence for these clients. To decrease the costs of care and to improve the quality of life, many clients with chronic obstructive pulmonary disease (COPD) and neuromuscular diseases are candidates for home ventilatory support programs.

Chalikian and Weaver (1984) report encouraging survival statistics for people on home ventilator programs, up to 11 years according to one study, with an overall 3-year survival rate of 67%, dependent on age and diagnosis. A second study over a 34-month period reported a survival rate of 73% for persons with restrictive pulmonary disease and 43% for persons with obstructive respiratory problems. The reduction in hospital days was 73% and 36% for the restrictive and obstructive disease groups, respectively.

Clients with obstructive respiratory disease will probably require positive-pressure ventilatory support; persons with neuromuscular diseases where decreased lung compliance is not a problem will be candidates for external negative-pressure ventilatory support. Positive-pressure respirators require an artificial airway, either a tracheostomy or endotracheal tube. Some positive-pressure ventilators (e.g., Bantam respirator, Thompson Respiration Products Inc.) can function with a noncuffed tracheostomy tube; the client will be able to speak using the air that leaks around the tube.

Noninvasive and Negative-Pressure Ventilatory Support

Persons with neuromuscular diseases that cause hypercapnia (excessive carbon dioxide in the blood), a decreased ability to perform self-care activities because of dyspnea, or sleep-related breathing problems are candidates for home ventilatory support using noninvasive devices. These include the rocking bed, exsufflation belt, or external negative-pressure ventilators, such as the Poncho (Puritan-Bennett, Emerson) or Pulmo-Wrap (Lifecare).

Negative-pressure ventilators function on the principle of the iron lung. A machine similar to a vacuum cleaner generates negative pressure, causing a sucking action on the thorax. Light-weight, portable negative-pressure ventilators are available that envelop the thorax rather than the whole body as does the tank-type ventilator. The ventilators feature a rigid chest grid that attaches to a back plate. A wrap with a drawstring for the neck and elastic and Velcro closures for the extremities envelops the chest apparatus (Fig. 72-1).

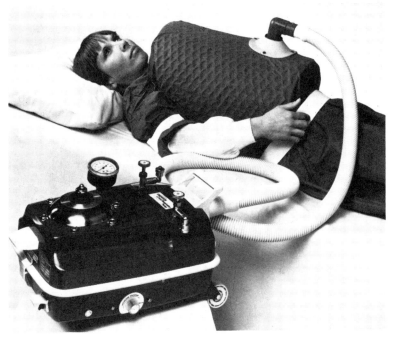

Figure 72.1
Negative-pressure ventilator (Emerson Chest Respirator Model 33-CRE).
(Courtesy of the JH Emerson Company, 22 Cottage Park Ave., Cambridge,
Massachusetts 02140)

The advantages of negative-pressure ventilators are their relatively small size
and ease of use and the ability to use them without a tracheostomy or endotracheal tube. They perform best in clients who have relatively compliant lungs
and who are able to control their secretions, such as people with spinal injuries
or disorders of the central nervous system. The Poncho and Pulmo-Wrap ventilators feature both control and assist modes. An electronic flow sensor that is
attached to the front of the person's nostril senses airflow and triggers the ventilator to assist spontaneous inspiratory effort. These newer negative-pressure
ventilators are superior to older tank-type ventilators that distribute negative
pressure over the entire body rather than just the thorax and cause tank shock
(pooling of blood in the extremities).

**Invasive
Positive-Pressure
Ventilators**

Clients who have tracheostomies or endotracheal tubes will require positive-
pressure ventilation. Most positive-pressure ventilators used in the hospital are
too complex for use in the home. The Emerson IMV ventilator has been found to
be suitable for home ventilation because it is relatively simple to use and troubleshoot. Using a Venturi system powered by an oxygen concentrator with the
Emerson ventilator will reduce the cost of oxygen. Otherwise an oxygen blender
powered by an air compressor and a cylinder of oxygen will be required.

A portable backup ventilator will be required for emergencies and for people
who are ambulatory or in wheelchairs (e.g., Life Products or Thompson portable
ventilators). These ventilators can be mounted on the back of a wheelchair and
powered with an automobile battery or they can be mounted on a cart with
wheels (Fig. 72-2).

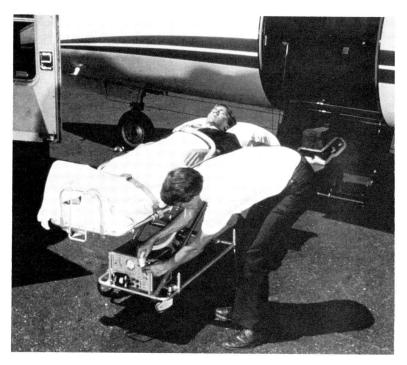

Figure 72.2
Client being transported using a positive-pressure ventilator. (Courtesy of Life Products, Inc.)

Selecting Candidates for Mechanical Ventilation in the Home

Clients with a strong desire to live at home, who are self-motivated, and who have supportive families are the best candidates for home ventilation. The teaching program must be completed in the hospital before discharge. When the client goes home, the home health nurse will assess the level of knowledge of the client and family and reinforce the client's knowledge of respiratory techniques, both routine and emergency. Sending the client home on pass overnight before discharge decreases the caregiver's anxiety about the responsibility of providing care.

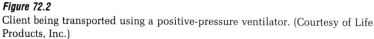

Assessment of Self-Care Potential

Client/Family Assessment

- Determine whether the client and family have the desire for the client to live at home with a ventilator. Assess whether the family is supportive and the client self-motivated.
- Determine whether a family member will be available to provide care if the client cannot perform self-care activities and if total care is required. Will a family member have to give up employment to attend to the client? Is this economically feasible? Will more than one family member be available for training? If the client requires total care, this is desirable.
- Determine whether other family members can provide respite care or whether this care will be available through an institution in the community. Can full-time nursing care in the home be obtained periodically to provide respite care? This is more desirable because the client will be able to stay in familiar surroundings.
- Determine whether the client or family member has the manual dexterity and eye–hand coordination required to perform respiratory techniques.

- Determine whether the client has adequate third-party coverage. Provide insurance counseling. Depending on the equipment and personnel required, the cost for a home ventilator program ranges from $1,000 to $5,000 monthly, as compared with the cost of hospital care, which costs from $12,000 to $20,000 monthly. If full-time nursing care will be required, this will cost from $15,000 to $16,000 monthly. Obtain a written commitment from the third-party provider before beginning the training program.
- Assist the client to assess the services of the available home vendors. (See Technique 73, Oxygen Administration.)

Physical Assessment

- Prior to beginning the training program in preparation for discharge home, assess whether the client is medically stable and whether there are other life-limiting diseases. Check that the client is stable on the ventilator and that the chest x-ray is clear (depending on the individual client). Check that blood gases are maintained within an optimal range. Determine whether the client will require supplemental oxygen or whether room air will suffice. Obtain baseline physical assessment data.
- Determine the amount of involvement that will be required by the family and the care that the client will be able to perform without assistance. This depends on the reason the client requires mechanical ventilation (e.g., neuromuscular disorder, COPD, post-trauma, or quadriplegia). The quadriplegic will be able to perform minimal self-care, whereas the person who requires only periodic ventilation will be self-sufficient in many activities.
- Determine whether the client will require invasive or noninvasive ventilatory support. Assess whether the client will be totally ventilator-dependent or whether ventilatory support will be required periodically (e.g., during sleep).
- When the client is transferred to the home ventilatory program, assess the level of knowledge of the caregiver. Base subsequent teaching and reinforcement on this information.

Environmental Assessment

- Assess the home for the best location for the client and equipment. This will depend on whether the client requires full-time ventilator support as opposed to periodic support (e.g., at night or during respiratory distress). Determine whether the client will be mobile in a wheelchair, with or without a portable ventilator. If the person is totally ventilator-dependent and bedridden, consider setting up the ventilator in the living room to enable the client to participate in normal family activities. The ventilator must be close to power and water supplies.
- If the client requires a wheelchair, check that it has a platform on the back for a portable ventilator.
- Assess the environment for cleanliness and air pollution (e.g., flowering plants or smokers in the family). General household cleaning practices must be adequate because, in the transition from hospital to home, many sterile techniques are replaced with clean techniques. This is acceptable practice because there is less risk of nosocomial infections at home.
- If the client is ventilator-dependent and uses a wheelchair, check the home for wheelchair access. Assess the width of doorways and the presence of stairs. Determine whether the client will have access to the bathroom for elimination and bathing or shower facilities.
- Prior to discharge from the hospital, check that the family has notified the electric company and community emergency agencies (e.g., fire department paramedics) that a ventilator-dependent person is in the home.
- If the client lives in an area where frequent power outages could be a problem, determine that sufficient battery power will be available to maintain the ventilator and suction equipment.

Planning Strategies

Potential Nursing Diagnoses

Breathing pattern, ineffective

Gas exchange, impaired: chronic respiratory problem, inability to clear secretions

Airway clearance, ineffective: chronic respiratory problem

Coping, ineffective family/individual: chronic disease, home ventilator program

Infection, potential for: related to home ventilator program

Expected Outcomes

Maintenance of adequate ventilatory support

Promotion of adequate gaseous exchange

Prevention of complications of ventilatory support such as airway obstruction or mechanical failure

Effective family/individual coping with chronic respiratory problem and home ventilator program

Health Promotion Goals

• The client and family will
  Manage a supplemental oxygen system and home ventilator program safely (See Technique 73, Oxygen Administration.)
  Perform routine and emergency respiratory techniques, including tracheostomy care, suctioning, chest physical therapy, medication administration (aerosol), and basic cardiopulmonary resuscitation, as appropriate
  Troubleshoot the ventilator when necessary. Maintain a backup portable ventilator with battery power and/or a manual resuscitator as appropriate
  Maintain the ventilator and equipment properly to ensure correct functioning and prevention of bacterial growth

Equipment

Ventilator (portable or stationary)

Oxygen source

Air compressor (for medication delivery)

Humidifier, distilled water

Alarm system

Ventilator tubing and valves (nondisposable) × 2 (one set for backup during cleaning)

Backup portable ventilator

Battery (backup power)

Manual resuscitator

Portable suction machine (electric, with battery backup)

Suction equipment

Interventions/Health Promotion

ACTION	*RATIONALE/AMPLIFICATION*
1. Check the ventilator for correct functioning. Drain condensation from all tubes.	Use the manufacturer's operator manual. Drain the tubes into a bucket or other receptacle, rather than back into the humidifier. This can be a source of infection.
2. Check and fill the humidifier as necessary.	Use distilled water in the humidifier.

ACTION	*RATIONALE/AMPLIFICATION*

3. Periodically analyze the oxygen concentration the client is receiving.

4. Measure the delivered tidal volume.

5. Check that all alarms are functioning correctly.

6. Auscultate breath sounds.

Related Care

1. Change the ventilator set-up and humidifier every 24 hours. Clean the tubings and humidifier reservoir in a weak vinegar solution. Rinse the equipment and hang to dry over the bathtub or in a similar area.	Vinegar deters bacterial growth in respiratory equipment.
2. Place tubing on the top rack of the dishwasher during the drying cycle (optional). When the tubings are dry, store them in a clean plastic bag.	The heat during the cycle kills most bacteria and decontaminates the tubing.
3. Suction the airways as necessary, or assist the client to do this.	The person will not be able to breathe effectively if the airways are not clear of mucus. This also reduces the risk of atelectasis or infection.
4. If the client has an artificial airway, provide a means of communication. If a "talking" tracheostomy tube is in place, the client will be able to communicate. People with regular tracheostomy tubes or laryngectomees will be able to communicate using an artificial larynx. A pencil and paper may also be useful. If the client lacks muscle tone, a picture board showing common needs can be used.	A "talking" tracheostomy tube has holes in the outside cannula so that some air can be diverted through the vocal cords. An artificial larynx enables the client to develop a mechanical voice by vibrating as the client changes the position of the vocal cords. This will require some instruction and encouragement.
5. Assist the client to perform mouth care. Not being able to swallow saliva is a problem for people with artificial airways.	
6. If the client has a cuffed tube (e.g., tracheostomy or endotracheal), maintain the cuff correctly.	Caring for cuffed tubes correctly prevents tissue breakdown and necrosis.
7. Change the tracheostomy or laryngectomy tube as necessary (see Technique 76, Tracheostomy Care).	

Education/ Communication

- Teach the client and family to

    Develop a daily routine for checking the ventilator

    Maintain the ventilator and oxygen equipment correctly

    Observe safety precautions for the use of oxygen

    Troubleshoot the ventilator. Place the client on the backup ventilator before adjusting the problem ventilator.

    Suspect ventilator failure if the client's condition suddenly begins to deteriorate

    Manually inflate the lungs using an Ambu bag if both ventilators malfunction

    Contact the home health nurse immediately if problems develop with the equipment. Transport the client by ambulance to the nearest emergency room in the event that the physician or nurse cannot be located. If the client is respirator-dependent, the lungs must be inflated manually.

    Manage the artificial airway (tracheostomy, laryngectomy) competently, if appropriate. (See Technique 76, Tracheostomy Care.) Assist the client with postural drainage, percussion and vibration, and suctioning as necessary.

    Observe and report changes in the client's sputum. This may indicate a respiratory infection.

    Report any symptoms of a respiratory infection (e.g., purulent sputum, dyspnea, or an elevated temperature)

    Request that people who are ill, particularly with upper respiratory tract infections, not come in contact with the client

    Remove irritants from the air as much as possible (e.g., cigarette smoke, pollens, or aerosol sprays). An air conditioner will be helpful in areas where smog is a problem. Change the air conditioner filters frequently.

Referrals and Consultations

- Instruct the client to report any problems with the ventilator immediately to the home health nurse. Provide a 24-hour emergency number for the family.
- Refer the client or family to the respiratory care vendor in the event of equipment malfunction.

Evaluation of Health Promotion Activities

Quality Assurance/ Reassessment

- Periodically observe the caregiver's respiratory care techniques, including airway management techniques and equipment maintenance.
- Observe the condition of the stoma if a tracheostomy or laryngectomy is present.
- Observe for signs of a respiratory infection. Culture the sputum if an infection is suspected. Initiate prompt treatment in consultation with the physician, because a respiratory infection will compromise the client's respiratory system.
- Periodically complete a general physical assessment, with emphasis on respiratory status. Obtain arterial blood gases as required.

DOCUMENTATION

Charting for the Home Health Nurse

Progress of the client/family in assuming responsibility for the ventilator program

The ability of the family member to initiate emergency care if necessary

Competency in maintaining the equipment and in caring for the client

Adequacy of the service provided by the respiratory care vendor

Psychological responses of the client and family, normalizing of relations between family members, and inclusion of the client in family activities. If the client is relatively stable, a portable ventilator can be strapped to a wheelchair to assist with mobility. Short trips by car can also be made using a portable ventilator.

Health Teaching Checklist

Name of Care Provider _____

Relationship to Client _____ Telephone #_____

Taught by _____ Date _____

	EXPLAINED	DEMONSTRATED
Ventilator set-up	_____	_____
Schedule on/off ventilator	_____	
Daily plan of care	_____	
Supplies, where to purchase	_____	
Infection control precautions	_____	_____
Routine ventilator/equipment maintenance	_____	_____
Troubleshooting	_____	_____
Power failure procedures	_____	_____
Emergency phone numbers	_____	
Basic cardiopulmonary resuscitation	_____	_____
Oxygen safety	_____	
Suctioning techniques	_____	_____
Chest physical therapy	_____	_____
Importance of adequate nutrition and fluid intake	_____	
Importance of active/passive exercise	_____	

Product Availability

Portable backup positive-pressure ventilators

Life Products (Boulder, Colorado)

LP-3 control mode
LP-4 control and assist modes, intermittent mandatory ventilation (IMV), high- and low-pressure alarm, high-pressure limit

Thompson Respiration Products (Boulder, Colorado)

Thompson M25B: variable I:E ratio, easy to carry, location of controls minimizes accidental alterations (Easier-to-connect Bennett PR-2 valve and tubing can be substituted for the Thompson exhalation valve.)

Positive-pressure ventilator

M3000 Minilung, 3000XA (control, assist, or IMV modes, patient-operated call alarm works whether respirator is on or off) (Thompson Respiration Products)

Emerson IMV (JH Emerson, Cambridge, Massachusetts)

Negative-pressure ventilators

Poncho cuirass (Puritan-Bennett, Emerson)

Pulmo-Wrap (Lifecare)

Maxivent, converts from negative-pressure to positive-pressure ventilator (Thompson Respiration Products)

Distilled water (available at all grocery stores)

Selected References

Benvenuti CS: Independence for the quadriplegic: The Bantam respirator. Am J Nurs 79(5):918–920, May, 1979

Chalikian J, Weaver T: CE mechanical ventilation, where it's at, where it's going. Am J Nurs 84(11):1373–1379, November, 1984

Darovic GO: Ten perils of mechanical ventilation . . . and how to hold them in check. RN 46(5):37–42, May, 1983

Gilmartin M, Make BJ: Mechanical ventilation in the home. Current Reviews in Respiratory Therapy 7(18):139–143, 1985

Zori SJ: CE mechanical ventilation: Bringing the patient into focus. Am J Nurs 84(11):1384–1388, November, 1984

73 Oxygen Administration

Background

Oxygen Supply

Oxygen is commonly administered in the home by persons who require supplemental oxygen for respiratory problems such as chronic obstructive pulmonary disease (COPD). The use of oxygen in the home requires a physician's prescription. Oxygen systems for home use include cylinders or tanks, oxygen concentrators, and liquid oxygen systems.

Oxygen concentrators separate and concentrate oxygen from room air. They are available in table-top models or larger floor models that can be equipped with castors for mobility. Liquid oxygen systems store oxygen in a liquid state under pressure. As the liquid warms it becomes a gas. Stationary home units, weighing about 70 lb, should be kept in a cool, well-ventilated area (Figs. 73-1 and 73-2). An indicator alerts the user when to call for a refill. Light-weight portable canisters that last for about 16 hours can be refilled from the home unit.

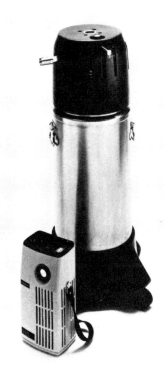

Figure 73.1
Inspiron 8500 liquid oxygen system. (Courtesy of Inspiron Corporation, Rancho Cucamonga, California)

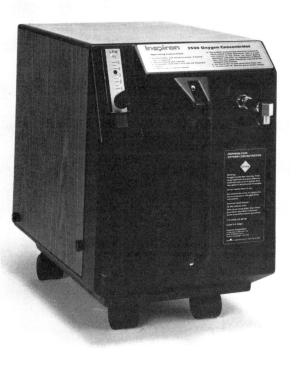

Figure 73.2
Inspiron 3500 Oxygen concentrator. (Courtesy of Inspiron Corporation, Rancho Cucamonga, California)

Most commonly, oxygen cylinders are used. Stationary tanks (G and H cylinders) stand about 5 feet high and weigh about 150 lb when full. D and E cylinders are portable, weighing from 10 lb to 17 lb, depending on the construction. The life of a tank of oxygen depends on the size of the tank and the flow rate (Table 73-1). A gauge alerts the user to the amount of oxygen remaining in the cylinder.

Table 73-1. OXYGEN FLOW RATES AND CYLINDER SIZE

FLOW RATE IN LITERS/MINUTE	H CYLINDER—HOURS OF USE	E CYLINDER—HOURS OF USE
1	100	10
2	50	5
3	33	3.3
4	25	2.5
5	20	2

Oxygen-Administration Devices

Oxygen is administered using either a nasal cannula or a Venturi mask (Fig. 73-3). A cannula is more convenient because it does not have to be removed for eating or drinking. Depending on the flow rate and the person's breathing pattern, a nasal cannula can deliver an oxygen concentration of approximately 24% to 44%. The Venturi mask will, because of its design, deliver the exact concentration of oxygen prescribed. The mask mixes room air with oxygen and comes with a variety of adaptors to deliver between 24% and 60% oxygen. Check the manufacturer's instructions for the specific liter flow of oxygen. Use a humidifier with either the cannula or mask to add moisture to the dry oxygen before it reaches the lungs.

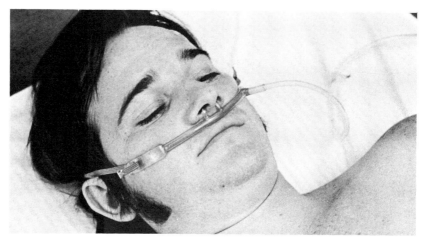

Figure 73.3
Nasal oxygen cannula. The client must breathe through the nose to benefit from this method.

Assessment of Self-Care Potential

Client/Family Assessment

- Assess whether the family is willing and able to assist the client with a home oxygen program.
- Determine whether the cost of oxygen and equipment will be paid by Medicare or other third-party payor.
- Assist the client to assess equipment and oxygen suppliers:
  Do they supply an explanation of billing if it is requested?
  Does the company bill Medicare or private payors directly or will the client receive a bill?

Do they provide assistance to set up and maintain the equipment and teach the client to use it properly?

Do they provide technical service and replacement parts?

Do they offer a 24-hour emergency service?

Will equipment no longer needed be promptly removed?

If equipment is rented, will they apply rental toward purchase? Renting oxygen equipment for a month before buying is a good idea to determine which equipment will be most beneficial.

Does the company maintain communication with the client, physician, or home health nurse?

Do they provide regular follow-up visits?

• Determine whether the client plans to rent an oxygen concentrator. The equipment will rent for a flat fee per month. Determine the amount of oxygen the client will require. If you estimate more than 8 to 10 cylinders per month, an oxygen concentrator will be more cost-effective. Expect an increase in the monthly electric bill.

Physical Assessment

• Determine the reason that the client requires supplemental oxygen (e.g., COPD, cancer of the lung). Obtain arterial blood-gas determination before beginning oxygen therapy.

• Obtain a respiratory history (e.g., smoking, environmental irritants, work-related irritants such as asbestos or strong chemicals).

• Assess the client's respiratory status during each visit, including breath sounds, respiratory effort, and skin color.

Environmental Assessment

• Determine that storage is available for oxygen cylinders or for the liquid oxygen system away from direct heat or sunlight, and that oil, grease, or other flammable materials are not stored near the system. Check that liquid oxygen, if used, is stored in a well-ventilated area, because some oxygen will evaporate when the unit is not being used.

• Determine whether open flames (e.g., gas stoves) will be at least 10 feet away from the oxygen source.

• Check that electrical equipment is properly grounded and that proper 3-pronged plugs are used for electrical appliances near the oxygen system.

Planning Strategies

Potential Nursing Diagnoses

Gas exchange, impaired: respiratory problem requiring supplemental oxygen

Breathing pattern, ineffective: respiratory problem requiring supplemental oxygen

Injury, potential for: due to home oxygen system

Knowledge deficit: management of home oxygen system

Expected Outcomes

Maintenance of adequate arterial oxygen level

Safe administration of supplemental oxygen

Understanding of the maintenance of a home oxygen system and the rationale for supplemental oxygen administration

Health Promotion Goals

• The client and family will
Administer and maintain a home oxygen system safely

Equipment

Oxygen source
Flow meter
Cannula or Venturi mask
Connecting tubing
Humidifier
Distilled water

Interventions/Health Promotion

ACTION

RATIONALE/AMPLIFICATION

1. Assemble and test the equipment:
   - Fill the humidifier with distilled water and attach it to the flow meter.
   - Attach the flow meter to the oxygen source.
   - Turn on the oxygen flow to check the function of the humidifier.
   - Connect the mask or cannula to the system and test.

2. Place the administration device on the client.

   Nasal prongs should be inserted so that the curve follows the natural curve of the nasal passages (see Fig. 73-3). Tubing is placed around each ear and secured under the chin. An oxygen mask should cover the mouth and nose. Adjust the metal band to fit the bridge of the nose. Secure the mask behind the head with the elastic band.

3. Set the flow meter to the prescribed rate.

4. Determine that the client is tolerating the oxygen.

Related Care

Daily Maintenance

1. Remove the cannula or mask from the humidifier and wipe it clean with warm water. Dry with a paper towel or clean cloth.

   Keeping all oxygen equipment clean prevents bacterial growth.

2. Remove the humidifier from the oxygen source. Empty the remaining distilled water, and wash the container with warm, soapy water. Rinse and dry.

   This prevents proliferation of bacteria. Disposable humidifiers should not be cleaned with soapy water but should be replaced weekly.

3. Refill the humidifier with distilled water and reconnect it to the oxygen source.

ACTION

RATIONALE/AMPLIFICATION

4. If the humidifier is not to be used immediately, let it air dry and reconnect it to the oxygen source. Refill it before use.

Weekly Maintenance

1. Remove the mask or cannula and tubing from the humidifier. Wash in warm, soapy water. Rinse completely by running warm water through the tubing using a small jug. Hang the tubing over a towel rail in the bathroom to air dry. Store the dry mask and tubing in a clean plastic bag.

If oxygen is required continually, use a new oxygen mask or cannula. Equipment can be rotated while one set is being cleaned. Dry equipment completely before storage to prevent bacterial growth.

2. If the client is using extra-long oxygen tubing, replace it monthly.

The extra-long tubing is difficult to clean properly.

3. Clean filters for an oxygen concentrator (if in use) weekly according to the manufacturer's instructions.

Education/ Communication

• Teach the client and family to

Only use the oxygen as directed. Too much oxygen will cause as many problems as too little oxygen.

Store oxygen equipment away from direct heat, open flames, grease, oil, or flammable material. Oxygen will support combustion and cause material to burn faster.

Order replacement oxygen tanks when the pressure gauge reads 500 psi or one-quarter full

Keep a backup portable oxygen cylinder available in the event of power failure or for travel, if the client is using an oxygen concentrator

Adjust the flow rate prior to putting on the cannula or mask. This prevents receiving a blast of oxygen and enables a quick check of the system to see that it is functioning correctly.

Secure the oxygen cylinder on a cart or stand to prevent falls and subsequent injury

Dust the cylinder only with a cotton cloth to prevent possible sparks, and not to cover the cylinder with material of any kind

Avoid using aerosols around the oxygen equipment to prevent fire. (Aerosols should never be used near a person with respiratory problems, since they can cause respiratory irritation.)

Avoid clothing or night dresses of nylon material and woolen blankets, which might cause sparks or static electricity

Keep open flames away from oxygen. Enforce no-smoking rules within 10 feet of the equipment. Place a sign in the room to remind visitors.

Avoid skin, eye, and clothing contact with the liquid from a leaking oxygen system

Avoid using electrical appliances (e.g., razors, hair dryers) while using oxygen

Always keep distilled water capped and refrigerated. Purchase distilled water in small quantities.

Special Instructions for People With Chronic Respiratory Problems

- Teach the client and family to

Give up smoking and not to allow smoking in the home

Avoid over-the-counter medications without consulting with the physician or nurse. They may conflict with prescribed medications. Aspirin can contribute to the symptoms of asthma.

Stress the importance of a healthful diet and exercise in the client's overall health status

Plan ahead if travel is anticipated:

Schedule travel so that rest will be possible to conserve energy.

Notify airline personnel of travel arrangements if oxygen will be required en route. (Cabin pressures in commercial aircraft simulate 10,000 feet above sea level. Some persons with respiratory problems experience difficulty above 5,000 feet.)

Check the altitude of the destination.

Arrange for respiratory equipment waiting on arrival, or contact a local vendor to supply equipment.

Check the quality of the air at the destination (smog, pollen, excessive heat or cold, dryness).

Carry medications personally in case luggage is delayed.

Carry a Medic-Alert card.

Stress the importance of frequent housecleaning. This can remove irritants and allergens. Use a damp cloth for dusting at least 3 times a week.

Avoid furnishing the house with carpet whenever possible. Use synthetic curtains rather than miniblinds, which gather dust. Wash drapes regularly.

Avoid using cleaning products with strong odors. These are respiratory irritants.

Control the home temperature to about 70°F (21.1°C) during the day, and 65°F (18.3°C) at night. Hot air irritates mucus membranes. Cold air precipitates bronchospasm.

A fan blowing on the client can make the client feel more comfortable.

Remove irritants and allergens from the home (e.g., flowering plants, animals, aerosols, chemicals with strong odors, or cigarette smoke).

Referrals and Consultations

- Refer the client to the American Lung Association for literature on respiratory disorders.
- Obtain a phone number for 24-hour emergency service for equipment and oxygen.

Evaluation of Health Promotion Activities

Quality Assurance/ Reassessment

- Evaluate the safety precautions employed by the client and family in the use of oxygen each time a visit is made.
- Check that the equipment is being maintained correctly.
- Determine that the client uses the oxygen only as prescribed.
- Reassess respiratory status and monitor arterial blood gases as required. Monitor for oxygen toxicity, which can mimic hypoxia. Evaluate for hypoxia, dyspnea, tachycardia, cyanosis, decreased sensorium, and restlessness.
- Check nasal mucosa for irritation if using nasal prongs. Switch to oxygen mask for a period of time if this is a problem. Check for dry mouth. This is a problem, particularly with central heating.

DOCUMENTATION

Charting for the Home Health Nurse

Competency of the client and family in using oxygen equipment

Liter flow and route prescribed

Respiratory assessment and condition of mucous membranes

Adherence to safety precautions

Adequate maintenance of oxygen equipment

Respiratory assessment

Ability to purchase or rent the required equipment

Psychological responses of the family and client regarding lifestyle or body-image changes with a chronic illness

Health Teaching Checklist

Name of Care Provider _____

Relationship to Client _____ Telephone # _____

Taught by _____ Date _____

	EXPLAINED	DEMONSTRATED
Use of oxygen and equipment, including liter flow and route	_____	_____
Sequencing of respiratory techniques	_____	_____
Side-effects of oxygen therapy (oxygen toxicity)	_____	
Safety precautions	_____	_____
Storage and maintenance of oxygen/equipment	_____	_____
Auscultation of breath sounds (if applicable)	_____	_____
Teaching hand-outs	_____	
Lifestyle alterations for chronic respiratory problems (asthma, bronchitis, chronic obstructive pulmonary disease [COPD])	_____	
Planning for travel	_____	
Environmental alterations	_____	
Supplier/vendor information	_____	
Insurance counseling	_____	
Community resources	_____	
24-hour emergency number	_____	

Product Availability

Oxygen flow meters
  Hudson Oxygen
  OEM Medical
  Ohmeda
  Puritan-Bennett Corporation

Oxygen humidifiers
  Airlife Inc.
  Inspiron Corporation
  Respiratory Care Inc.
  Travenol Laboratories, Inc.—Medical Products Division

Oxygen-administration devices
Airlife Inc.
Hudson Oxygen
Inspiron Corporation
Puritan-Bennett Corporation

Client instruction booklet

Christmas Seal League of Southwestern Pennsylvania: Self-Help: Your Strategy for Living with COPD. Distributed by Bull Publishing Co., P.O. Box 208, Palo Alto, CA 94302; (415) 322-2855

Selected References

Burton GG, Hodgkin JE: Respiratory Care, 2nd ed. Philadelphia, JB Lippincott, 1984

Hamilton H: Procedures. Springhouse, PA, Intermed Communications, 1983

McPherson SP: Respiratory Therapy Equipment, 3rd ed. St Louis, CV Mosby, 1985

74   Pressure Breathing Treatments

Background

Incentive Spirometry

This technique involves the use of a volume-measuring device (incentive spirometer) to improve the tidal volume and prevent atelectasis. It will also strengthen the client's cough and ability to expectorate. It can be used in place of intermittent positive-pressure breathing (IPPB) if the client is capable of producing an adequate tidal volume unassisted. Keep a record of the attempts to encourage the client to improve each subsequent attempt. Follow the manufacturer's instructions to assist the client in using the device (see Technique 68, Breathing Exercises and Chest Physiotherapy).

Hand-Held Nebulizer Therapy

Hand-held nebulizers are an effective device for delivering aerosolized medications to clients who are capable of producing an adequate tidal volume. They can be combined with an incentive spirometer to allow the care provider to document volumes as well as deliver medication. A compressor will be required for this type of therapy. This technique is less complicated for the care provider and client than IPPB therapy.

Intermittent Positive-Pressure Breathing

Intermittent positive-pressure breathing using a respirator increases the tidal volume for clients who cannot voluntarily do deep breathing exercises. If the client can initiate the inspiration, the machine will provide positive pressure to produce the desired tidal volume. IPPB is appropriate to deliver aerosolized medications if a hand-held nebulizer is not effective.

Assessment of Self-Care Potential

See Technique 73, Oxygen Administration.

Planning Strategies

Potential Nursing Diagnoses

Gas exchange, impaired

Injury, potential for

Breathing pattern, ineffective

Airway clearance, ineffective

Expected Outcomes

Improved oxygenation (PaO_2)

Prevention of atelectasis

Decreased congestion of the bronchial mucosa

Reduction of episodes of bronchospasm (IPPB)

Absorption of prescribed medications

Improved expectoration

Health Promotion Goals

- The client and family will
  Administer breathing treatments as often as directed
  Administer breathing treatments before meals
  Sequence breathing treatments before postural drainage and before chest physiotherapy

Equipment

HAND-HELD NEBULIZER

Compressor

Flow meter

Medications (as ordered)

Saline

Hand-held nebulizer

Mouthpiece, connecting tubing

76-inch section, corrugated plastic tubing

Tissues

IPPB

Oxygen source

IPPB machine

Breathing circuit (tubing set-up)

Mouthpiece

Noseclips, if needed

Medications (as ordered)

Tissues

Interventions/Health Promotion

ACTION	*RATIONALE/AMPLIFICATION*
Compressor With Hand-Held Nebulizer	
1. Connect breathing circuit and mouthpiece to the IPPB machine. Insert medications/saline in the medication cup on the breathing circuit. Turn the machine on (Fig. 74-1).	The physician may order medication to be delivered using the IPPB machine. This will be mixed with saline according to the strength required. Saline alone may also be used.

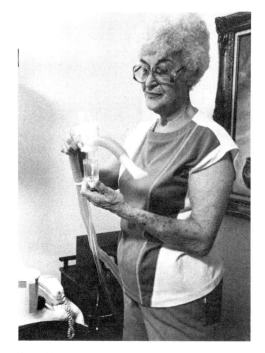

Figure 74.1

ACTION

2. Adjust the nebulizer if necessary.

3. Place the client in a sitting position.

4. Instruct the client to close lips tightly around the mouthpiece and to take a slow, deep breath. Hold the breath for a few seconds, and exhale slowly with lips pursed. Use a noseclip if the client has difficulty not breathing through the nose (Fig. 74-2).

RATIONALE/AMPLIFICATION

The nebulizer humidifies the inspired air. Observe for mist flowing from the mouthpiece.

This allows greater lung expansion. If the client remains in bed, raise the head to at least 45 degrees.

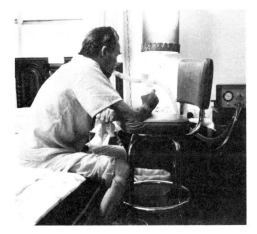

Figure 74.2

ACTION	**RATIONALE/AMPLIFICATION**
5. Complete the treatment.	This usually takes 10 to 20 minutes depending on the client's breathing pattern.
6. Instruct the client to remove the mouthpiece to cough. Turn off the machine if the client needs to rest.	The client will not obtain the full benefit from the medication if the machine is turned on during breaks.
7. When the treatment is completed, turn off the compressor. Rinse medication cup and mouthpiece. Dry with a paper towel and reassemble the equipment.	

Intermittent Positive-Pressure Breathing

1. Connect the breathing circuit to the IPPB machine. Add medication/saline to the cup as ordered. Turn the machine on and observe the nebulizer for mist.	Observing for mist will ensure that the nebulizer is functioning correctly and that the client will obtain full benefit of the medication.
2. Instruct the client to close lips tightly around the mouthpiece. Inhale through the mouth and relax once the machine is triggered (Fig. 74-3). Exhale slowly through the mouthpiece. Remove the mouthpiece to cough. Turn off the machine if the client needs to rest.	The machine cycle will automatically fill the lungs.

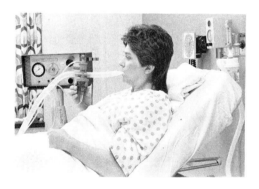

Figure 74.3

3. Complete the treatment.	This usually takes 10 to 20 minutes.
4. Provide a mouthwash if desired.	

Related Care

Incorporate breathing treatments with breathing exercises and chest physiotherapy.	Prevent nausea by avoiding breathing treatments immediately following mealtimes.

Daily Maintenance

1. Following the last treatment of the day, dismantle the breathing circuit from the machine. Clean in warm, soapy water using a soft brush as necessary. Rinse with running water.	If the tubing from the machine contains moisture, clean it also.

ACTION	RATIONALE/AMPLIFICATION
2. Soak in a solution of 1 cup white vinegar and 4 cups of water for at least 30 minutes. Remove the equipment from the vinegar solution and hang to air dry.	This discourages bacterial growth, which could lead to a respiratory infection. Over a bath or shower is ideal for air drying the tubings so that they can drip.
3. When the equipment is dry, store it in a plastic bag.	This keeps the equipment free from dust.

Weekly Maintenance

Wipe the machine with a damp cloth. Keep the machine in an area free from dust between treatments.

Periodic Maintenance

1. Change filters on the machine every 6 months following the manufacturer's instructions.	
2. If the client has a Bennett AP-4 or 5, check that the valve drum is clean and free from dust. Follow manufacturer's instructions.	The machine will not function correctly if this is not done.
3. Check IPPB tubing assembly exhalation valve for moisture. Dry it if this is a problem.	The valve will stick if it is wet.

Education/ Communication

- Teach the client and family to
  Administer breathing treatments before meals to prevent nausea or vomiting
  Administer breathing treatments before postural drainage and chest physiotherapy to enhance the effect of these procedures
  Discontinue breathing treatments and notify the home health nurse if side-effects are a problem
  Use a nose clip if breathing through the mouthpiece is a problem
  Check all connections to make sure they are tight. The machine will not function correctly if connections are not tight
  Check the tubing and breathing circuit for any kinks or other obstructions
  Discard any medication that remains at the end of the treatment
  Turn off the machine while resting during the treatment to prevent wasting the medication
  Remove the mouthpiece before coughing
  Maintain the equipment correctly
  Have on hand two complete sets of tubing so that one can be used while the other is cleaned
  Keep machine and equipment off the floor where dust can be a problem
  Be sure that the compressor or IPPB machine has a three-pronged plug to prevent electric shock. Observe safety precautions for the use of oxygen. (See Technique 73, Oxygen Administration.)
  Make homemade saline solution if saline is used with treatments (Table 74-1)

Table 74-1. HOMEMADE SALINE SOLUTION

INGREDIENTS

¼ teaspoon table salt (not iodized)
1 cup distilled water
Mason jar

METHOD

Mix salt and distilled water in the jar. Screw the lid on loosely. Place the jar in a pot of water to ¾ the height of the jar. Bring the water to a boil and boil for 25 minutes to sterilize the saline. Turn off the heat and leave it on the stove to cool. When cool, remove the jar and secure the lid. Store the saline in the refrigerator. Remove only what is necessary for each treatment, and do not return any unused saline to the jar. Discard any solution left at the end of the week and make it fresh. Discard the solution if it becomes cloudy.

Evaluation of Health Promotion Activities

Quality Assurance/ Reassessment

- Periodically observe the client's technique, and check that the equipment is being maintained correctly.
- Evaluate for side-effects of IPPB: dizziness, nausea or vomiting, rapid pulse rate, palpitations, or increased dyspnea. The symptoms will vary with the prescribed medication. These can occur with nebulizer therapy, but are more likely with IPPB.
- Determine that the client uses breathing treatments only as prescribed.
- Reassess respiratory status. Monitor periodic blood gases if applicable.

DOCUMENTATION

Charting for the Home Health Nurse

Competency of the client and family in administering IPPB/nebulizer therapy

Adherence to safety precautions while using oxygen

Adequate maintenance of equipment

Respiratory assessment

Side-effects experienced with IPPB/nebulizer therapy (if applicable)

Ability to purchase or rent the required equipment

Psychological responses of the family and client regarding lifestyle or body-image changes that occur with a chronic respiratory problem

Health Teaching Checklist

Name of Care Provider _____

Relationship to Client _____ Telephone #_____

Taught by _____ Date _____

	EXPLAINED	DEMONSTRATED
Procedure for using breathing device	_____	_____
Safety precautions	_____	_____
Adverse side-effects of treatment and medications used	_____	
Maintenance procedures	_____	_____
24-hour emergency phone number	_____	
Referral/vendor information	_____	
Insurance/Medicare counseling	_____	

Product Availability

IPPB machines
  Bird Products/3M
  Puritan-Bennett Corporation
IPPB breathing circuits and hand-held nebulizers
  Airlife Inc.
  Hudson Oxygen
  Inspiron Corporation
  Puritan-Bennett Corporation

Selected References

Burton G, Hodgkin J: Respiratory Care: A Guide to Clinical Practice, 2nd ed. Philadelphia, JB Lippincott, 1984

McPherson SP: Respiratory Therapy Equipment, 3rd ed. St Louis, CV Mosby, 1985

Spearman CB et al: Egan's Fundamentals of Respiratory Therapy, 4th ed. St Louis, CV Mosby, 1982

75   Suctioning

Background

Surgical procedures, pain, and chronic medical problems such as muscular dystrophy reduce the client's ability to cough effectively. Failure to clear the respiratory tract effectively results in hypoxia, hypercapnia (increased CO_2), and respiratory infections. People who are unable to mobilize secretions unaided will require suctioning. If the person can cough secretions into the pharynx, suctioning may be limited to the mouth and pharynx. A laryngectomy or tracheostomy will facilitate suctioning the trachea, but creates more potential for respiratory infections. Blind endotracheal suctioning may be required if the person cannot mobilize secretions and does not have an artificial airway in place. This technique requires more skill and will usually be performed by the respiratory therapist or home health nurse.

Measures to Mobilize Secretions

Encourage the person in deep breathing and coughing as much as possible because any entry into the upper respiratory tract is an opportunity for infection. Ambulation or frequent movement in bed will also assist in mobilizing secretions. Maintaining an adequate fluid intake will assist in liquefying secretions so that the airway can be cleared more easily. If secretions are tenacious, a few drops of sterile saline can be instilled into the artificial airway (or suction catheter in the event of blind endotracheal suctioning) to liquefy secretions.

Infection-Control Measures

To prevent nosocomial infections while the client is in the hospital, strict sterile technique is necessary. In the home environment, there is less chance of respiratory infection because the client is exposed to the same organisms on a daily basis. Organisms that are resistant to antibiotics are found in the hospital, but they usually would not be present in the home. In addition, the difficulty in teaching sterile technique to family members, as well as the prohibitive cost of sterile supplies, demands a different approach for airway care in the home. Teach the client and family to use a clean technique, emphasizing correct handwashing. Cold sterilization can be used for resterilizing suction catheters, particularly if the client has a tracheostomy on a long-term basis. Cleaning catheters and suction equipment in soap and water is usually all that is necessary if correct handwashing techniques are used.

Assessment of Self-Care Potential

Client/Family Assessment

- Determine the willingness and ability of family members to assist the client in respiratory techniques.
- Assess whether the family can meet the expenses of the equipment required. Determine whether equipment will be rented or purchased (e.g., suction machine).
- Assess the client for body-image changes, particularly if artificial airways are in place. Assess the ability of the client and family to accept these changes.
- Assess the knowledge level of the client and family and the amount of teaching that will be required. Determine the frequency of visits that will be necessary to teach and to supervise respiratory care for the client.

Physical Assessment

- Assess skin color for cyanosis, indicating hypoxemia. Use adequate lighting. In dark-skinned or tanned individuals check for cyanosis of mucous membranes or loss of reddish undertones in the skin.
- Inspect the person for evidence of difficult respirations (sternal retraction, use of accessory muscles to breathe).
- Assess the person for gurgling or noisy respirations, indicating secretions in the respiratory tract. Auscultate the lung fields for the presence of crackles.
- Determine whether the client can clear the airway by coughing.
- Determine the size catheter that will be required. It should be large enough to remove secretions but not large enough to occlude the airway. Size 16 French is appropriate for most adult clients. Infants require 8 to 10 French, and children 10 to 12 French.
- Observe the color and consistency of secretions. Blood-streaked sputum indicates mucosal trauma from suctioning. Whitish or greenish sputum or an offensive smell can indicate a respiratory infection.
- During suctioning, particularly blind endotracheal suctioning, check the client periodically for pulse abnormalities. Hypoxia can cause premature ventricular contractions noted by irregularity in the pulse. Vagal stimulation can cause extreme bradycardia.

Environmental Assessment

- Assess the home for the presence of respiratory irritants such as dust, pollen, or chemicals. Investigate cleaning techniques. Damp dusting and vacuuming will be less irritating to the client than dry dusting and sweeping. Determine whether aerosols, which are potential irritants, are used in the home. Blooming house plants can also be a problem.
- Assess the home for cleanliness. Clean techniques cannot be carried out if the environment and family habits do not promote cleanliness.
- Ascertain a place in the home where suctioning equipment can be cleaned or soaked. Running water will be required. Catheters and suction tubing will need to be hung to drain.

Planning Strategies

Potential Nursing Diagnoses

Airway clearance, ineffective: inability to cough respiratory secretions

Gas exchange, impaired: retained respiratory secretions

Infection, potential for

Knowledge deficit: suctioning techniques and infection-control precautions

Expected Outcomes

Effective airway clearance

Effective gas exchange in the alveoli

Prevention of hypoxia and hypercapnia

Prevention of respiratory infection

Increased knowledge of safe suctioning techniques

Health Promotion Goals

- The client and family will
  Promote measures to reduce the requirement for suctioning
  Suction the respiratory tract as necessary to maintain a clear airway, using a clean technique
  Employ measures to maintain the arterial oxygen content prior to and during suctioning

Equipment
Suction machine with battery pack
Supplemental oxygen equipment (optional)
Suction catheters
Sterile water-soluble lubricant (for blind endotracheal suctioning only)
Connecting tube and Y connector
Water in a disposable bathroom cup
Sterile normal saline in syringe (3 ml) (optional)
Clean examination gloves (optional)
Mirror (if necessary)

Interventions/Health Promotion

ACTION

RATIONALE/AMPLIFICATION

1. Check the operation of the suction machine.

If the amount of suction is adjustable, the pressure should not be lower than −120 cm water pressure for adults or −60 cm water pressure for pediatric clients.

2. Wash hands. Pour clean tap water in a fresh, disposable, bathroom cup. Attach the connecting tubing to the suction machine. Attach the Y connector to the connecting tubing.

Don clean examination gloves if desired. Do not allow water to stand between suctioning because this will encourage bacterial growth. The Y connector will enable fingertip control of suctioning to prevent trauma to the respiratory mucosa from excessive buildup of pressure. If polyethylene catheters with built-in fingertip control are used, the Y connector may be omitted. Controlling suction by clamping the catheter between the fingers rather than using fingertip control causes excessive buildup of pressure.

3. If supplemental oxygen is available, administer to the client for a few minutes before suctioning.

Administering oxygen before suctioning decreases the possibility of hypoxia during suctioning.

4. Select a catheter and attach it to the Y connector. Perform blind endotracheal suctioning or suction the artificial airway as indicated.

Blind Endotracheal Suctioning (ETS)

1. Place the client in a sitting position. Lubricate the tip of the catheter with sterile lubricant.

This position facilitates endotracheal suctioning. Lubricant facilitates passing the catheter and decreases trauma to the mucous membranes. Use only water-soluble lubricant. Inhalation of oil-based products can cause granulomatous pneumonia.

ACTION

RATIONALE/AMPLIFICATION

2. Insert the catheter with a downward angle through the nostril and into the nasopharynx (Fig. 75-1). Advance the catheter slowly. Stop at any sign of obstruction.

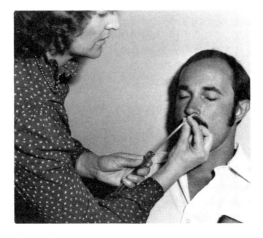

Figure 75.1
Blind endotracheal suctioning. (Photograph by Keith Mitchell, Medical Media, Veterans Administration Medical Center, Amarillo, Texas)

3. When the catheter is in the oropharynx, ask the client to take a slow, deep breath.

The client usually gags when the catheter reaches the oropharynx. A deep breath causes the epiglottis to retract and allows the catheter to pass through the vocal cords and into the trachea.

4. Ask the client to continue to take deep breaths through the mouth while slowly advancing the catheter as far as possible. Withdraw the catheter 1 cm to 2 cm.

Deep breaths reduce the gag reflex and the feeling of choking. Do not apply suction while inserting the catheter to prevent damage to the mucous membranes. Advancing the catheter in this manner should place the tip just above the carina level. This can be confirmed by listening for breath sounds through the catheter. The client *can* breathe through the catheter while it is in place. The client will also be unable to speak if the catheter is passed through the vocal cords.

5. Withdraw the catheter slowly while rotating it between the fingers and applying intermittent suction. If secretions are tenacious, instill approximately 5 ml of sterile normal saline through the catheter. Suction for 10 to 15 seconds only.

Continuous suction can cause the mucosa to be drawn into the eye of the catheter. Sterile saline helps to thin secretions.
Limiting suctioning attempts to 15 seconds reduces hypoxia caused by suctioning air from the trachea.

ACTION	RATIONALE/AMPLIFICATION
6. Allow the client to rest before repeating the procedure. Give supplemental oxygen if appropriate. Rinse the catheter by suctioning a few milliliters of water between attempts if necessary.	The procedure is exhausting to the person. Oxygen administration allows the arterial oxygenation to return to the presuction level.
7. Suction the oropharynx and mouth after the tracheal suctioning is complete, if necessary. Suction water through the catheter and connecting tubing to rinse. Disconnect the catheter and soak it in a soap and water solution. Turn off the suction machine. Leave the connecting tubing and Y connector attached to the suction machine, and coil conveniently for future use.	Use the clean catheter to suction the trachea. Suctioning the mouth first introduces additional bacteria into the trachea.

Suctioning a Tracheostomy or Laryngectomy

ACTION	RATIONALE/AMPLIFICATION
1. Disconnect the ventilator (if appropriate). Place the connector on a clean towel on the client's bed or on lap if the person is seated.	
2. Introduce the catheter into the tracheostomy or laryngectomy tube. Use sterile water-soluble lubricant to moisten the catheter tip if insertion is difficult. Withdraw the catheter slowly while rotating the catheter and applying intermittent suction. Apply suction only while withdrawing the catheter.	A tracheostomy will usually have a tube in place. Once a laryngectomy has healed, the person will only insert a tube periodically to dilate the stoma. The technique is similar whether or not there is a tube in place. If the person is on a respirator, a cuffed tube will usually be required. Using intermittent suction prevents excessive buildup of pressure and resultant mucosal damage (Fig. 75-2).

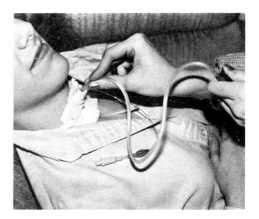

Figure 75.2
Suctioning a tracheostomy using fingertip control to prevent excess pressure in the suction catheter.

ACTION

3. Instill approximately 5 ml of sterile saline into the airway if secretions are tenacious. Limit suctioning attempts to 15 seconds.

4. Reconnect the ventilator if the client is being ventilated. Suction a few milliliters of water to rinse the catheter. Repeat the procedure if necessary. Rinse the catheter and suction the mouth and pharynx if necessary. Rinse the tubing with water.

5. Turn off the suction machine. Disconnect the catheter from the connector and place it in soap and water to soak. Coil the tubing conveniently for future use.

RATIONALE/AMPLIFICATION

This thins the secretions so they can be suctioned or coughed. Limiting suctioning attempts prevents hypoxia.

The client may be able to remove secretions from the mouth with a tissue. If not, the mouth may be suctioned after suctioning the trachea. Suctioning the mouth first introduces bacteria into the trachea.

Related Care

1. Clean catheters after use:
   • Place catheters immediately into soap and water solution to soak.
   • Each day, soak the suction tubing and Y connector in soap and water.
   • Rinse the catheters and tubing in clean water and hang to drip dry. Store in plastic bags until ready to use.

2. If preferred, use a germicide to disinfect catheters:
   • Rinse catheters with water after soaking in soap and water.
   • Use 1 oz of Control 3 to 1 gallon of water. Soak catheters and tubing in the solution. Rinse with water and hang to dry. Place in plastic bags until ready for use.

3. Ambulate the client as often as possible, or encourage active or passive exercise in bed. Turn the immobile client every 2 hours. Encourage coughing and deep breathing every 2 hours or more frequently if necessary. Teach the client to use an incentive spirometer or to blow up balloons if appropriate. (See Technique 68, Breathing Exercises and Chest Physiotherapy.)

4. Encourage oral fluids.

Secretions will be difficult to remove if allowed to dry.

Placing a towel over the shower door is an ideal place to dry the catheters.

The active ingredient in Control 3 is dimethylbenzylammonia chloride 10%. Discard the solution every 14 days.

Exercise and deep breathing will assist the client to mobilize secretions.

Increased fluid intake makes secretions more liquid.

ACTION	*RATIONALE/AMPLIFICATION*
5. Avoid persons with respiratory infections.	An upper respiratory infection will increase mucus production. Allowing secretions to accumulate will encourage the development of respiratory infections.
6. Use a humidifier to increase the humidity in the room if beneficial for a tight, dry cough.	Increased humidity helps liquefy secretions. *Do not use a teakettle or open pan of water on an electric plate in the client's room.* There is danger of burning the client.
7. Auscultate the client's lungs periodically to determine whether secretions are accumulating.	Fluid in the respiratory tract will be indicated by moist crackles.
8. Raise the head of the bed as much as possible to facilitate lung expansion. Turn unresponsive clients from side to side to encourage mucus to drain from the mouth rather than to occlude the airway.	If an unresponsive client is allowed to remain supine, mucus or regurgitated stomach contents will occlude the airway.

Education/Communication

- Teach the client and family to
  Suction the client only if necessary. It is preferable for the person to cough secretions. Provide assistance in removing secretions from the mouth with a tissue or wet paper towel as necessary. Any suctioning attempt carries the risk of introducing an infection and damaging the respiratory tract.
  Avoid persons with respiratory infections to prevent transmitting a respiratory infection to the client
- Teach the client to
  Suction the tracheostomy or laryngectomy using a small makeup mirror. While the client is seated, place the mirror on a TV table so that the airway can be visualized (Fig. 75-3).
- Tell the client and family to report changes in secretions, which can indicate a respiratory infection.

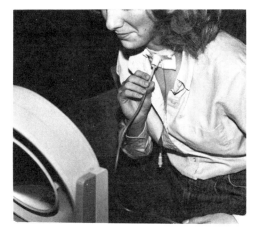

Figure 75.3
Client is able to suction herself using a small makeup mirror to aid visualization.

| **Referrals and Consultations** | International Association of Laryngectomees, 219 East 42nd Street, New York, NY 10017; (212) 467-3700 |

Evaluation of Health Promotion Activities

Quality Assurance/ Reassessment

- Periodically observe the caregiver's suctioning technique.
- Obtain a sputum culture using a sterile suction catheter and sterile gloves if a respiratory infection is suspected. Refer the client to the physician.

DOCUMENTATION

Charting for the Home Health Nurse

Progress of the client/family in assuming responsibility for suctioning the client

Psychological responses of the family and client regarding the respiratory problem; the ability of the family to support the client

Color, amount, consistency, and odor of respiratory secretions

Respiratory assessment findings

Ability of the family to purchase or rent the required equipment; availability of third-party coverage

Records Kept by the Client/Family

Frequency of suctioning

Color, amount, consistency, and odor of respiratory secretions

Periodic vital signs to monitor for temperature elevation indicating possible respiratory infection

Health Teaching Checklist

Name of Care Provider _____

Relationship to Client _____ Telephone # _____

Taught by _____ Date _____

	EXPLAINED	DEMONSTRATED
Measures to liquefy and mobilize secretions	_____	
Incorporation of breathing exercises, chest physiotherapy, and postural drainage with suctioning	_____	_____
Checking breath sounds	_____	_____
Suctioning techniques	_____	_____
Prevention of hypoxia	_____	_____
Changes in secretions that should be reported	_____	
Equipment maintenance	_____	_____

Product Availability

Humidifiers are available at large grocery stores and pharmacies. They are relatively inexpensive. In areas where hard water is a problem, consider using distilled water, which is available at grocery stores, or rainwater, which can be stored in empty plastic milk jugs that have been cleaned with soap and hot water.

Red rubber suction catheters that can be reused are recommended for home use. They are available from medical-supply companies listed in the yellow pages of the telephone book or from home health equipment agencies. Suction machines and suction equipment are available from the same sources. Disposable polyethylene catheters are also available. They may be cleaned and reused but will not last as long as the red rubber catheters. The sterile polyethylene catheters are more expensive.

Control 3 is available through medical-supply companies. An 8-oz bottle will last up to 16 weeks and costs about $12.

Small makeup mirrors are available in grocery and department stores at minimal cost.

Clean examination gloves are available in pharmacies and at medical-supply companies.

National respiratory care vendors are

Glassrock Home Health Care

Abby

Travacare

Literature:

Lauder E: Self-Help for the Laryngectomee, 1983–84 ed. Available from the author, 11115 Whisper Hollow, San Antonio, TX (also available in Spanish)

Selected References

Fuchs PL: Streamlining your suctioning techniques. Part 1. Nasotracheal suctioning. Nursing '84 14(5):55–61, May, 1984

Fuchs PL: Streamlining your suctioning techniques. Part 3. Tracheostomy suctioning. Nursing '84 14(7):39–43, July, 1984

76   Tracheostomy Care

Background

A tracheostomy is a surgical opening into the lower part of the neck extending into the trachea. The opening (stoma) is maintained by inserting a tracheostomy tube. The person then breathes through this tube. Most tracheostomy tubes consist of three parts: the outer cannula (with or without a cuff to keep it in place); the inner cannula; and the obturator, which is inserted into the outer cannula while the tube is inserted into the stoma and is then replaced with the inner cannula (Fig. 76-1). It is vital that the tube be kept patent at all times, and, on at least a daily basis, the inner cannula is removed and cleaned to remove encrusted secretions that can block the tube.

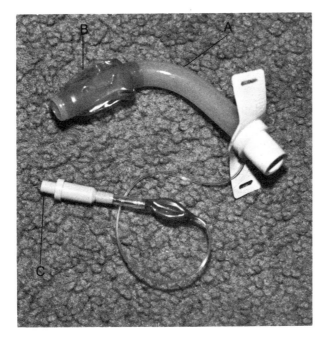

Figure 76.1
Disposable plastic tracheostomy tube. (A) Outer cannula. (B) Cuff. (C) Port for inflating cuff.

Most tracheostomy tubes have a cuff that is inflated to provide an airtight seal for people who require positive-pressure ventilation. Because constant pressure from the cuff can interrupt the blood supply to the trachea, only inflate the cuff if the client will be on a ventilator. Otherwise, leave it deflated. If the person requires positive-pressure ventilation, a soft cuff that does not require periodic deflation should be used for managing a tracheostomy at home. Routinely refer the client to the physician to replace the tracheostomy cuff every 90 days to prevent the development of cuff problems that could result in an emergency situation. "Talking tracheostomy tubes" are ideal for clients who will require long-term management with a tracheostomy. The design of these tubes allows air to flow through the vocal chords during exhalation so that the person is able to speak. If a regular tube is in place and the cuff is deflated, the person can speak by occluding the tube with a finger during exhalation. If the tube is occluded with a specially designed plug for periods of time, the cuff will be deflated and the person will be able to speak normally.

Strict sterile technique is used in caring for a tracheostomy while a person is in the hospital. Substitute clean techniques for sterile techniques in managing respiratory care at home. Emphasize effective handwashing. Clean techniques are appropriate for home care because antibiotic-resistant organisms are not usually present in the home, and there is no risk of nosocomial infection. In addition, teaching sterile technique to the caregiver may not be feasible and increases the cost of home care considerably.

Assessment of Self-Care Potential

Client/Family Assessment
- Determine the willingness and the ability of family members to assist the client to provide self-care. Assess the amount of care that the client can perform unassisted. Assess the amount of care that will be required from the respiratory therapist or home health nurse.
- Assess the ability of the family to pay for long-term respiratory care services, particularly if the person is on a ventilator. Determine if third-party payment is available and whether insurance counseling has been provided.
- Explore respiratory product vendors with the family to determine the most appropriate vendor.
- Assess whether the client's altered body image has been accepted by the client and family.
- Determine what specific supplies will be needed and whether these will be supplied by the home health agency or purchased locally by the family.

Physical Assessment
- Assess the tube for patency. Observe the client for adequate oxygenation and respiratory distress.
- Assess the condition of the stoma and surrounding skin. Check for excoriation of the skin due to excessive secretions.
- Note the characteristics and amount of secretions to monitor for respiratory infections.
- Check vital signs (particularly temperature) to monitor for infection.

Environmental Assessment
- Check the home for the presence of respiratory irritants. Remove as many irritants as possible from the environment.
- Observe the home environment for cleanliness. If standard sanitary practices are not followed, clean respiratory techniques cannot be implemented.
- Check for adequate handwashing facilities adjacent to where tracheostomy care will be given. Check that a fresh supply of clean handtowels will be available.
- Check that adequate lighting is available. Determine if a reading lamp could be used to supplement lighting.

Planning Strategies

Potential Nursing Diagnoses

Airway clearance, ineffective: artificial airway

Infection, potential for

Home maintenance management, impaired: artificial airway

Knowledge deficit: tracheostomy care

Self-concept, disturbance in: body image due to artificial airway

Social isolation: loss of/change in vocalization due to artificial airway

Expected Outcomes

Maintenance of patent airway

Prevention of respiratory infection

Reintegration into social support systems to the level desired

Attainment of optimal level of self-care

Acceptance of body-image changes

Mastery of alternative communication techniques

Health Promotion Goals

- The client and family will
  Assume care of the tracheostomy
  Use infection-control practices to prevent respiratory infection
  Accept body-image changes

Equipment

2 disposable kitchen cups (5-oz size) or

2 small bowls

Hydrogen peroxide

Saline or distilled water

Pipe cleaners or small brush

Twill tape

4 × 4s or nonstick dressing (Telfa)

Suction equipment

6-ml syringe (if cuff is to be deflated)

Brown paper bag for used 4 × 4s

Interventions/Health Promotion

ACTION	RATIONALE/AMPLIFICATION
1. Place the client in a semi-Fowler's position. Wash hands thoroughly. Assemble the equipment convenient to the client on a table or TV tray. Pour hydrogen peroxide and saline or distilled water into 2 receptacles. Open the paper bag to receive soiled articles.	
2. Suction the tracheostomy before giving tracheostomy care. If the client is on mechanical ventilation, disconnect the ventilator and place the connector on a clean towel.	If the client is ventilator-dependent, give tracheostomy care quickly to prevent hypoxia.
3. Remove the inner cannula. Place it in the peroxide and clean it with the brush or pipe cleaners. Rinse it in the saline or distilled water. Replace the inner cannula, taking care to lock it into the correct position. Reconnect the ventilator if the client is being ventilated.	Peroxide effectively cleans organic matter from the cannula.

ACTION	*RATIONALE/AMPLIFICATION*
4. Using a 4 × 4 soaked in peroxide, gently remove exudate from around the stoma. Rinse the area with saline or distilled water on a 4 × 4. Pat the area dry with a 4 × 4. Note the condition of the skin.	Removing exudate from the skin prevents excoriation.
5. Unless excessive amounts of exudate are a problem, leave the area open. If secretions are a problem, cut a slit in a 4 × 4 and place around the tube. A small piece of Telfa (nonadhesive dressing) can also be used to dress the stoma.	Scissors that are not used for any other purpose should be used to cut the 4 × 4s used for dressings. Clean the scissors with an alcohol sponge before cutting the dressing. Telfa is easier to remove if secretions have dried and the procedure is uncomfortable for the client. Telfa is considerably more expensive than the 4 × 4s.
6. Remove the tracheostomy ties and replace them with clean tape. Knot the ties rather than tying in a bow to prevent accidentally untying them.	While the ties are changed, another family member can hold the tracheostomy tube in place to prevent accidental decannulation. Have the person wash hands first. If the tube has an inflated cuff, this also will hold the tube in place. An alert, cooperative client can hold the tube in place also. If the client is restless and uncooperative, replace the new ties before cutting the old ties away with scissors.
7. If the cuff is inflated, suction the airway. Deflate the cuff and suction again before reinflating the cuff.	Use the prescribed amount of air to reinflate the cuff. If unsure of the amount, inflate the cuff until minimal resistance is met. Listen for an air leak when the person is again connected to the ventilator. A minimal air leak will not affect ventilation, but if a large leak is present, inflate the cuff a little more. If a cuff pneumometer is available, do not exceed 20 mm Hg of pressure in the cuff. Greater pressures cause necrosis of the trachea.
8. Perform tracheostomy care on a daily basis, or more often if managing secretions is a problem. Manipulate the tracheostomy tube as little as possible during the procedure to prevent discomfort to the client, irritation to the stoma, and the introduction of bacteria.	Any manipulation of the tube or stoma predisposes the client to infection.
9. Discard soiled articles in the paper bag. Wash hands.	

Related Care

1. Frequently check that the ties are secure and that they are not tight enough to obstruct circulation.

ACTION   **RATIONALE/AMPLIFICATION**

2. Routinely check the pressure in the cuff if it is inflated, using a minimal leak technique or pneumometer. When visiting the client, cuff pressure can be checked with a sphygmomanometer (Fig. 76-2). This will guide the family regarding the amount of air to insert.

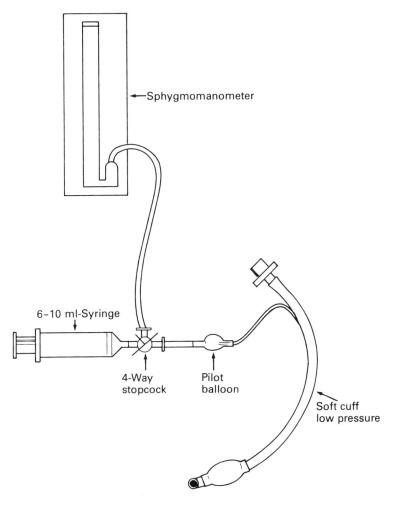

Figure 76.2
Checking the cuff pressure using a sphygmomanometer.

3. Suction only when necessary. Encourage deep breathing and coughing.

Any entry into the airway predisposes the client to infection by introducing bacteria, as well as causing trauma to the mucosa.

4. Clean reusable bowls and tube-cleaning brush by washing in a dishwasher or using hot, soapy water and rinsing with tap water.

**Education/
Communication**

- Teach the client and family to

Have an extra tracheostomy tube available to replace in the stoma in case of accidental decannulation. Before a client is discharged, the stoma will be well formed, which makes reinsertion of the tube easier. Unless a client is respirator-dependent, inserting the tube will not be an emergency. If the client is respirator-dependent, teach a family member how to reinsert the tube. The caregiver could insert a new tube when the tube is due for routine replacement under the supervision of the physician. This would give the person confidence in the event of a problem.

Inflate the cuff according to the client's needs. Check the cuff pressure with a sphygmomanometer or use a minimal leak technique to inflate the cuff.

Give mouth to tracheostomy resuscitation should a respiratory arrest occur. This is appropriate only if the cuff is inflated. If the cuff is deflated, cover the tube with the finger and give mouth-to-mouth resuscitation.

Prevent food or medication from entering the tracheostomy. If this occurs, suction immediately.

Place a small makeup mirror on a table in front of the client to facilitate doing tracheostomy care unassisted (See Technique 75, Suctioning.)

Be careful when taking a tub bath or shaving, so that water does not get into the tube. Cover the tube with an appliance to prevent water from entering the trachea while showering. (See Technique 71, Laryngectomy Care.)

Protect the tracheostomy from dust, dirt, and lint with a gauze pad, laryngectomy bib, or high-necked clothing. (See Technique 75, Laryngectomy Care.)

Protect the skin around the tracheostomy from irritation by performing tracheostomy care daily or more often if secretions are increased. Adapt Stomahesive (designed for ostomy care) to protect excoriated skin (Fig. 76-3).

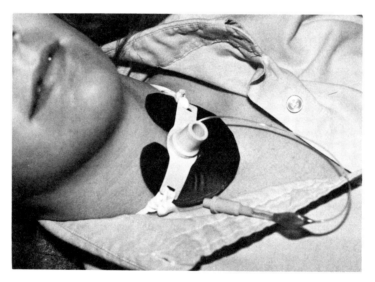

Figure 76.3
Protect the skin around the tracheostomy with Stomahesive. Cut Stomahesive in the shape of a C to fit around the tube. Cut small slits along the inside edge so that the Stomahesive will lie flat around the tube, and apply it to the person's skin. This will act as a barrier to secretions and allow healing.

In winter avoid cold air entering the tube directly. Use high-necked clothing or a light scarf.

Avoid persons with respiratory infections. Remove respiratory irritants from the home (e.g., pollen, dust, aerosols, pets). Use damp dusting or vacuuming to clean, as opposed to sweeping, dry dusting, and using aerosols.

If a tracheostomy is temporary, follow the precautions mentioned until the tracheostomy has healed. Keep the area clean and dry. Replace Steristrips or tape approximating the edges of the stoma should they become excessively soiled. Expect some secretions to leak from the stoma until healing is complete.

Referrals and Consultations

- Instruct the client or family to report any signs of respiratory infection to the home health nurse (purulent sputum, increased volume of secretions, elevated temperature and increased respirations, respiratory distress).
- Refer a pediatric client to a home-bound education program through the local school district if appropriate.
- Provide 24-hour emergency numbers for the caregiver should professional help be required.

Evaluation of Health Promotion Activities

Quality Assurance/ Reassessment

- During visits, observe the caregiver's technique for performing tracheostomy care.
- Determine the client's progress in assuming self-care activities if appropriate.

DOCUMENTATION

Charting for the Home Health Nurse

Adequacy of caregiver's technique

Respiratory assessment

Character of stoma and surrounding skin

Cuff pressure if appropriate

Acceptance of the tracheostomy by the client/family

Adaptation of the client to changes in activities of daily living (ADL)

Additional teaching needs

Records Kept by the Client/Family

Vital signs including temperature

Character and amount of sputum

Condition of the stoma and surrounding skin

Problems encountered when giving tracheostomy care

Health Teaching Checklist

Name of Care Provider _____

Relationship to Client _____ Telephone #_____

Taught by _____ Date _____

	EXPLAINED	DEMONSTRATED
Tracheostomy care technique	_____	_____
Strategy for accidental decannulation	_____	
Cuff management	_____	_____
Communication (e.g., talking tracheostomy or other)	_____	
Emergency phone numbers (24-hour coverage)	_____	
Infection-control precautions	_____	_____
Special precautions	_____	_____
Problems to report	_____	

Product Availability

Tracheostomy tubes can be obtained from medical-supply companies listed in the yellow pages of the telephone book.

Stomahesive or similar products are available at pharmacies that stock ostomy supplies.

Distilled water and hydrogen peroxide are available at grocery stores and pharmacies. Saline is available at pharmacies for contact lens care. If it is purchased in a squirt bottle, this is ideal for rinsing the inner cannula. Alternately, saline can be made at home. (See Technique 74, Pressure Breathing Treatments, for recipe.) Telfa and 4 × 4s are also available at pharmacies.

Twill tape suitable for tracheostomy ties can be obtained from stores selling dressmaking supplies.

Selected Reference

Brannin PK: Respiratory diseases and management. In Hudak CM, Lohr T, Gallo BM: Critical Care Nursing, 3rd ed, pp 191–227. Philadelphia, JB Lippincott, 1982

Appendices

Resources for Home Health Care

Accent on Living Magazine
Box 700
Bloomington, IL 61701

Administration on Aging
Office of Human Development
330 Independence Ave, SW
Washington, DC 20201

Aging Magazine
Office of Human Development
200 Independence Ave, SW
Washington, DC 20201

American Association of Retired Persons
1909 K Street, NW
Washington, DC 20049

Federal Council on Aging
330 Independence Ave, SW
North Bldg, Room 4620
Washington, DC 20201

International Federation on Aging
1909 K Street
Washington, DC 20049

International Senior Citizens Association, Inc.
17753 Wilshire Blvd
Los Angeles, CA 90025

Mature Living Magazine
For Mature Christian Adults
Materials Services Dept, MSN 108
127 Ninth Avenue North
Nashville, TN 37234

Modern Maturity Magazine
215 Long Beach Blvd
Long Beach, CA 90802

National Clearinghouse on Aging
Administration on Aging
DHEW Building, Room 4146
330 Independence Ave, SW
Washington, DC 20201

National Council on the Aging
1828 L Street
Washington, DC 20036

National Council of Senior Citizens
1511 K Street, NW
Washington, DC 20005

National Institute on Aging
9000 Rockville Pike, Bldg 31
Bethesda, MD 20014

Senior Citizens Service Organizations
(Check yellow pages for local groups)

Travel Information Service
Moss Rehabilitation Hospital
12th Street and Tabor Road
Philadelphia, PA 19141

50 Plus Magazine
150 East 58th Street
New York, NY 10022

Arthritis

Arthritis Foundation
1314 Spring Street, NW
Atlanta, GA 30309

Arthritis Information Clearinghouse
Box 9782
Arlington, VA 22209

Canadian Arthritis and Rheumatism Society
45 Charles Street East
Toronto, Ontario M4G 3V9
Canada

National Institute of Arthritis and Metabolic Diseases
Bethesda, MD 20014

Cancer

American Cancer Society, Inc.
National Office
777 Third Avenue
New York, NY 10017
  Local programs may include: Reach to Recovery (post-mastectomy adjustment),
  Road to Recovery (radiation therapy), Dialogue (radiation therapy), I Can Cope
  (family adjustment to the diagnosis of cancer)

Cancer Information Clearinghouse
National Cancer Institute
Office of Cancer Communications
Building 31, Room 10A-18
Bethesda, MD 20205

Diabetes

American Diabetes Association
2 Park Ave
New York, NY 10016

Diabetes Forecast Magazine
American Diabetes Association
Box 6782
Church Street Station
New York, NY 10249

Medic-Alert Foundation International
Box 1009
Turlock, CA 95380

Disease-Specific Organizations

Alzheimer's Disease and Related Disorders Association, Inc.
360 North Michigan Ave
Suite 1102
Chicago, IL 60601

Amyotrophic Lateral Sclerosis Society of America
12011 San Vincente Boulevard
Los Angeles, CA 90049

Herpes Resource Center
Box 100
Palo Alto, CA 94302

Muscular Dystrophy Associations of America, Inc.
810 Seventh Ave
New York, NY 10019

National Association for Sickle-Cell Disease, Inc.
945 S Western Ave
Suite 206
Los Angeles, CA 90006

National Epilepsy League
6 N Michigan Ave
Chicago, IL 60602

National Hemophilia Foundation
Room 903
25 W 39th Street
New York, NY 10018

National Multiple Sclerosis Society
205 East 42nd Street
New York, NY 10017

United Cerebral Palsy Associations, Inc.
66 East 34th Street
New York, NY 10016

United Ostomy Association
1111 Wilshire Blvd
Los Angeles, CA 90017

Financial Assistance

American Association of Retired Persons
1909 K Street, NW
Washington, DC 20049

Equal Employment Opportunities Commission
2401 East Street, NW
Washington, DC 20506

Health Insurance Association of America
1850 K Street, NW
Washington, DC 20006

Social Security Administration
1875 Connecticut Ave, NW
Room 1120
Washington, DC 20009

United States Social Security Administration
Division of Disability Operations
6401 Security Blvd
Baltimore, MD 48453

Nutrition

The American Dietetic Association
430 North Michigan Ave
Chicago, IL 60611

American Home Economics Association
2010 Massachusetts Ave, NW
Washington, DC 20036

Lifeline Letter (Home TPN)
Oley Foundation
Albany, NY 12208

National Dairy Council
6300 River Rd
Rosemont, IL 60018

National Research Council
Food and Nutrition Board
2101 Constitution Ave, NW
Washington, DC 20037

Nutrition Foundation
489 Fifth Ave
New York, NY 10017

Pediatric

Association for Children with Learning Disabilities
4156 Library Road
Pittsburgh, PA 15234

Child Health Affairs
Department of Health and Human Services
5600 Fishers Lane
Rockville, MD 20852

Child Welfare League of America, Inc.
67 Irving Place
New York, NY 10003

La Leche League International
9619 Minneapolis Ave
Franklin Park, IL 60131

National Easter Seal Society for Crippled Children and Adults
2023 West Ogden Ave
Chicago, IL 60612

National Foundation–March of Dimes
Box 2000
White Plains, NY 10602

National Institute of Child Health and Human Development
NIH
9000 Rockville Pike
Bethesda, MD 20014

Scouting for Handicapped
Education Relationships Service
Boy Scouts of America
North Brunswick, NJ 08902

Shriner's Hospital for Crippled Children
323 N Michigan Ave
Chicago, IL 60601

Professional and Service Organizations

American Medical Association
535 North Dearborn Street
Chicago, IL 60610

American Nurses' Association
2420 Pershing Rd
Kansas City, MO 20005

Centers for Disease Control
Atlanta, GA 30333

Consumer Product Information Service
Public Documents Distribution Center
Pueblo, CO 81009

National Organization for Women
Action Center
425 13th Street, NW
Washington, DC 20004

National Safety Council
444 North Michigan Ave
Chicago, IL 60611

Occupational Safety and Health Administration
200 Constitution Ave, NW
Washington, DC 20001

Office of Consumer Services
US Department of Health and Human Services
Washington, DC 20201

Public Affairs Pamphlets
381 Park Ave
New York, NY 10016

Salvation Army
National Headquarters
120 W 14th Street
New York, NY 10011

Respiratory and Coronary

American Heart Association
7320 Greenville Ave
Dallas, TX 75231

American Lung Association
1740 Broadway
New York, NY 10019

American Telephone and Telegraph Company (laryngectomee aides)
1776 On the Green
Morristown, NJ 07960

Cardiac Data Corporation
1280 Blue Hills Ave
Bloomfield, CT 06002

Cardiocare
Division of Medtronic, Inc.
425 East 61st Street
New York, NY 10021

Cardiopace
3181 SW Sam Jackson Park Road
Portland, OR 97201

Communicaid (R)
1560 West William Street
Decatur, IL 62522

Dart Medical
500 Hogsback Road
Box 212
Mason, MI 48854

Instromedix
10950 SW 5th Ave
Beaverton, OR 97005

Intermedics, Inc.
Box 617
Freeport, TX 77541

International Association of Laryngectomees
777 Third Ave
New York, NY 10017

MedAlert
1 Penn Plaza
Brooklyn, NY 11236

National Asthma Center
875 Avenue of the Americas
New York, NY 10001

National Heart and Lung Institute
9600 Rockville Pike, Bldg 31
Bethesda, MD 20014

Pacemaker Diagnostic Clinic
4020 Newberry Road
Gainesville, FL 32607

Pacesetter
12884 Bradley Ave
Sylmer, CA 91342

Pulse International
Association of Pacemaker Patients, Inc.
Box 54305
Atlanta, GA 30308

United Medical Corporation
Cardio Data Systems
56 Haddon Ave
Box 117
Haddonfield, NJ 08033

Self-Care

Advocates for the Handicapped
77 West Washington Street
Room 402
Chicago, IL 60602

Alexander Graham Bell Association for the Deaf, Inc.
The Volta Bureau
3714 Volta Place, NW
Washington, DC 20007

American Association for the Education of the Severely Handicapped
1600 West Armory Way
Seattle, WA 98119

American Association of Workers for the Blind, Inc.
1511 K Street, NW
Washington, DC 20005

American Blind Bowlers Association
150 North Bellair Ave
Louisville, KY 40206

American Coalition of Citizens with Disabilities
Room 817
1346 Connecticut Ave, NW
Washington, DC 20036

American Foundation for the Blind
15 West 16th Street
New York, NY 10011

American Occupational Therapy Association, Inc.
6000 Executive Blvd
Rockville, MD 20852

American Physical Therapy Association
1156 15th Street, NW
Washington, DC 20005

American Printing House for the Blind
1839 Frankfort Ave
Box 6085
Louisville, KY 40206

American Red Cross
National Headquarters
17 & D Streets, NW
Washington, DC 20006

American Speech and Hearing Association
1081 Rockville Pike
Rockville, MD 20852

American Wheelchair Bowling Association, Inc.
2424 N Federal Highway #109
Boynton Beach, FL 33435

Amputees' Service Association
Box A-3819
Chicago, IL 60690

Architecture and Transportation Barriers Compliance Board
Washington, DC 90049

Association of Handicapped Artists, Inc.
503 Brisbane Blvd
Buffalo, NY 14203

Audio Book Company
14937 Ventura Blvd
Sherman Oaks, CA 91403

Bathing Aids to the Handicapped
Box 1956
Greeley, CO 80632

Blind Outdoor Leisure Development
National Office
533 East Main
Aspen, CO 81611

Bureau of Education for the Handicapped
US Office of Education
Washington, DC 20202

Canadian Paraplegic Association
153 Lyndhurst Ave
Toronto, Ontario M4G 3V9
Canada

Canadian Rehabilitation Council for the Disabled
Suite 2110
1 Yonge Street
Toronto, Ontario M5E 1E8
Canada

The College Guide for Students with Disabilities
ABT Publications
55 Wheeler Street
Cambridge, MA 02138

Computers for the Physically Handicapped
7602 Talbert Ave
Huntington Beach, CA 92647

Congress of Organizations of the Physically Handicapped
7611 Oakland Ave
Minneapolis, MN 55423

Disabled American Veterans
3725 Alexandria Pike
Cold Spring, KY 41076

Federal Office for Handicapped Individuals
US Department of Health and Human Services
200 Independence Ave, SW
Washington, DC 20201

Federation of the Handicapped
211 West 14th Street
New York, NY 10011

Green Pages: A Directory of Products and Services for the Handicapped
641 West Fairbanks
Winter Park, FL 32789

Goodwill Industries of America
9200 Wisconsin Ave
Washington, DC 20014
    See also local Goodwill Industries

Guiding Eyes for the Blind
Yorktown Heights, NY 10598

Handicapped Artists of America, Inc.
8 Sandy Lane
Salisbury, MA 01950

Hearing Dogs
Administrator of Special Programs
American Humane Association
Box 1266
Denver, CO 80201

Help Yourself Aids
Box 15
Brookfield, IL 60513

Homebound Book Service
359 McLean Blvd
Paterson, NJ 07509

Independence Factory
Box 597
Middletown, OH 45042

Information Center for Individuals with Disabilities, Inc.
20 Park Plaza, Suite 330
Boston, MA 02116

Institute of Rehabilitation Medicine
New York University Medical Center
400 East 34th Street
New York, NY 10016

International Association of Rehabilitation Facilities
5530 Wisconsin Ave
Suite 955
Washington, DC 20015

Library of Congress
Division for the Blind and Physically Handicapped
Washington, DC 20542

National Amputation Foundation
12-45 150th Street
Whitestone, NY 11357

National Association of the Deaf
814 Thayer Ave
Silver Spring, MD 20910

National Association of the Physically Handicapped
2 Meetinghouse Road
Merrimack, NH 03054

National Center for a Barrier-Free Environment
1425 H Street, NW
Suite 600
Washington, DC 20005

National Center for Law and the Handicapped, Inc.
1235 North Eddy Street
South Bend, IN 46617

National Commission on Architectural Barriers for Rehabilitation of the
    Handicapped
Social and Rehabilitation Services
Washington, DC 20201

National Congress of Organizations of the Physically Handicapped
1627 Deborah Ave
Rockford, IL 61103

National Council for Homemaker–Home Health Aide Services, Inc.
67 Irving Place
New York, NY 10003

National Federation of the Blind
1346 Connecticut Ave, NW
Washington, DC 20036

National Federation for Dentistry for the Handicapped
1121 Broadway, Suite 5
Boulder, CO 80302

National Health Information Clearinghouse
235 Park Avenue South
11th Floor
New York, NY 10003

National Institute on Adult Day Care
National Council on the Aging
600 Maryland Avenue, SW
West Wing 100
Washington, DC 20024

National Paraplegia Foundation
333 North Michigan Ave
Chicago, IL 60601

National Rehabilitation Association
1522 K Street, NW
Washington, DC 20005

National Society for the Prevention of Blindness
79 Madison Ave
New York, NY 10016

National Wheelchair Athletic Association
40-24 62nd Street
Woodside, NY 11377

National Wheelchair Basketball Association
Office of the Commissioner
110 Seaton Building
University of Kentucky
Lexington, KY 40506

New England Spinal Cord Injury Foundation, Inc.
369 Elliot Street
Newton Upper Falls, MA 02164

North American Riding for the Handicapped Association
℅ Leonard Warner
Box 100
Ashburn, VA 22011

Office for Handicapped Individuals
US Department of Health and Human Services
Office of the Secretary
Washington, DC 20201

Office of Disease Prevention and Health Promotion
US Department of Health and Human Services
Washington, DC 20201

Paralyzed Veterans of America, Inc.
4330 East West Highway, Suite 300
Washington, DC 20014

Reader's Digest
Large-Type Edition
Box 241
Mt Morris, IL 61054

Registry of Interpreters for the Deaf, Inc.
Box 1339
Washington, DC 20013

Rehabilitation International
432 Park Ave South
New York, NY 10016

Rehabilitation Services Administration
US Department of Health and Human Services
Washington, DC 20402

Society for Advancement of Travel for the Handicapped
26 Court Street
Brooklyn, NY 11242

Technical Aids to Independence, Inc.
12 Hyde Road
Bloomfield, NJ 07003

Telephone Pioneers of America
Frank B. Jewett Chapter
Bell Tel Lab
600 Mt Ave
Murray Hill, NJ 07974

United States Ski Association
Central Division
Handicapped Skiers Committee
Wm. E. Stieler, CHM
6832 Marlette Rd
Marlette, Michigan 48453

Vocational and Educational Opportunities for the Disabled
Insurance Co of North America
Human Resources Center
Willets Road
Albertson, NY 11507

Vocational Guidance and Rehabilitation Services
2239 East 55th Street
Cleveland, OH 44103

Volunteer Services for the Blind, Inc.
919 Walnut Street
Philadelphia, PA 19107

2 Teaching/Learning Principles and Strategies

The client or an assistant must perform the recommended health-care procedures in the absence of the nurse. Teaching and learning, therefore, are essential aspects of home health-care delivery.

Generally, learning has been shown to take place more effectively if

The learner participates actively in the process. Therefore, return demonstrations, "learning by doing," discussion of feelings and attitudes, and client participation in designing the teaching–learning sessions increase the probability of learning.

The vocabulary being used by the instructor is easily understood by the client. It therefore becomes essential that "medical jargon" be kept to a minimum and that the language be that of the client. Developmental and educational levels must also be considered when planning the process of teaching.

The overall content to be learned is broken down into increments that are manageable to the client. This allows the client to progress at an individual rate. In addition, the client does not become overwhelmed with vast amounts of facts and details.

Client/family successes are positively reinforced. In designing reinforcement, client assessment must be performed to ensure that rewards intended to be positive reinforcers are perceived as such by the client.

Client/family basic life needs (according to Mazlow) are met. The implication is that teaching would not be effective if basic life needs are not first met.

The client/family member understands the value of the content. Therefore, client/family perceptions related to the content to be taught should be assessed prior to teaching the content.

Excessive stress is not present. While a low level of stress is necessary to learning, higher levels of stress impede learning. Some time should be taken prior to teaching to assess client/family stressors currently present.

A positive relationship is developed between the teacher and learner

The teacher is perceived as a credible source by the learner

The teaching–learning session is not rushed. Timing should be dependent on the client/family's available time for the session and on the attention span of the learner. Extremes (excessive rushing or taking too much time) should be avoided.

Environmental distractions are eliminated. Reduce excessive noise, temperature extremes, and unnecessary interruptions.

There are no value/cultural conflicts with the content to be learned

Developing a Teaching Plan

Assessment of learner
    Developmental level
    Vocabulary and educational level
    Motivation to learn
    Values/attitudes toward content
    Present knowledge related to the content
    Perception of benefit/importance of content
    Any sensory deficit that might impede learning or indicate a need for altering the method of teaching
    Perception of environmental stimuli that might be a conflict to learning

Planning
- Develop expected outcomes.
- Develop health-care modifications (short-term goals):
  - Organize content into increments manageable to learner.
  - Plan logical sequence of content presentation.
  - Design stages for providing rewards for successes: design method of reinforcement.

Intervention
- Present content at educational, developmental, and vocabulary level of learner.
- Control environment to enhance learning: reduce unnecessary interruptions, reduce noise levels, and reduce excessive cold or heat if possible.
- Provide comfortable seating. Provide adequate lighting.
- Present content without sense of "rush" or "taking too much time," and at a time convenient to client/family.
- Make content meaningful in terms of client values/attitudes.
- Encourage client/family participation in the process to the extent possible.

Evaluation of learning
- Base evaluation of content on expected outcomes and short-term goals or health-care modifications.
- Observe return demonstration of skills.
- Periodically visit the home during client/family performance of procedure and observe its performance.
- Provide documentation checklists or forms for client to maintain to document progress.

Home Health Certification and Plan of Treatment

DEPARTMENT OF HEALTH AND HUMAN SERVICES HEALTH CARE FINANCING ADMINISTRATION	FORM APPROVED OMB No. 0938-0357

HOME HEALTH CERTIFICATION AND PLAN OF TREATMENT

1. Patient's Name and Address	2. Patient's HI Claim Number
	3. Medical Record Number

4. Dates: Start of care and verbal order for SOC	5. Certification Period: From: To:

6. Home Health Agency Name and Address	7. Principal Diagnosis: Narrative, Dates of Onset/Exacerbation, ICD-9-CM Code □□□.□□
	8. Surgical Procedure(s) Relevant to Care: Narrative, Date, ICD-9-CM Code □□□.□□

9. Other Pertinent Diagnosis—Narrative, Dates of Onset/Exacerbation, ICD-9-CM Code(s)

□□□.□□   □□□.□□

□□□.□□   □□□.□□

10.

Functional Limitations		Activities Permitted	
□ Amputation	□ Ambulation	□ Bedrest	□ Crutches
□ Bowel/Bladder	□ Mental	□ Complete	□ Cane
(incontinence)	□ Speech	□ BRP	□ Wheelchair
□ Contracture	□ Vision	□ Up as tolerated	□ Walker
□ Hearing	□ Respiratory	□ Transfer Bed/Chair	□ No Restrictions
□ Paralysis	□ Other (Specify)	□ Exercises Prescribed	□ Other (Specify)
□ Endurance		□ Partial Weight Bearing	
		□ Independent at Home	

11. Safety Measures:

12. Orders for Services and Treatments (Specify Modality, amt/freq/dura)	13. Medications: Dose/Frequency/Route (N) New (C) Changed

14. Mental Status:	□ Oriented	□ Forgetful	□ Disoriented	□ Agitated
	□ Comatose	□ Depressed	□ Lethargic	□ Other

15. Nutritional Requirements:

16. Medical Supplies & DME Ordered	17. Allergies

18. Goals/Rehabilitation Potential/Discharge Plans	19. Significant Clinical Findings/Summary from each discipline

20. Prognosis: □ Poor   □ Guarded   □ Fair   □ Good   □ Excellent

21. Attending Physician's Name and Address	22. PHYSICIAN CERTIFICATION: I □ certify □ recertify that the above home health services are required and are authorized by me with a written plan for treatment which will be periodically reviewed by me. This patient is under my care, is confined to his home, and is in need of intermittent skilled nursing care and/or physical or speech therapy or has been furnished home health services based on such a need and no longer has a need for such care or therapy, but continues to need occupational therapy.
23. Attending Physician's Signature and Date	

Form HCFA-485(U4) (4-85)   PROVIDER

DEPARTMENT OF HEALTH AND HUMAN SERVICES
HEALTH CARE FINANCING ADMINISTRATION

FORM APPROVED
OMB No. 0938-0357

MEDICAL UPDATE AND PATIENT INFORMATION

1. Patient's Name	2. HIC No.	3. Sex ☐ M ☐ F

4. Date of Birth	5. Medicare Covered? ☐ Yes ☐ No	6. Period Covered or Certification Period From: Through:

7. Provider Name and Number	8. Place of Treatment, If Other Than Home (Name and Address)

9. Are services related to any accident or employment related injury? ☐ Yes ☐ No	10. Date and Reason Agency Last Contacted Physician	11. Is the patient receiving additional medically reasonable and necessary skilled care pursuant to a Physician's Plan of Treatment paid for by other than Medicare? ☐ Yes (Specify) ☐ No

12. Dates of Last Inpatient Stay From: To:	Type of Facility	13. Date Physician Last Saw Patient

14.
SPECIFIC SERVICES AND TREATMENTS (CODES ON REVERSE)

TOTAL VISITS	SERVICES	SPECIFIC TREATMENT ORDERS	FREQUENCY AND DURATION	TX CODE

15. Updated Information: New Orders/Treatments/Clinical Facts

16. Functional Limitations/Rehabilitation Potential/Goals (Each Discipline)

17.
HOME-BOUND

A. Reason Home-bound—Narrative:

B. Indicate any times when Home Health Agency made a visit and the patient was not home and reason why if ascertainable	C. Specify any known medical and/or non-medical reasons the patient regularly leaves home and frequency of occurrence

18. Is there an available, able and willing care giver? ☐ Yes (Specify) ☐ No	19. Unusual Home/Social Environment

20. Does your Agency have any supplementary plans of treatment on file from a physician other than the referring physician or from other specialists for care being given the patient by your agency? ☐ Yes ☐ No   If Yes, Please explain briefly.

21. Other DME Available for Use	22. Signature of Nurse or Therapist Completing or Reviewing Form	Date

Form HCFA-486(U3) (4-85)   PROVIDER

561

DEPARTMENT OF HEALTH AND HUMAN SERVICES
HEALTH CARE FINANCING ADMINISTRATION

FORM APPROVED
OMB No. 0938-0357

PLAN OF TREATMENT/ MEDICAL UPDATE AND PATIENT INFORMATION
ADDENDUM

1. Patient's Name

2. Patient's HI Claim Number

3. Provider Number

4. Period Covered

From: To:

CERTIFICATION/PLAN OF TREATMENT (*CONTINUED*)	MEDICAL UPDATE/PATIENT INFORMATION (*CONTINUED*)

4   Medications Commonly Used in the Home*

DRUG NAME AND CLASSIFICATION	PURPOSE, ROUTE, DOSAGE	SIDE-EFFECTS	NURSING IMPLICATIONS
Acetaminophen, a non-narcotic analgesic and antipyretic	For mild pain or fever, 325 mg to 650 mg PO or rectally q 4 hr or prn not to exceed 2 gr daily	Severe hepatotoxicity with large doses; skin—rash, urticaria	Interactions: Warfarin: may increase hypothrombombinemic activity Cholestyramine: inhibits acetaminophen's absorption Implications: has no significant anti-inflammatory effect. Excessive alcohol ingestion may increase hepatotoxicity. Check all of client's nonprescription drugs: many have acetone and/or alcohol included.
Aspirin, a non-narcotic analgesic	For arthritis, 2.6 gr to 5.2 gr PO daily; for mild pain or fever, 325 mg to 650 mg PO or rectally q 4 hrs prn; for thromboembolic disorders, 325 mg to 650 mg PO daily or bid	Prolonged bleeding time; tinnitus and hearing loss; nausea and vomiting, occult bleeding; abnormal liver function studies; skin rash, bleeding	Interactions: Urine acidifiers: increased blood levels of aspirin Urine alkalizers: decreased blood levels Corticosteroids: enhanced salicylate elimination Oral anticoagulants and heparin: increased risk of bleeding Implications: contraindicated with GI bleeding, GI ulcer, or any bleeding disorder. May cause increase in SGOT, SGPT, alkaline phosphatase, and bilirubin. May produce false negative results with Testape and Clinistix, and false positives with Clinitests. Advise clients to observe for bleeding gums, petechiae, significant GI bleeding.
Apresoline (Hydralazine), an antihypertensive	For essential hypertension: alone or in combination with other antihypertensives Dose: initially 10 mg PO qid; maximum dose: 200 mg daily IM: 20 mg to 40 mg repeated as necessary, usually every 4 to 6 hours IV: 20 mg to 40 mg repeated as necessary, generally every 4 to 6 hours	Headaches, peripheral neuritis, dizziness CV: orthostatic hypotension, tachycardia, arrhythmias, angina, palpitations, sodium retention GI: nausea, vomiting, diarrhea, anorexia Skin: rash Other: lupus erythematosus-like syndrome, weight gain	Interactions: Diazoxide: may cause severe hypotension Implications: use with caution if the client is taking other antihypertensives, or if the client has cardiac disease. Monitor vital signs frequently. Reduce orthostatic hypotension by changing positions slowly. Give with meal to increase absorption. Observe for sore throat, muscle and joint aches, fever, skin rash (symptoms of lupus erythematosus-like syndrome).

*NOTE: This list of medications is not intended to be an exhaustive list of medications used in home health. Rather, it is a selection of drugs indicated by practicing home health nurses to be commonly used ones. Other medications are listed with the related procedures (*i.e.*, laxatives are listed under "enemas").

As recommended by Medicare, and as a safety and time-saving measure, appropriate medication information cards should be taken when making home visits. Minimal information should include drug purpose, usual dosages, side-effects, interactive effects, and nursing implications.

It is understood that medical research and usage create continual change. Thus, new drugs and changes in other aspects of medication administration are continually being made, making current practice obsolete.

DRUG NAME AND CLASSIFICATION	PURPOSE, ROUTE, DOSAGE	SIDE-EFFECTS	NURSING IMPLICATIONS
Aldomet, Dopomat (methyldopa), an antihypertensive	For sustained hypertension. Take 250 mg PO bid or tid in first 48 hours. Increase as needed every 2 days. Entire daily dose may be given in the evening or at bedtime. Maintenance: 500 mg to 2 g daily in 2 to 4 divided doses	Thrombocytopenia, hemolytic anemia Headache, asthenia, dizziness, weakness, decreased mental acuity, psychic disturbances, sedation Orthostatic hypotension, bradycardia, myocarditis, aggravated angina, weight gain, edema Stuffy nose, dry mouth Hepatic necrosis Diarrhea, pancreatitis	Interactions: Norepinephrine, amphetamines, antidepressants (tricyclic), pheothiazines: possible hypertensive effects Implications: Weigh daily. Give total dose at bedtime. Change positions slowly to avoid orthostatic hypotension.
Benadryl (diphenhydramine), an antihistamine and antitussive	Treat allergy symptoms, rhinitis, motion sickness, antiparkinsonism 25 mg to 50 mg PO tid or qid; or 10 mg to 50 mg deep IM or IV up to 500 mg daily For nonproductive cough, 25 mg PO q 4 hr (not to exceed 100 mg daily)	Drowsiness, confusion, vertigo, headache Palpitations Nasal stuffiness, diplopia Nausea, vomiting, diarrhea, constipation Dysuria, urinary retention Urticaria	Interactions: With CNS depressants, increased sedation Implications: do not consume alcohol while taking Benadryl. Do not drive or perform other hazardous activities. Take with milk to reduce GI distress. Coffeee or tea may reduce drowsiness.
Brompton's Cocktail Contains varying amounts of methadone or morphine; cocaine or amphetamine; syrup or honey; gin or alcohol	Severe chronic pain of terminal cancer 10 ml to 20 ml of mixture q 3 to 4 hr if morphine is a component; q 6 to 12 hr if methadone is a component. Adjust dosages at 48- to 72-hour intervals. Maximum dosage depends on client response.	Nausea, vomiting, constipation Urinary retention Sedation, somnolence, clouded sensorium, euphoria, convulsions with large dosages Hypotension, bradycardia	Interactions: With alcohol, CNS depressants, additive effect Implications: keep client as pain-free as possible. Often effective when narcotic analgesics alone do not provide relief. If cocaine is a component, swish solution in mouth since it is absorbed through oral mucosa. Administer around the clock to relieve client of anticipation of pain. To prevent nausea, sometimes use in combination with phenothiazines. Mixture is stable for 4 weeks at room temperature. Refrigerate to increase stability to 8 weeks.
Coumadin (warfarin sodium), an anticoagulant	Inhibits vitamin K–dependent activation of several clotting factors Prevention and treatment of deep vein thrombosis, rheumatic heart disease with valve damage, atrial arrhythmias Dosage: adults, 10 mg to 14 mg orally for 3 days, then calibrated according to prothrombin times Usual maintenance dose: 2 mg to 10 mg orally daily	Fever and skin rash, hemorrhage, uterine bleeding, diarrhea, cramps, nausea	Interactions: Observe client carefully for bleeding if taking thyroid, heparin, steroids, influenza vaccine, sulfonamides, quinidine, indomethacin, salicylates, barbiturates Implications: Observe for bleeding: nursing infants of mothers on anticoagulant therapy, elderly clients, persons on vitamin K (coumadin can be neutralized by vitamin K) Observe gums for bleeding, watch for bruises, tarry stools, hematuria or hematemesis, heavy menses Instruct the client to avoid over-the-counter drugs containing salicylates and to use an electric razor and soft toothbrush

DRUG NAME AND CLASSIFICATION	PURPOSE, ROUTE, DOSAGE	SIDE-EFFECTS	NURSING IMPLICATIONS
Diabinese (chlorpropamide), an oral antidiabetic agent	For stable, maturity-onset nonketotic diabetes uncontrolled by diet alone 250 mg PO daily with breakfast or in divided doses if GI disturbance occurs Dosage may be increased according to client need to 750 mg daily	Nausea, heartburn, vomiting Tea-colored urine Bone marrow aplasia Prolonged hypoglycemia Rash, facial flushing, pruritus	Interactions: Increased hypoglycemic effect with anabolic steroids, oral anticoagulants, chloramphenicol, salicylates, sulfonamides, phenylbutazone Prolonged hypoglycemic effect and masking of symptoms of hypoglycemia with beta blockers, clonidine Decreased response with thiazide diuretics, glucagon, corticosteroids Implications: Avoid alcohol. Observe for signs of renal insufficiency.
Darvon, Dolene, Darvon-N (propoxyphene), analgesics	For mild to moderate pain 65 mg PO q 4 hr prn (Darvon) 100 mg PO q 4 hr prn (Darvocet-N, Darvon-N)	Headache, excitement, dizziness, sedation, euphoria Nausea, vomiting, constipation Psychological and physical dependence	Interactions: none significant Implications: Do not take if history of narcotic addiction Avoid activities requiring an alert state until CNS response to drug has been established. Limit alcohol intake.
Digoxin (cardiac glycoside)	Increases force of myocardial contraction Slows heart rate Prolongs refractory period of the AV node Adults: for maintenance, 0.125 to 0.5 mg orally daily Children over 2 years: for maintenance, 0.02 mg/kg orally daily divided into 12-hour doses	Toxicity: fatigue, headache, vertigo, malaise, dizziness, stupor, paresthesias, generalized weakness Increased severity of congestive heart failure, arrhythmias, hypotension Yellow-green halos around visual images, blurred vision, light flashes	Interactions: Antacids (kaolin-pectin) create decreased absorption of digoxin. Schedule doses as far apart as possible. Loop diuretics and thiazides predispose to digitalis toxicity. Anticholinergics increase absorption of oral digitalis. Implications: check radial and apical pulse prior to administration; if pulse less than 60 beats/minute, call nurse or physician prior to taking. Instruct client/family regarding symptoms of toxicity.
Heparin, an anticoagulant	Accelerates formation of antithrombin III–thrombin complex. Inactivates thrombin and prevents conversion of fibrinogen to fibrin. Adults: 5,000 units subcutaneously every 12 hours. The dosage is highly individualized.	Hemorrhage with excessive dosage, prolonged clotting time, thrombocytopenia Fever, chills, pruritus, burning of feet, urticaria, arthralgia, rhinitis	Interaction: Salicylates: produces increased anticoagulant effect Implications: Inspect client for petechiae, nosebleeds, bruises, tarry stools, bleeding gums, hematuria, hematemesis. Give low-dose injections sequentially between the iliac crests of the lower abdomen deep into subcutaneous tissue. Inject slowly, leaving needle in place 10 seconds following injection. Do not massage area after needle is withdrawn. Alternate injection sites.
Lasix (furosemide), a loop diuretic	Enhances water absorption by inhibiting reabsorption of sodium and chloride at the proximal portion of the ascending loop of Henle Adults: 20 mg to 80 mg PO daily in morning; second dose in 6 to 8 hr; dose increased until desired response is achieved: up to 600 mg daily Infants, children: 2 mg/kg daily, increased as needed up to 6 mg/kg daily	Transient deafness with rapid injection, hypokalemia, hypochloremic alkalosis; fluid and electrolyte imbalance, hypocalcemia, hyperglycemia, impairment of glucose tolerance Dermatitis Leukopenia, thrombocytopenia, volume depletion, orthostatic hypotension	Observe elderly clients closely: they are especially susceptible to excessive diuresis. Advise clients to change positions slowly. Avoid excessive exercise in hot weather. Give in morning to prevent nocturia. Monitor vital signs during rapid diuresis.

DRUG NAME AND CLASSIFICATION	PURPOSE, ROUTE, DOSAGE	SIDE-EFFECTS	NURSING IMPLICATIONS
Nitroglycerin, an antianginal	Reduces the heart's demand for oxygen One sublingual tablet immediately on indication of anginal attack May repeat every 5 minutes for 15 minutes Apply transdermal disk to hairless site once daily	Headache, weakness, dizziness Orthostatic hypotension, flushing, palpitations, fainting Nausea, vomiting Cutaneous vasodilation	Avoid alcoholic beverages. Implications: store in cool, dark place. Replace supply every 3 months. When terminating transdermal patch, do so gradually. Use caution when wearing transdermal patch near microwave: burns can result. Monitor blood pressure and intensity and duration of response. Take at first sign of attack. Moisten with saliva and place under tongue to absorb. Rest. If no relief, nurse or physician should be called.
Orinase (tolbutamide), an oral antidiabetic agent	Stable maturity-onset diabetes uncontrolled by diet and previously untreated Initially 1 g to 2 g PO daily; may be adjusted to maximum 3 g daily	Bone marrow aplasia Nausea, heartburn, hypoglycemia Rash, pruritus, flushing	Interactions: Salicylates, chloramphenicol, oral anticoagulants, phenylbutozone, sulfonomides, anabolic steroids: increased hypoglycemic activity Corticosteroids, thiazide diuretics, glucagon: decreased hypoglycemic response Implications: avoid moderate to large alcohol intake
Ismelin (guanethidine sulfate), an antihypertensive	For moderate to severe hypertension: used in combination with other antihypertensives Initially, 10 mg PO daily; can be increased weekly or at monthly intervals Usual dose: 25 mg to 50 mg daily	Dizziness, bradycardia, orthostatic hypotension, congestive heart failure, arrhythmias Nasal stuffiness, diarrhea	Interactions: Levodopa, alcohol: may increase hypotensive effect Ephedrine, tricyclic antidepressants, amphetamines, norepinephrine: may inhibit antihypertensive effect Implications: Avoid strenuous exercise. Hot showers may cause hypotensive response. Change positions slowly.
Thorazine (chlorpromazine), a phenothiazine antipsychotic	For psychosis 500 mg daily PO in divided doses, increasing to 2 g; or 25 mg to 50 mg IM q 1 to 4 hr prn	Transient leukopenia, extrapyramidal reactions, sedation, dizziness, orthostatic hypotension, tachycardia, ECG changes, blurred vision, constipation, urinary retention, menstrual irregularity, inhibited ejaculation, dark urine, jaundice, abnormal liver functions, sterile abscess, weight gain	Interactions: Antacids: inhibit absorption of oral phenothiazines: do not take doses closer than every 2 hours. Anticholinergics: increased anticholinergic activity Implications: Use sunscreening agents and protective clothing to avoid photosensitivity responses. Avoid alcohol or other depressing agents. Change positions slowly.

5   Isolation Precautions

Please note that the guidelines from the Centers for Disease Control (CDC) relate to the hospital setting. Since many persons with communicable disease and infective conditions are cared for in the home, it is expected that the professional nurse will use judgment and a sound knowledge base of disease transmission in determining how to translate the CDC guidelines into the home setting. The following categories are offered as a contribution to that knowledge base.

Important: Good handwashing is essential in all types of isolation. Handwashing has been shown to be the single most important means of preventing the spread of infection. Handwashing should be done for a minimum of three minutes using soap and friction (see Technique 35, Handwashing).

Category: Strict

REQUIREMENTS

ROOM	VENTILATION	APPAREL	ARTICLES	DISEASES*
Private; should not share with other family members	Some conditions require special ventilation.	Masks, gowns, gloves are indicated for direct care or contact.	Contaminated articles must be left in the room or bagged in paper bags and boiled or soaked in bleach to clean and disinfect.	Diphtheria, pneumonic plague, smallpox,* varicella (chickenpox), zoster

Category: Contact

REQUIREMENTS

ROOM	VENTILATION	APPAREL	ARTICLES	DISEASES*
Private; may share room with siblings or others with the same disease or condition	Normal room air	Masks for those who come in close contact; gowns or aprons if soiling is likely; gloves for touching infective materials	Contaminated articles must be left in the room or placed in paper bags and the contents boiled or soaked in bleach to clean and disinfect.	Respiratory infection in infants and children, diphtheria (cutaneous), group A Streptococcus, endometritis, herpes, impetigo, influenza in infants and young children, certain multiply-resistant bacterial infections, pediculosis, viral pneumonia, rubella, scabies, draining infected wounds

Category: Respiratory

REQUIREMENTS

ROOM	VENTILATION	APPAREL	ARTICLES	DISEASES*
Private; may share room with others with similar condition	Normal room air	Masks for those who come in close contact; no gowns or gloves	Articles that come in contact with respiratory secretions should be bagged and disinfected by boiling or soaking in bleach.	Measles, meningitis, meningococcal pneumonia, meningococcemia, mumps, whooping cough, pneumonia *(Hemophilus influenzae)* in children

Category: Tuberculosis (AFB Isolation)

REQUIREMENTS

ROOM	VENTILATION	APPAREL	ARTICLES	DISEASES*
Private; door kept closed; may share with others with same condition	Special ventilation required	Masks only if client is coughing and cannot be relied on to cover mouth	Articles are rarely involved in the transmission of tuberculosis; articles should be cleaned and disinfected or discarded.	Tuberculosis

Category: Enteric Precautions

REQUIREMENTS

ROOM	VENTILATION	APPAREL	ARTICLES	DISEASES*
Private room is needed only if the client has poor hygiene habits; may share the room with others who have the same condition	Normal room air	Masks are not indicated; gowns or aprons only if soiling is likely; gloves only when touching infective materials	Articles that have come in contact with infective materials should be bagged and cleaned by boiling or by soaking in bleach or other disinfectant.	Amebic dysentery, cholera, acute diarrhea, enterocolitis, enteroviral infection, gastroenteritis, type A viral hepatitis, viral meningitis, poliomyelitis, typhoid fever, viral pericarditis, myocarditis, or meningitis

Category: Drainage/Secretion Precautions

REQUIREMENTS

ROOM	VENTILATION	APPAREL	ARTICLES	DISEASES*
Private room is not indicated.	Normal air	Masks are not needed; gowns or aprons only if soiling is likely; gloves only when touching infective materials	Articles contaminated with infective material should be discarded or bagged and decontaminated by boiling or soaking in bleach or a disinfectant	Abscess, burn infection, conjunctivitis, infected decubitus ulcer, skin infections, wound infections

Category: Body/Fluid Precautions

REQUIREMENTS

ROOM	VENTILATION	APPAREL	ARTICLES	DISEASES*
Private room if hygiene is poor (*i.e.*, if person does not wash hands after handling infective material)	Room air	No masks; gown or apron if soiling of clothing with blood or body fluids is likely; gloves if touching blood or body fluids	Articles contaminated with blood or body fluid should be bagged and decontaminated by boiling or soaking in bleach or disinfectant	Acquired immune deficiency syndrome, arthropod-borne viral fevers (yellow fever, Colorado tick fever), hepatitis B, hepatitis non-A, non-B, leptospirosis, malaria, relapsing fever, syphilis

Selected Conditions That Do Not Require Isolation*

Nondraining abscess

Actinomycosis

Liver abscess

Botulism

Bronchitis (adult)

Candidiasis

Nondraining cellulitis

Common adult colds

Gonorrhea

Histoplasmosis at any site

Hookworm

Infectious mononucleosis

Influenza, adult

Legionnaires' disease

Leprosy

Neutropenia

Pharyngitis, adult

Pinworm

Reye's syndrome

Rheumatic fever

Ringworm

Tapeworm

Tetanus

Trench mouth

Urinary tract infection

* For a complete list of diseases and conditions, please consult the CDC Guidelines, which are available from the Centers for Disease Control, Atlanta, GA 30333.

Selected Reference

Garner JS, Simmons BP: CDC guidelines for the prevention and control of nosocomial infections. Am J Infect Control 12(2):103–166, 1984

6   Environment for the Visually Impaired

Background

Visual acuity diminishes gradually with some disabilities and as age advances. The rates of change are variable and therefore cannot be totally predicted. Since the changes are gradual, unconscious adaptation in daily living processes occurs, initially creating little disability. However, as the vision deficit increases, and the client is no longer able to perceive the cues that formerly supplemented for minor visual deficits, marked functional disability occurs. Remedies to alter the functional disability lie in two areas: (1) surgery or corrective lenses and (2) environmental adaptation. The second is easily accomplished and can often assist in reducing the functional disability.

Reduced color discrimination and intolerance of glare are two major visual problems that develop with aging. Thus, shapes become indistinct, colors appear to be duller than they are, and objects become indistinguishable from each other. A result is that furniture becomes an unperceived obstacle, dark doorways are indistinguishable, and many other items lose their identifiable characteristics.

In addition to reduced color discrimination, reduced depth perception and increased perception of glare often cause false interpretations of the presence of steps or slippery spots. As the client takes measures to negotiate the perceived steps or slippery spots, imbalance and falls occur.

Many of these visual changes necessitate compensatory measures that can be at least partially accomplished by alterations in the environment. The goals are to avoid accidents, enhance communication, and maintain functional abilities.

Assessment

Client

- Assessment of the client's vision should be done in the environment in which the client will be residing. In addition, visual assessment should be done in the work/school environment or any other setting where the client will be spending large portions of time.
- Assess the ability to distinguish colors, particularly those of edges of furniture, doorways, rugs, tables, and other items that could cause injury if bumped into.
- Assess distance vision and close vision. Assess the distinction between distant and far objects and the client's perception of the distance of objects.
- Assess the acuity of the other senses and the client's abilities to use other senses to compensate for visual loss.
- Assess the client's sense of balance and coordination to ensure prevention of falls caused by a combination of visual perceptual difficulties and poor coordination and/or balance.
- Assess the client's short-term memory to ensure that placement of furnishings and other household items will not be forgotten.
- Assess the client's ability to distinguish edges of steps.

Environmental Assessment

- Assess the color of furniture in relation to the immediate background and surroundings. Attention should be directed to color contrast that is easy for the client to detect.

- Assess the color of doors and doorframes in relation to adjacent walls, with attention directed to color contrast.
- Assess the quality and type of lighting in rooms that will be used by the client for the following factors: if the light is direct or indirect; if it is overhead and causes "glare-spots" reflecting off the floor that could be misinterpreted as wet spots; and if the lighting is incandescent or fluorescent (which produces less glare).
- Assess the floors to determine if there are throw-rugs or other items that could cause stumbling and/or falls, and to determine if the floor is highly waxed and slippery, thus creating a hazard.
- Assess the position of open windows in relation to the chair normally used by the client to determine if the bright light of the window will be behind the person speaking to the client, thus causing additional glare.
- Assess the steps and/or stairs for slippery surfaces and for the presence of handrails to assist in negotiating the stairs.

Environmental Alterations

- Rearrange the furniture so that there is maximum color contrast around the objects.
- If the doors and walls are indistinguishable to the client, arrange to have the doorframes painted with a contrasting color distinguishable to the client.
- Replace incandescent lighting with fluorescent lighting.
- Cover windows causing needless glare with sheer curtains.
- Remove highly polished surfaces from the floor.
- Remove throw-rugs and other indistinguishable items that are potentially hazardous.
- Advise the family to refrain from frequent furniture rearranging so the client will not have to continually reorient to the surroundings.
- Clearly mark the edges of steps with contrasting color if the client has difficulty distinguishing the edges.
- Inquire if handrails can be installed beside steps and stairs.

Equipment Available

Journals and books with large print can be obtained.

If reading material desired by the client is not available in large print, a closed-circuit television can be obtained. This device is used to read materials that would otherwise be too small to see. The reading material is inserted under the screen, and the letters are magnified and projected on a screen to be seen by the client.

A Snelling chart and/or color discrimination test booklet to test the client for vision acuity can be obtained from the state commission for the blind. Some states require certification to perform vision screening. For information regarding this, consult the state commission for the blind, or the local public health department.

Magnifiers. Hand-held magnifiers are available ranging from single-lens magnifiers small enough to carry in the pocket to complex designs with lights and two to three lenses.

Stand magnifiers are available for persons who experience difficulty in holding a magnifier steady or when the person wants to have both hands free (i.e., to do embroidery). The lenses are larger in the standing magnifiers and can be obtained with a built-in light source.

Headborne magnifiers. This is the magnifier of choice for those already wearing eyeglasses. The magnifier is attached to the glasses. The client can have several lenses to use, as appropriate, or can get one permanently attached to the eyeglasses.

Field expanders. These devices are intended for the person whose visual field is severely restricted. The major disadvantage of this device, however, is that as the field is increased, the acuity of the images also decreases.

Telescopic aids. These are helpful for persons having distance visual difficulties. Both hand-held and headborne telescopes are available.

Many other devices ranging to very expensive devices are being developed. Information regarding availability and current research and development can be obtained from the American Foundation for the Blind, through the state commission for the blind.

Appropriate Referrals

Referral should be made to the State Commission for the Blind for assistance with recommendations regarding assistive environmental alterations and assistive devices.

Referral to the Social Security Office will assist in determining legal blindness and in securing financial assistance if needed.

Primary Goals

The primary goal of securing any device and of altering the environment relates to *client independence and quality of life.* Teaching and assistive emphasis should be placed on the client's *strengths* rather than *weaknesses.* The family and significant others should be involved in the counseling and teaching regarding rehabilitation.

Selected References

Mellor M: Aids for the 80s. New York, American Foundation for the Blind, 1982

Independent Living Aids Inc., (Brochure) 11 Commercial Court, Plainview, NY 11803

7 Self-Help Devices

Background

Even though a person has a degree of disability, independence can be maintained or increased by using appropriate self-help devices and by altering the environment to make it more "functional."

Many self-help devices are available commercially. Others can be purchased at dime stores or hardware stores. Often the best self-help devices are those improvised by the family or nurse to meet the specific needs of an individual client. If unable to improvise or purchase an item needed, consultation with an occupational therapist often helps to locate a self-help device, to improvise one, or to gain assistance in overcoming the limitation.

Listed below are only some of the devices available.

Grooming Devices

A long-handled comb: curved handle or built-up handle to enlarge it*

Built-up handle hair brush*

Extension mirror to be fit around client's neck. These can also be purchased with a magnifying mirror. They are available in department stores.

Fingernail brush. Mounts with two suction cups to adhere to cabinet or sink top. Allows the client to clean fingernails with the use of only one hand. This model can also be used in the kitchen for a vegetable brush.

Dressing Aids

Sock and stocking aids. These have long handles or straps, allowing the client to put on socks and stockings from a sitting position.

Long-handled shoe horn with built up handle.* These provide ease of putting on shoes in a sitting position.

Elastic shoelaces. These permit shoes to be tied once. They come in various lengths and colors and allow lace shoes to be slipped on without tying.

Combination button aid and zipper pull. Built-up handle and wire loop on one end allow one-handed buttoning. Hook on the other end allows for zipper pull.

Dressing stick. This 24-inch stick with hooks on both ends assists in pulling up trousers, underclothing, and so on, for the client unable to bend.

Eating Aids

Dishes. Dishes are available with one side built up to allow food to be pushed up and trapped on cutlery. Entire sets of dishes are available in Melamine in attractive designs. A homemade plate guard can also be attached to the plates used by the client.

Cutlery. Handles can be built up by use of plastic foam curlers or narrow foam rubber pipe insulation, or they can be purchased with wood built-up handles.

Securing of straws: A bulldog clip can be secured to the edge of the glass and a straw inserted through the hole on the clip handle and into the liquid.

* All built-up handles can be made by applying foam rubber curlers or pipe insulation or by applying bicycle handles.

Cutting board. The corner of a cutting board can be built up with small pieces of wood or other material. It can be used to anchor bread for buttering or other items needing to be anchored.

A jar opener can be mounted in the kitchen for ease of opening jars with one hand.

Drinking cups. Large-handled mugs can be purchased. In addition, cups are available with non-spill tops and with large handles and holders that can be shaped to fit tumblers, soft-drink cans, and so forth.

A non-slip material (similar to that used in bathtubs) applied under dishes can be used at the table to prevent their slipping.

An adjustable cuff can be purchased that can be applied to the hand and various sizes of handles can be secured in the cuff. This is appropriate for persons having little or no grip.

Tablecloth clamps, purchased at the dime store and applied to the dining table, secure the table cloth and prevent it from slipping.

Non-slip placemats are available in various colors.

Large-handled vegetable peeler, large-handled food grater, and one-handed slicing knife and frame for slicing bread are available commercially.

A two-sided suction holder (for holding soap; available in the dime store) can also be used under plates and other dishes to hold them in place.

Communication and Security

Automatic night lights are available.

Magnifiers of various magnitudes and sizes are commercially available.

Telephones can be amplified for adjustable volume control. Big button telephones are available with hands-free speaker.

Wiring can be done in the home for hearing-impaired clients to allow a lamp to flash on and off when a doorbell or telephone rings.

Radio-controlled switches are available for remote control (up to 40 feet away) of lights, small appliances, and television.

Clothing

Regular gowns and pajama tops can be seamed down the back and attached with velcro or ties, for ease of application.

Large terrycloth and vinyl bibs with "gutters" to catch crumbs and spills are available or can be made.

Reachers

Simple long tongs (used for barbecue) often suffice to reach items beyond arm's length.

Other reachers have magnetic tips, easy gripping devices, and adjustable "jaws."

Wheelchair and Walker Accessories

A basket or bag can be applied to the front of a walker for carrying small items.

A small holder with a squeeze clamp to be applied to the front of the wheelchair, below the armrest, is available for carrying small items that fall easily.

A cup or soft-drink-can holder can be applied by using a squeeze clamp to the front of the wheelchair below the armrest.

A lap board (available in dime stores) assists the wheelchair client to write and eat.

Furniture*

Shower safety can be accomplished by renting, purchasing, or improvising a stool for the client to sit on that has suction cups on each leg to prevent falling or slipping (Fig. A-1). In addition, a hand-held shower head, or one mounted at client's height, will provide ease of showering.

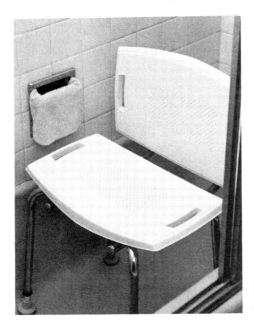

Figure A-1
Chair with suction tips for use in a shower or tub.

Toilet risers are available to elevate the toilet seat for ease of sitting and rising (Fig. A-2).

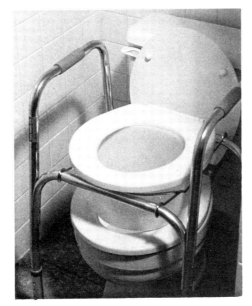

Figure A-2
Toilet riser of adjustable height.

If the client has difficulty sitting and rising from ordinary chairs, a stable box can be constructed and covered with padding (2 to 5 inches high, and contoured to fit the seat). This is stabilized on the chair by ties to the back (or some other mechanism) and increases the height of the seat to comfort level.

If the chair seats are too high for the client to sit comfortably, add a short footstool to the front so the client's feet can comfortably reach the footstool.

* All items that cannot be made in the home can be rented or purchased from local home health equipment agencies. In addition, agencies specializing in self-care items exist. Items can be purchased through mail order from some of these (one example is Health Care Products from Dixson, Inc., PO Box 1449, Grand Junction, Colorado 81502, telephone 800-443-4926).

8

Glossary of Common Medical Terms

Aeration: the process of gaseous exchange in the blood in which oxygen is replenished in the tissues

Afebrile: absence of abnormal temperature elevation

Alignment: the proper relationship of one body part to another

Alopecia: abnormal hair loss

Anaphylaxis: an acute allergic reaction

Anemia: a deficiency of red blood cells or hemoglobin

Anesthesia: loss of sensation

Anorexia: loss of appetite

Anoxia: reduction of oxygen in the body tissues to an abnormal level

Anterior: toward the front

Antiseptic: an agent that inhibits the growth of certain microorganisms

Anus: the terminal ending of the rectum

Aphasia: inability to express oneself properly through speech, or loss of verbal comprehension

Arrhythmia: irregular heart action

Asepsis: absence of pathogenic microorganisms

Asphyxia: a decrease of the amount of oxygen and an increase in the amount of carbon dioxide in the body as a result of respiratory interference

Axilla: the armpit

Bilateral: affecting both sides

Biopsy: the removal of small tissue parts for examination

Bradycardia: abnormally slow heartbeat

Calculus (Calculi, pl): stone

Coma (Comatose): abnormally deep stupor

Contracture: a permanent shortening of a muscle with distortion of the body part

Contusion: a bruise

CPR: cardiopulmonary resuscitation, efforts to restore respirations and heartbeat in an apparently deceased person

Cyanosis: bluish discoloration of the skin and nail beds due to reduced oxygen in the blood

Decubitus ulcer: an open lesion on the skin caused by prolonged pressure

Diarrhea: liquid feces

Dilate (dilation): expansion of the size of an opening

Distal: farthest from the center or midline of the trunk

Dysphagia: difficulty swallowing

Dyspnea: difficulty or labored breathing

Edema: swelling

Emaciated: excessively thin or lean

Embolus: a blood clot that has moved from its point of origin and is obstructing a blood vessel

Emesis: vomitus; the liquid contents of the digestive tract that are forcefully expelled through the mouth and nose

Epistaxis: nosebleed

Febrile: pertaining to fever

Feces: the waste contents of the bowel

Fever: abnormally high body temperature above 98.6°F

Fissure: a deep fold or groove in an organ

Flatulence (flatus): gas in the stomach or intestines

Gait: the way a person walks

Genitals: external reproductive organs

Hematuria: blood in the urine

Hemoptysis: blood in the sputum

Hemorrhage: abnormal escape of blood from the blood vessels

Hemorrhoids: distended veins in the rectum

Hypertension: abnormally high blood pressure

Hyperthermia: abnormally high body temperature

Hypotension: abnormally low blood pressure

Hypothermia: abnormally low body temperature

Incoherent: unintelligible

Incontinence: inability to retain urine

Intramuscular: within the muscle

Jaundice: yellowish tinge to the skin due to the presence of bile pigments in the blood

Lateral: to the side away from the midline

Lethargic: sluggish; stuporous

Lithotomy: lying on the back, knees flexed, hips externally rotated

Mastitis: inflammation of the breast

Nausea: a feeling of the need to vomit

Necrosis: death of an area of skin or bone that is surrounded by healthy tissue

Nocturia: urination during the night

NPO: nothing by mouth; no food or fluids should be consumed

Obese: extremely fat

Oral: referring to the mouth

Pathogen: a disease-producing microorganism

Perineum: area between anus and posterior aspect of genitals

Petechiae: pinpoint red spots on the skin

pH: a symbol used to express alkalinity or acidity

Posterior: toward the back

Postural: affected by the posture or the attitude or position of the body

PRN: as needed

Prone: lying on the abdomen with the face downward

Proximal: closer to the midline of the trunk

Pruritus: intense itching

Purulent: containing pus

Rectum: the distal portion of the large intestine

Sanguineous: bloody drainage

Serosanguineous: watery drainage with blood

Serous: watery drainage

Spasm: an involuntary convulsive muscular contracture

Sputum: a substance ejected from the mouth containing a mixture of saliva, mucus, and sometimes pus

Stuporous: a condition of near or complete unconsciousness

Supine: lying on the back with the face upward

Suppuration: the formation of pus

Tachycardia: an excessively rapid pulse or heart rate, over 100 beats per minute in the adult

Thrombus: a clot

Unilateral: affecting one side

Vertigo: feeling of dizziness

9

Common Weights and Measurements

1. Converting from one form of measurement to another
   The basic equivalents are:

   $$60 \text{ mg} = 1 \text{ gr}$$
   $$1 \text{ mg} = \frac{1}{60} \text{ gr}$$
   $$0.060 \text{ g*} = 1 \text{ gr}$$
   $$1 \text{ g} = 15 \text{ gr}$$
   $$30 \text{ g} = 1 \text{ oz}$$
   $$1 \text{ ml} = 15 \text{ m (mimums)}^{\dagger}$$
   $$30 \text{ ml} = 1 \text{ fluid oz}$$

   * g = gram and gr = grain

   † Both 15 m and 16 m are commonly used. There are exactly 15.43 m in 1 ml.

2. Conversion table

| APOTHECARY UNITS | | METRIC UNITS | | HOUSEHOLD UNITS |
Weight	Liquid	Weight	Liquid	
1 gr	1 minim	0.064 g	0.01 ml	1 drop
15 gr	15 minims	1 g	1 ml	15 drops
1 dram or 60 gr	1 fl dram or 60 minims	4 g	4 ml	1 tsp or 60 drops
1 oz	1 fluid oz	30 g	30 ml	2 Tbsp
1 lb	12 oz	375 g	375 ml	1.5 cups
	1 pint	500 g	500 ml	2 cups
	1 quart	1 kg	1 liter or 1000 ml	4 cups
	1 gallon	4 kg	4 liters or 4000 ml	16 cups

4. Converting temperatures
   Centigrade to Fahrenheit: C degrees × 1.8 + 32 = F degrees
   Fahrenheit to Centigrade: (F degrees −32) × .5556 = C degrees

5. Converting pounds to kilograms
   Pounds to kilograms: pounds divided by 2.2 = kilograms
   Kilograms to pounds: kilograms × 2.2 = pounds

10

Common Household Measurements

1 tsp = ⅛ fl oz or 1 dram
4 tsp = 1 Tbsp
1 Tbsp = ½ oz or 4 drams
16 Tbsp (liquid) = 1 cup
12 Tbsp (dry) = 1 cup
1 cup = 8 fl oz
1 glass = 8 fl oz or ½ pint
16 fl oz = 1 lb
1 pint = 1 lb or 2 cups
1 quart = 4 cups
1 gallon = 16 cups

11   Common Medical Abbreviations

Abd	abdomen	F	Fahrenheit
ac	before meals	F cath	Foley catheter
ad lib	as desired	FHT	fetal heart tones
amb	ambulate	fl	fluid
amt	amount	fract	fracture
ant	anterior	ft	feet
approx	approximately	G in W	glycerin in water
ASHD	arteriosclerotic heart disease	gal	gallon
		GB	gallbladder
ax	axillary	GC	gonorrhea
bid	twice a day	GI	gastrointestinal
BM	bowel movement	g	gram
BP	blood pressure	gr	grain
C	centigrade	gt	drop
$\bar{c}$	with	GU	genitourinary
CA	cancer	gyn	gynecology
cap	capsule	H	hypodermic
cath	catheter	h	hour
cc	cubic centimeter	hgb	hemoglobin
CHF	congestive heart failure	hct	hematocrit
cm	centimeter	H_2O	water
CO_2	carbon dioxide	hosp	hospital
comp	compound	hr	hour
cont	continued	hs	hour of sleep
CPR	cardiopulmonary resuscitation	ht	height
		ID	intradermal
CVA	cerebrovascular accident	IM	intramuscular
diab	diabetic	inter	between
diag	diagnosis	I&O	intake and output
diam	diameter	IPPB	intermittent positive-pressure breathing
dil	diluted		
disc	discontinued	irrig	irrigation
dr	dram	iss	one and one-half
D/W	distilled water	IV	intravenous
Dx	diagnosis	kg	kilogram
EENT	eye, ear, nose, and throat	L	liter
elix	elixir	lt	left
et	and	lat	lateral
etc	and so on	lb	pound
exam	examination	lg	large

liq	liquid
LLL	lower left lobe (lung)
LP	lumbar puncture
LUL	left upper lobe
M	male; thousand
m	minim; meter
max	maximum
mcg	microgram
mEq	milliequivalent
mg, mgm	milligram
MI	myocardial infarction
mid	middle
min	minute; minimum
ml	milliliter
mm	millimeter
mo	month
N	normal
neg	negative
neuro	neurological
no	number
noct	nocturnal (night)
non. rep.	do not repeat
NPO	nothing by mouth
N/S	normal saline
N&V	nausea and vomiting
o	orally
O_2	oxygen
occ	occasional
o.d.	once daily
oint	ointment
op	operation
ophth	ophthalmology
opt	optimal
ortho	orthopedic
OS	left eye
OT	occupational therapy
oto	otology
OU	both eyes
oz	ounce
P	pulse
$\bar{p}$	after or post
palp	palpable
Pap	Papanicolaou smear test
pc	after meals

PEARLA	pupils equal and reactive to light and accommodation
PIH	pregnancy-induced hypertension (toxemia)
PKU	phenylketonuria
pH	hydrogen concentration
PO	per os (by mouth)
pos	positive
postop	postoperatively
prep	preparation
preop	preoperatively
prn	whenever necessary
prog	prognosis
prot	protein
pt	pint
PT	physical therapy
pulv	powder
PVC	premature ventricular contraction
q	every
qid	four times a day
qh	every hour
q2hr, q3hr	every 2 hours; every 3 hours, etc.
qod	every other day
qn	every night
q.n.s.	quantity not sufficient
q.s.	quantity sufficient
qt	quart
R	rectal
resp	respirations, respiratory
RLL	right lower lobe (lung)
Rx	therapy; treatment
$\bar{s}$	without
SC	subcutaneous
sig	write or label
sm	small
sol	solution
SOS	may be repeated once if urgently needed
spec	specimen
sp. gr.	specific gravity
stat	immediately
subling	sublingual (beneath the tongue)

supp	suppository	TPR	temperature, pulse, and respiration
sympt	symptom	tsp	teaspoon
T	temperature	ung	ointment
T&A	tonsillectomy and adenoidectomy	vag	vaginal
tab	tablet	VD	venereal disease
TAT	tetanus antitoxin	vit	vitamin
Tbsp	tablespoon	vol	volume
tid	three times a day	VS	vital signs
tinct	tincture		

Index

Numbers followed by f indicate a figure; t following a page number indicates tabular material.